THE SOBER REVOLUTION

THE SOBER REVOLUTION

*Appellation Wine and the
Transformation of France*

JOSEPH BOHLING

CORNELL UNIVERSITY PRESS
ITHACA AND LONDON

First published 2018 by Cornell University Press

Printed in the United States of America

Library of Congress Cataloging-in-Publication Data

Names: Bohling, Joseph, 1978– author.
Title: The sober revolution : appellation wine and the transformation of France / Joseph Bohling.
Description: Ithaca : Cornell University Press, 2018. | Includes bibliographical references and index.
Identifiers: LCCN 2018015873 (print) | LCCN 2018016576 (ebook) | ISBN 9781501716058 (epub/mobi) | ISBN 9781501716065 (pdf) | ISBN 9781501716041 | ISBN 9781501716041 (cloth; alk. paper)
Subjects: LCSH: Wine industry—France—History—20th century. | Wine and wine Making—Marks of origin—France—History—20th century.
Classification: LCC HD9382.5 (ebook) | LCC HD9382.5 .B64 2018 (print) | DDC 338.4/76632009440904—dc23
LC record available at https://lccn.loc.gov/2018015873

To my family,
for loving me absolutely

CONTENTS

FIGURES AND TABLES

Figures

Tables

ACKNOWLEDGMENTS

Books, like good wine, come from a particular place. This one began at the University of Iowa, where I wrote my senior thesis on the late nineteenth-century phylloxera crisis in France that devastated the vines and the people who cultivated them. Sarah Farmer was the first to fire my interest in history and suggest a thesis topic on wine. Other professors at the University of Iowa also inspired me. Many thanks to Jeff Cox, Sarah Hanley, Elizabeth Heineman, and Mark Peterson for giving my life some direction. Good teachers really do have a positive and long-lasting impact.

After college, I left one heartland for another, this time in southern France, the old hub of industrialized viticulture. I spent a year in Uzès and another in Montpellier improving my language skills and getting to know the people and wines of this area. Although so much of this book is focused on political matters in Paris, I haven't forgotten what makes the people of this region unique. Like many American travelers, I received my first taste of *terroir* in Provence, especially while feasting with Fred Xabada and his family over lamb and lots of gigondas. Memories abound of the celebrated *dimanche*—those long Sundays of cooking, eating, drinking, and socializing—that give people reason to pause. Such days seem hard to sustain in this century, but I hope that they prevail.

When I moved to Berkeley, the activism of Raj Patel and Michael Pollan made me increasingly aware of how consumers become ensnared in larger systems, free to make choices but not necessarily choices of their own making. I had the privilege of studying with a long line of talented teachers and scholars, among them Susanna Barrows, Tom Laqueur, Stanley Brandes, Jonah Levy, Daniel Sargent, Tyler Stovall, and Peggy Anderson. The late Susanna Barrows was my mentor early on. She invited me into her homes in Berkeley and Paris and always knew how to orchestrate an evening of delicious food and deep conversation. Whenever I have writer's block or a class doesn't go well, I often think about what Susanna would have done, but this, I know, is futile because her genius was intuitive, unfettered, and elusive. Tom Laqueur, one of the great cultural historians of his generation, pushed me away from cultural history to learn political economy; although I resisted the idea at first, I now credit him for transforming the way I see culture. A special thanks to Alan Karras for employing me as a lecturer in UC-Berkeley's International and Area Studies program for two years. This was a period of rapid intellectual growth for me, as I had the opportunity to teach many of the classic texts of political economy and fine-tune my knowledge of the history of capitalism. I'm grateful to all of the students who listened to me, exchanged ideas with me, and refined my thinking.

At Berkeley, I had the privilege of being part of a large cohort of graduate students who pushed me to be a better scholar. Those were exciting times. The future seemed wide open as we helped one another develop our respective fields. Eliah Bures, Chad Denton, Grahame Foreman, Stephen Gross, Siti Keo, Jacob Mikanowski, Mark Sawchuk, and Alex Toledano waded through early versions of this book, when the ideas were inchoate and the prose was unpolished. Thank you for making me see things more clearly. Many others made graduate school life more enjoyable, among them Rob Nelson, Megan Pugh, Annie Ruderman, Chris Shaw, and Sarah Zimmerman. Some in my cohort stayed in academia and others left, whether willingly or after putting up a fight with a tough job market. It has been disheartening to see university doors close to so many brilliant scholars, but it does make me happy to see my Berkeley friends doing so well no matter the path that they're on.

I can't thank my Portland State University (PSU) colleagues enough for making the history department such a pleasant and stimulating working environment. Tim Garrison has been an incredibly humane department chair. Any time a problem has arisen, he has been quick to come up with a solution. The junior faculty in my department welcomed me into their writing group when I arrived at PSU, which has been an immense help in making me think about how scholars outside of my field read my work. Thanks to Desmond Cheung, Patricia Goldsworthy-Bishop, Catherine McNeur, Laura Robson, and Jenn Tappan for their constructive criticisms, and for making work life at PSU so enjoyable. I'm also thankful for the intellectual exchange and moral support from Richard Beyler, Jim Grehan, ChiaYin Hsu, David Johnson, John Ott, and Ken Ruoff. The history department is fortunate to have a group called The Friends of History, which, among other things, invites historians to campus to present their work, provides financial support for faculty research trips, and helps create a vibrant intellectual community in the halls and classrooms at PSU. I am grateful to the Friends of History and especially Lou Livingston for their continued generosity and support. Working at PSU would not be the same without them. Jeff Brown and Andrea Janda have kept the department administration smooth and steady. On top of that, Andrea has been a great help with questions of style, and our frequent discussions about gardening always bring me a little peace of mind, even though my theories of gardening still far exceed my practice of it.

Many scholars have supported my work even when they were under no obligation to do so. After Susanna Barrows's untimely death, Phil Nord mentored me as if I was one of his own students. Over the years, he has brought greater clarity to my work, and urged me to play for bigger stakes. Out of sheer generosity and a genuine commitment to his field, he continues to counsel me to this day. Alain Chatriot has been with this project since day one. During my fieldwork, Alain shepherded me through the archives, kept me informed on scholarly trends in France, and introduced me to like-minded scholars. Today, he remains one of my harshest critics and warmest colleagues. I wouldn't know Alain if Patrick Fridenson hadn't welcomed me into his scholarly network. Like Alain, Patrick has been with this project since early on and I thank him for all the opportunities that he has created for me in France. Herrick Chapman has become a reliable advisor who has helped me etch out a place in the French history community. Off and on for several years now, Owen White has graciously exchanged material and ideas, sometimes at critical moments in this project's development. Owen's willingness to share the territory exemplifies what is best about the community of French historians in the United States.

Other scholars have helped out in one way or another, either by commenting on this work, by putting me in touch with other scholars, by opening a door, or simply by providing good cheer. Thanks to Michael Bess, Venus Bivar, Bertrand Dargelos, Marie-France Garcia-Parpet, Patricia Goldsworthy-Bishop, Kolleen Guy, Scott Haine, Jessica Hammerman, Steve Harp, Jeff Horn, Rick Jobs, Gilles Laferté, Pau Medrano Bigas, Giulia Meloni, Mary Ashburn Miller, Phillip Naylor, Didier Nourrisson, Éric Panthou, Sue Peabody, Rod Phillips, Sara Pritchard, and Barbara Traver.

During the fieldwork for this book, I logged countless hours in French archives. Many archivists facilitated my research, too many to list here, but I would like to thank them collectively for their help and hospitality. I also called on about twenty "sober revolutionaries" to ask them questions about their experiences. A high point for me was being invited to Edgard Pisani's home to talk about agricultural politics and the creation of the Common Agricultural Policy in the early 1960s. Although Pisani has recently passed away, some of the people I interviewed are still living, and I thank them for their time and for opening their homes to me.

Research is as costly as it is enriching. Among the institutions that made this book possible is the Alcohol Research Group in Emeryville, California, which provided me with three years in which my sole responsibility was to write and to attend a weekly seminar. That kind of comfort doesn't come along very often, and so I'm grateful to the wonderful group of researchers there for welcoming me into their company. The Institute of International Studies at UC-Berkeley, through a Reinhard Bendix Memorial Fellowship, also helped fund a fifteen-month research stay in France. More recently, PSU's Friends of History has defrayed the costs of research trips to Paris, which has been invaluable in allowing me to finish this project and start a new one.

At Cornell University Press, many thanks to Mahinder Kingra, my editor, for taking on this project with such enthusiasm. Carmen Torrado Gonzalez, Karen Laun, and Bethany Wasik have made the production process smooth. Martin Schneider read closely and carefully in his copyediting.

The anonymous reviewers provided expert criticisms and helped focus some of my arguments. Thanks to Ella Indarta for making the map, a project that was far more challenging and political than I imagined. Some ideas or passages from this book originally appeared in two articles published in *French Historical Studies* and *French Politics, Culture, and Society*. I'm grateful to these journals for granting me permission to reprint those ideas and passages here.

Many friends kept me sane during this project and gave me a good reason to take a break from my work. Thanks to those who have drunk wine and talked wine with me, often late into the night. Talking seriously about wine, about different vintages and different philosophies and approaches to working the land and making wine, is a true pleasure. Such experiences are far too ephemeral and occur too infrequently in one lifetime, but I'm most grateful to have the memory of them. The following people showed me that wine drinking really does achieve something of consequence: Alain Chatriot, Luc Erdogan, Josh Eubank, Byron Fuller, Guillaume Gérard, and Alex Toledano. Andy Friedman, I hope that this book has a *soupçon of asparagus* and a *flutter of a nutty Edam cheese*, although it probably doesn't. Others, too, have been a joy to share a table with: Poppy Alexander, Annie Janusch, Kate Marshall, Ben Schrom, Simon and Judith Trutt, Greg Volk, and Sasha Wizansky. All of these people have helped me see the value of a multidimensional life. How lucky I've been!

To my family, I owe the most. My immediate and extended families have lived with my scholarly obsessions for a long time now, and they have tolerated too many absences and put up far too patiently with the slog of writing a book. Growing up in Iowa, I had a close relationship with all of my grandparents, who planted deep roots in the Midwest. They are no longer here for me to thank, and I could never repay them enough for imparting on me a sense of time, history, and identity. My whole life, my parents have encouraged me to follow my passions, and they've always done their best to make everything possible for me. I hope that I've made them proud. My brother has a way of making me take life less seriously, even though I know how serious he can be, and he unfailingly comes to the rescue with my occasional computer crises. Special thanks to my in-laws and the extended Burke and Gould families for taking me in and for giving me a taste of what it's like to be a Vermonter and a New Yorker.

They, too, take pride in place. Thanks to each and every one of you for loving me no matter what.

Finally, there's Maria, my *compagnon de route*. Did you know what you were in for when you took on me and this book? Maria has tolerated more about wine than anyone, not all of it, alas, as fun as drinking it. Through her steady presence and commitment to our partnership, my sacrifices have become hers. She has read more, criticized more, and nourished me more than anyone. Her example has improved me and this book. I understand the meaning of place much better now. Without Maria, there would have been no sober revolution.

Abbreviations

AOC	Appellation of Controlled Origin
	Appellation d'origine contrôlée
CAP	Common Agricultural Policy
CGB	General Confederation of Beet Growers
	Confédération générale des planteurs des betteraves
CGP	General Commissariat of the Plan
	Commissariat général du Plan
CGVA	General Confederation of Algerian Vine Growers
	Confédération générale des vignerons algériens
CGVM	General Confederation of Southern Vine Growers
	Confédération générale des vignerons du Midi
CNAO	National Committee of Appellations of Origin (CNAO)
	Comité national des appellations d'origine
CNDCA	National Committee for the Defense against Alcoholism
	Comité national de défense contre l'alcoolisme
CNPFV	National Committee for Wine Promotion
	Comité national de propagande en faveur du vin

CNVS   National Confederation of Wine and Spirits
           Confédération nationale des vins et spiriteux
CP   Peasant Confederation
           Confédération paysanne
EEC   European Economic Community
FAV   Federation of Vine Growing Associations
           Fédération des Associations viticoles
FNPFC   National Federation of Cider Producers
           Confédération nationale des producteurs de fruits à cidre
FNSEA   National Federation of Farmers' Unions
           Fédération nationale des syndicats d'exploitants agricoles
GI   Geographical Indication
HCEIA   High Commission for Studies and Information on Alcoholism
           Haut Comité d'étude et d'information sur l'alcoolisme
IFA   French Institute of Alcohol
           Institut français de l'alcool
INAO   National Institute of Appellations of Origin
           Institut national des appellations d'origine
INED   National Institute of Demographic Studies
           Institut national d'études démographiques
INSEE   National Institute of Statistics and Economic Studies
           Institut national de la statistique et des études économiques
IVCC   Institute of Industrial Wines
           Institut des vins de consommation courante
IWO   International Wine Office
ONSER   National Organization of Road Safety
           Organisme national de sécurité routière
SFMAV   French Society of Pro-Wine Doctors
           Société française des médecins amis du vin
SNBA   National Syndicate of Ambulating Distillers
           Syndicat national des bouilleurs ambulants
SNBC   National Syndicate of Home Distillers
           Syndicat national des bouilleurs de cru
UFC   Federal Union of Consumption
           Union fédérale de la consommation
VDQS   Delimited Wines of Superior Quality
           Vins délimités de qualité supérieur
VDT   (European) Table Wines
           Vins de table

VQPRD   (European) Quality Wines Produced in a Determined Region
        Vins de qualité produits dans des régions déterminées
WHO   World Health Organization
WTO   World Trade Organization

Note on Usage

Regions and Regional Wine

I follow the scholarly custom of capitalizing the names of wine regions and use lowercase for the wines that originate from these regions. Hence, Burgundy, Bordeaux, and Champagne refer to the regions, whereas burgundy, bordeaux, and champagne refer to wines from these regions.

Metric and American Equivalent

1 hectare = 2.47 acres
1 liter = 0.26 gallons
1 hectoliter = 26.42 gallons

Guide to Terms

Appellation wine
Also referred to in this book as luxury or "quality" wine. Wine that comes from state-approved grape varietals and vineyards in officially designated wine regions. Appellation wine is place-specific, as opposed to "industrial wine," which can come from anywhere. Most of the metropolitan policymakers discussed in this book assumed that appellation wine and quality wine were synonymous, an assumption that reflected and perpetuated class and racial biases against peasant and Algerian producers.

Beet grower
These cultivators often turned their beets into either alcohol or sugar. They were loosely allied with the industrial vine growers in obtaining state subsidies to cope with the problem of overproduction.

Cider producer
Farmers with an orchard, mostly in Brittany and Normandy, who turned their apples into cider. Cider producers joined forces with industrial

vine growers and beet growers in persuading the state to subsidize their surpluses.

Home distiller
Found throughout France, these farmers and gardeners distilled the fruits of their own property into brandy. Although much of their production took place on a small scale, home distillation was also a way for vine growers and cider producers to find outlets for their surpluses. The state allowed 10 liters of tax-free home-distilled brandy per year.

Industrial wine
Also referred to in this book as "ordinary wine," "table wine," or *vins de consommation courante*. Wine that came from high-yielding vines produced in the plains of the Languedoc that tended to be acidic and low in alcohol, was often deemed to be of inferior quality, and was blended by merchants with mass-produced, more alcoholic wines from Algeria and Italy. Consumers often preferred the wines that fell under this category, but state officials subordinated these wines as "ordinary" given their links to peasants in mainland France and settlers in French Algeria, two groups that policymakers wished to reform. Unlike appellation wines, which are branded with their place of origin and style of production, industrial wine used a corporate trademark such as Postillon or Préfontaines, not all that different from Coca-Cola.

Merchant
Middlemen or *négociants* who sourced grapes from different areas, usually with the purpose of making cheap industrial wine.

Plonk
English slang that denotes low-quality, standardized, industrial wine.

Technocrat
Otherwise known as an expert. Technocrats are trained in France's elite institutions and staff the government administration. Although they are often perceived and portrayed to be ideologically and politically neutral, technocrats entered the policymaking process with their own cultural assumptions and political agendas.

Terroir
A fluid term that loosely translates as "a sense of place." Appellation wines are typically seen as expressing *terroir*, a sense of how and where they are made.

Vine grower
Cultivator of vines, but not necessarily a winemaker. Although in appellation districts many vine growers also made their own wine, the vine growers of industrial wine, particularly in the Languedoc, often could not afford winemaking equipment and thus sold their grapes to merchants who blended them with the more alcoholic wines of Algeria and Italy.

The Sober Revolution

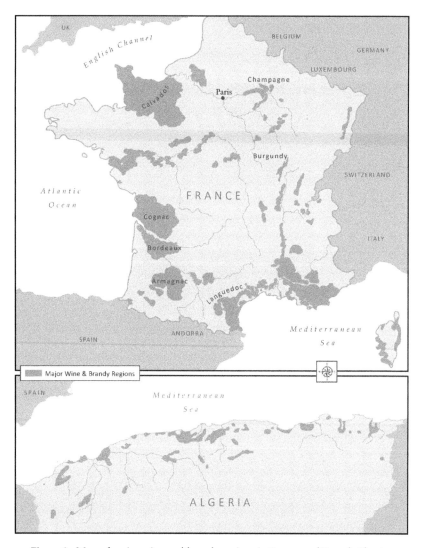

Figure 1. Map of major wine and brandy regions in France and French Algeria. Metropolitan policymakers generally did not distinguish among Algerian wine regions; for this reason these regions are not identified on the map.

INTRODUCTION

In 1957, Roland Barthes penned an essay exposing how the French enshrouded wine in myths—it quenched thirst, stimulated the mind, made the timid talkative, cured illness, and provided strength and nourishment—all the while blissfully ignoring the turmoil that arose from wine production.[1] For nearly half a century, France's wine industry—dominated in large part by two vast regions of single-crop grapevine plantings—had suffered from repeated surplus crises, falling prices, and social strife. In 1907, left-leaning peasant vine growers in the southern Languedoc region had staged one of the largest uprisings since the French Revolution and consequently obtained state subsidies to offset the challenges of overproduction.[2] Their struggle set the pattern for subsequent wine gluts. Between the 1930s and the 1950s, the Languedoc's woes were aggravated by the rapid expansion of industrialized viticulture in colonial Algeria, where European settlers had expropriated the land of an indigenous population that was poor, under-nourished, and restive.[3] French consumers unwittingly supported this state of affairs through their everyday wine-drinking habits.

Barthes's "Wine and Milk," which appeared at a critical juncture in post-1945 France, suggested that seemingly disparate events—war in Algeria, political instability in Paris, and habitual wine drinking—were connected, and for good reason. In 1954, Algerians ignited their war of independence from French rule. Because wine played such a vital role in the settlers' structure of wealth and power, the Algerian independence movement attacked the industry as a symbol of imperial oppression. At the same time in Paris, the Pierre Mendès France government notoriously campaigned against France's high rates of wine-related alcoholism by scaling back production and encouraging the French to drink milk. In a country with deeply held beliefs about the virtues of wine—most French people viewed it as a food, as a national icon, even as an *antidote* to alcoholism—Mendès France's milk drinking was taken as an insult. Such beliefs gave the wine industry democratic legitimacy and helped the Algerian and alcohol lobbies overthrow his government in short order. "Wine and Milk" signaled a new understanding of the problems stemming from France's political and imperial order; it also revealed the drinking mythologies that obstructed reform.

Barthes's observations mirrored a broad movement initiated after World War II to modify French myths about wine, a transformation I call "the sober revolution." During the economic boom known as the Thirty Glorious Years, a period in which agricultural industrialization prevailed, the French wine industry made a surprising transition from an orientation around mass production and consumption in Algeria and the Languedoc to an emphasis on artisanship, luxury, and distinction in metropolitan regions. France had long produced tiny amounts of luxury wine in regions like Bordeaux, Burgundy, and Champagne, but as France integrated into global markets after World War II, industry leaders fought to modernize the sector and expand luxury production in order to remain competitive with the established wine producers among their European neighbors as well as with the rapidly developing wine industries in the Americas. Production quantities stayed relatively consistent throughout this period, but much of the industrial wine was distilled and diverted into non-drinkable products, and luxury wine production and exports increased to compensate for the shrinking domestic market (figure 2). Statistics illustrate the change in wine-drinking

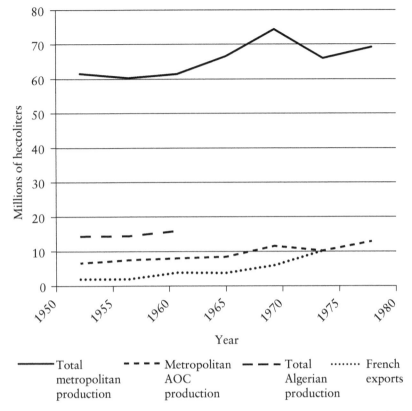

Figure 2. French wine production and exports, 1950–1980. Data from Marcel Lachiver, *Vins, vignes et vignerons: Histoire du vignoble français* (Paris: Fayard, 1988) and Leo A. Loubère, *The Wine Revolution in France: The Twentieth Century* (Princeton: Princeton University Press, 1990).

habits (figure 3).[4] Total wine consumption per individual over the age of fourteen fell 47 percent over the course of a generation, from 173 liters in 1960 to 90 liters in 1985, a trend that sets France apart from industrialized countries like the United States. Conversely, luxury wine consumption rose from about 13 liters per capita between 1960 and 1964 to nearly 24 liters between 1981 and 1985.[5] This shift toward luxury wine—which sober revolutionaries defined as produced and regulated in regionally specific places in mainland France—has continued and intensified in our own day.

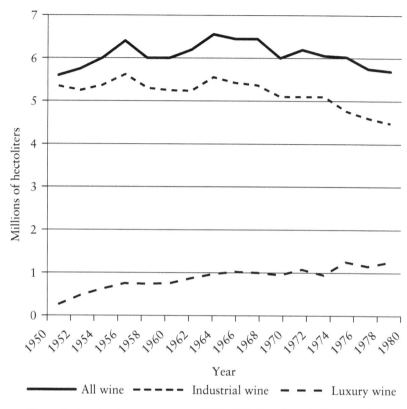

Figure 3. French wine consumption, 1950–1980. Data from Catherine Aubey and Daniel Boulet, "La consommation d'alcool en France régresse et se transforme," *Économie et statistique* 176 (April 1985).

Scholars have charted the origins of France's modern luxury wine industry in the first decades of the twentieth century but not its contested and contingent rise from the 1930s into the postwar years.[6] Explanations for its origins and rise focus almost exclusively on the supply side when, in fact, its consolidation depended as much on the state's ability to harness and cultivate new tastes among a new middle class that had more disposable income and access to a wider array of French and foreign goods than had previous generations.[7] The sober revolution and the modernization of the wine industry were two sides of the same "civilizing" project that attempted to engineer new market and social norms. For political reasons after 1945, most French people gradually altered their perceptions of wine from a food, a "taste of necessity," into a "taste of luxury."[8]

The sober revolution took place because different and sometimes antagonistic groups—demographers, doctors, economists, engineers, legal experts, politicians, statisticians, consumer activists, and the dynamic industries of luxury wine, automobiles, oil, insurance, and tourism—made a controversial connection between wine surpluses, on the one hand, and alcoholism and malnutrition, on the other, and saw these related problems as symptomatic of a flawed political and economic system. These sober revolutionaries joined forces in the High Commission for Studies and Information on Alcoholism (HCEIA). Established by Mendès France in November 1954, just after the onset of the Algerian War, the HCEIA resided in the office of the prime minister and claimed to serve the "general interests" of the nation above the particular concerns of any one sector, such as public health, agriculture, or the economy. The HCEIA advocated policies to wean consumers off Algerian and peasant wine and brandy in the name of public health, but its members' interests ran deeper, into restructuring wine production and the political and imperial order that supported it. In their view, wine surpluses and alcoholism represented problems with the distribution of power in state institutions, the inward orientation of the economy, and the shape and meaning of France as the country decolonized and pursued economic modernization.

Given the political power of the industrial vine growers and the protectionist policies that continued to sustain them well into the post-1945 era, the sober revolutionaries would not have succeeded without important structural changes. In 1958, the war in Algeria brought down the parliamentary-based Fourth Republic (1946–1958); it was replaced by an executive-based Fifth Republic (1958–present), which empowered technocrats to overcome parliamentary obstacles, reform the wine industry, and liberalize the economy.[9] Then, the decolonization of Algeria in 1962 diminished the amount of Algerian wine on the French market. Finally, the member-states of the European Economic Community (EEC) organized a common wine market in the 1960s, which eventually allowed the sober revolutionaries to mobilize France's European partner nations against the wine surplus problem in the Languedoc and against French myths about the virtues of daily wine drinking. With the exception of Italy, wine held less economic and cultural value to France's European partners.

The sober revolution consolidated France's luxury wine industry on both economic and ethical grounds. Criticisms of the wine industry as a source of economic inefficiency and public health problems incited reform-minded wine leaders in regions such as Bordeaux, Burgundy, and Champagne to refurbish the industry's image by promoting the work of the National Institute of Appellations of Origin (INAO), a state agency that local producer associations and government bureaucrats had established in 1935 to codify and regulate luxury vine growing, winemaking, and brandy-making practices.[10] The INAO relayed transparent information to consumers about the producer and the unique qualities of the place and methods of production, qualities that were said to be "local, loyal to, and consistent with tradition."[11] This "sense of place," often referred to as *terroir*, made these wines irreproducible elsewhere, an enticing prospect in an age of the mass (re)production of goods.[12] The INAO oversaw the development of two important place-based classification systems: the Appellation of Controlled Origins (AOC), created through a series of laws between 1905 and 1935, and the Delimited Wines of Superior Quality (VDQS), established in 1944 as a middle ground between industrial and luxury wine (figure 4). In recent years, the appellation system has become an international model used to defend local food systems against industrialized agriculture.

INAO leaders actively promoted an image of mainland France as the home of luxury wine, a strategy that simultaneously prepared the wine industry for global markets, marginalized the country's tormented history of industrial wine production and alcoholism, and questioned Algeria's status as an integral part of the metropole. Joseph Capus, a Bordeaux senator and one of the architects of the INAO, argued that appellation vineyards were "part of the national heritage" and that "the state [had] the same rights and obligations" toward them as it did toward "certain sites and historical monuments."[13] In this tradition of excellence that Capus summoned the state to protect, Algeria and the Languedoc—where "industrial workers" produced a "standardized liquid" to sell to merchants who made "neutral wine, without vice but also without virtue"— were nearly entirely absent, as were many other mainland peasants whose wine and brandy failed to conform to the INAO's definition of authenticity and quality.[14] Algeria, officially not a colony but an administrative part of France between annexation in 1848 and independence in 1962, was

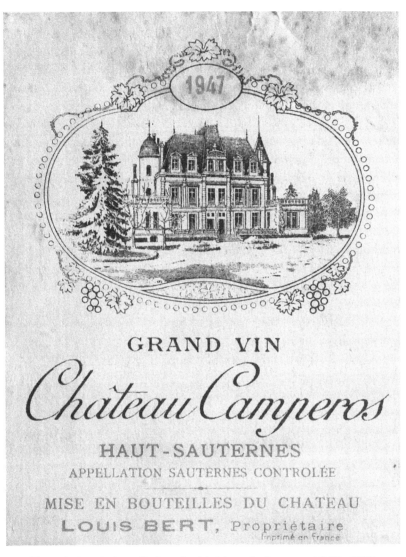

GRAND VIN

Château Camperos

HAUT-SAUTERNES

APPELLATION SAUTERNES CONTROLÉE

MISE EN BOUTEILLES DU CHATEAU

LOUIS BERT, Propriétaire

Imprimé en France

Figure 4. A typical appellation wine label from the Sauternes AOC in 1947. The label features the producer's name, the vineyard location, the AOC designation, and a bucolic image of a chateau.

denied AOC classification.[15] This reflected the metropolitan wine industry's rejection of the prevalent idea that "Algeria is France." Appellation
wines were to connect consumers to the producers and evoke bucolic
images of European France, not the pain and suffering found in Algeria
and the Languedoc. In doing so, the INAO uncoupled Algeria from the
metropole and created a framework for imagining a post-Algerian France;
once France had retreated from empire, it could help efface the intimate
relationship that had bound Algeria to France for over a century.

Today, considering the appellation system's success in laying claim to
authenticity, most wine and food enthusiasts probably take for granted
France's appellation system and the notion of *terroir* that it promotes,
seeing them as inherent parts of French wine and agriculture. On the
contrary, this success was never inevitable. After World War II, the
INAO was still a fledgling organization struggling to change the way
French producers, consumers, and government officials viewed wine
and brandy. The INAO had to contend with the fact that most French
people preferred drinking copious amounts of either locally made,
non-market wines and brandy or industrial wines—popularly known
as *pinard*, *gros rouge*, or "plonk." Industrial wines were blended from
high-yielding varietals that "made the vine piss" and that were grown in
different places, particularly the monocropping plains of the Languedoc
and Algeria.[16] These vines were cultivated by both peasants and large
landowners; indigenous laborers often worked the vineyards in Algeria.
Merchants (*négociants*) and wine companies dominated this industrial
wine system, as they bought grapes from various growers and mixed
them together, sometimes adding water, sugar, and chemicals to create
a consistent and cheap beverage, what one journalist called a "national
Coca-Cola" (figures 5 and 6).[17]

American scholarship has generally focused on France's luxury goods
production, in no small part because France has exported this image to
the world and because it distinguishes the country in a general way from
American attitudes and practices.[18] Yet there is not much evidence to suggest that French consumers cared where their wine came from. In the early
twentieth century, a vine-growing association in Burgundy admitted that
consumers were "more indifferent than we assume about the origin of the
wine that they drink."[19] In the 1950s, Barthes asserted that few consumers
knew that their wine was the "product of an expropriation" in Algeria.[20]

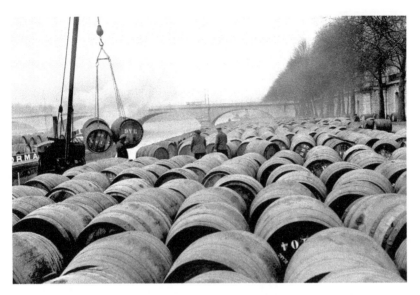

Figure 5. Unloading barrels of industrial wine on the banks of the Seine in Paris, c. 1938. Reprinted by permission of the Image Works.

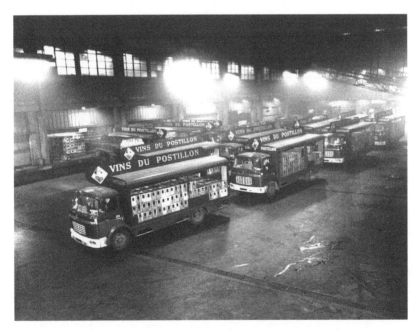

Figure 6. Transporting industrial wine by truck, c. 1955. Postillon was a major wine company in the middle decades of the twentieth century, comparable in status to the Coca-Cola Company. Photo by René-Jacques.

Until the 1960s and 1970s, France had yet to reach the level of urbanization and affluence that would allow most consumers to think differently about wine. In large parts of southern France and Algeria, high yields and the profit motive came before the artistry of winemaking; for most consumers, wine was an everyday beverage that fulfilled basic nutritional and social needs, not a luxury product that conjured up quaint images of the countryside and associated the drinker with deep pockets and educated tastes. Thus, most French consumers did not naturally gravitate toward luxury wines that were rooted in specific, regulated areas of production but were instead encouraged to do so to serve the interests of the modernist wing of the wine industry, the state, and other interest groups amid the political dynamics and uncertainties of sweeping change.

The story of the sober revolution challenges four assumptions of the Thirty Glorious Years narrative.[21] The first assumption is that the "economic miracle" was solely a postwar story. After the war, technocrats condemned the immobility of the Third Republic (1870–1940) and the Vichy regime (1940–1944) in order to distance themselves from past policy and legitimate their own leadership. Yet this behavior elides how heavily these technocrats borrowed from their predecessors. In fact, many of the postwar reformers of the wine industry had been active participants in the movements of the 1930s and early 1940s to strengthen the state's management of the economy. Instead of treating the Vichy regime as a parenthesis in French history, this book adds to scholarship that emphasizes important continuities in actors and public policy across the war.[22]

Attempts at regulating the wine industry exemplify this continuity. The appellation system and the related movements of state reform, anti-alcoholism, automobile tourism, the economic restructuring of Algeria, and European integration all had prewar roots. The major wine policy innovation after the war was to link problems of production to problems of consumption. Technocrats saw wine policy as symptomatic of the paralysis that had plagued earlier regimes, a strategy that helped them create a symbolic rupture with the past and build legitimacy for economic modernization. Ironically, these reformers accomplished their task by helping launch the appellation system as a new model of production that claimed to protect a celebrated tradition of luxury wine. Technocrats employed symbols of both rupture and continuity—modernity and nostalgic traditionalism—to legitimate their reforms.

The second assumption is that the Thirty Glorious Years created a happy consensus through top-down, state-sponsored economic growth.[23] Although a higher standard of living was doubtless appealing to a generation that had experienced economic depression and war, how to arrive at that new standard was hotly contested. The controversies surrounding the establishment of new wine regulations highlight how conflictive this process could be and how the opponents of state power were ultimately sidelined. The difficulties that the state faced in legitimating the appellation system meant that in most cases change was brought about by the government issuing decrees instead of Parliament passing laws. State officials still needed public consent; before issuing decrees, therefore, they considered the demands of social movements and consulted with powerful interest groups. Working together, these groups launched press campaigns to try to mold public opinion and to give their reforms a democratic air. Sober revolutionaries framed the wine problem in a way that would isolate their opponents, couching reforms not just in terms of economic interests but also in terms of consumer protection and national tradition. This entailed treating the appellation system as an authentic expression of French wine and brandy and blaming the industrial wine system for many of the country's economic and social ills, such as poor housing, alcoholism, automobile accidents, and violence in Algeria. The state may have spearheaded the modernization of the wine industry and the economy more generally, but its success depended on a hard-fought battle to win public consent by promoting consumer welfare and by refashioning France's historical memory as European through the appellation system.[24]

The third assumption is that the socioeconomic changes of the Thirty Glorious Years were largely a domestic story, too often neglecting putatively external events—namely, decolonization and European integration.[25] Historians have only begun to explore the ways in which Algeria's independence and the European common market spurred the state's drive to remake French economic and social life.[26] It is especially curious that economic historians of colonial Algeria have neglected the wine industry, the region's leading sector.[27] To Kristin Ross's assertion that cars and soap were the central tropes of France's post-1945 modernization, I would add wine, an important source of revenue and symbol of national identity.[28] The shift from an industrial to an appellation-based wine system would not have been possible without a broad alliance pushing for modernization as France withdrew from Algeria and integrated into the EEC.

The fourth assumption is that industrialization, concentration, and rationalization—characteristic trends of the Thirty Glorious Years—necessarily disadvantaged craftsmanship and small-batch production.[29] Scholars and food activists have rightly described the period as one of agricultural industrialization.[30] Yet the wine industry cut against the grain. The growth of the appellation system inverts the predominant trend in twentieth-century agriculture: against increasingly delocalized, industrialized foods, wine production became more localized. The appellation system provided an opportunity for vine growers to seize power from the merchants who controlled the industrial wine system and become competitive in global markets.[31] Through the appellation system and alliances with technocrats and other groups, small-scale producers could survive and thrive during an age that celebrated the ethos of bigger is better.

Chapter 1 overviews the rise of the merchant-controlled industrial wine system, demonstrating how it became intertwined with the parliamentary and imperial Third Republic. Through their allies in Parliament, the industrial wine lobbies received protection against international competition. By the economic depression of the 1930s, however, reform-minded industry leaders, economists, and politicians began to criticize the state for its inability to manage the surpluses that stemmed from this arrangement and that risked tarnishing the reputation of France's luxury wine sector. The authoritarian and openly racist Vichy regime supported the movement to regulate the wine industry and promote appellations by authorizing technocrats to carry out economic renewal. Yet the harsh conditions of the war and the occupation stood in the way of any lasting reforms. Black markets flourished, as state control collapsed. The chapter concludes that the economic and social problems arising from wine production in the Third Republic and the Vichy regime laid the foundations for the appellation system's consolidation after the war.

Chapters 2 through 5 move chronologically from 1945 to 1976, spotlighting how the struggles to localize production in the metropole became part of a broader push to integrate France into European and global markets, redistribute power from politicians to technocrats, develop new norms to enable economic expansion and ensure public health and safety, and market a metropolitan image of the French heritage to French and international consumers. Chapter 2 looks at how technocrats and export-oriented industries allied with public health activists in trying to reform the industrial wine system and liberalize the economy. Their movement contributed to socioeconomic development in the countryside and French Algeria. Yet in the parliamentary and imperial Fourth Republic, peasant and settler vine growers and allied politicians continued to subvert reforms that would have undermined their privileges.

Chapters 3 and 4 analyze how new alliances, new institutions, and uncontrollable events began to break the deadlock of reform after 1958. Chapter 3 examines how the coalition of technocrats and public health activists, having failed to tackle the industrial wine system head on in the early 1950s, drove a wedge through that system by loosely allying with the INAO. Working together, this coalition pursued the European settlers of Algeria and the home distillers, two groups that were becoming increasingly unpopular in the late 1950s as France faced war in Algeria and new competition in the EEC. These groups' wine and brandy competed with the appellation system's product and its representation of the national heritage.

Chapter 4 analyzes how the state negotiated the economic imperative of promoting wine tourism with the moral imperative of limiting drinking and driving. Automobile tourism provided an opportunity for France's vine growers to link notions of quality to distinct metropolitan places of production and to market a sanitized image of wine, but France's high rate of alcohol-related accidents contradicted the image that they were trying to sell of idyllic landscapes, happy peasants, and civilized consumption. The various movements against the industrial wine system benefited from and helped justify the Fifth Republic's more technocratic style of governance and its efforts to rebrand French wine as metropolitan.

Chapter 5 explains how the decolonization of Algeria and European integration solidified the appellation system. If this system had emerged in response to competition from Algeria, it flourished amid the competition presented by the European common market from the 1960s on. France's European partners helped dispel lingering myths about wine being food and about Algeria being France. Industrial wine would not disappear—a trip to any Monoprix supermarket today will attest to that—but the EEC would seize jurisdiction over it and Algerian imports would diminish. In the 1960s, France's identity as an agricultural and imperial nation was eclipsed by a new consumer society that in time would express an intense nostalgia for the authentic rural experiences of the metropolitan *terroirs*. Decolonization and European integration thus facilitated the localization of French wine production though the appellation system, a system that has in turn influenced agricultural production around the world, a topic picked up in the conclusion.

The sober revolution is a story about the state's battle for control over a central commodity in the nation's economic and social life as France modernized, decolonized, and entered more competitive global markets. This story, like any, has winners and losers. Regulations empowered those producers that they protected but excluded those whom state officials perceived as unproductive, unprofitable, unruly, and a public health nuisance. Regulations also had the effect of labeling as "alcoholic" or a "public enemy" any consumer who deviated from the new drinking norm that the state was working to impose.[32] The state marked the settlers of Algeria, the mainland peasants who made their own wine and brandy, and the consumers who drank low-end products as a form of Other lurking on the periphery of an authentic, metropolitan wine industry and nation.

Just after World War II, a jurist and politician tellingly drew a connection between the appellation system and nationality: in fact, "nothing holds the cachet of nationality more than the appellation of origin."[33] Granting appellations, like granting nationality, entailed a controversial process of selection; many vine growers and brandy makers—fierce individualists defiant of the state's unsolicited intrusion in their affairs—were excluded from the appellation system and official narratives of French excellence in wine production. As France urbanized and entered the postcolonial era, the state promoted a new mythology of wine that linked consumers to the region of production and to a rural experience that was historically hexagonal—the "Hexagon" being widely used by French people to refer to their country after 1962.[34] This new mythology conveniently ignored the appellation system's contribution to modernizing the economy, uprooting the peasantry, and treating Algeria as exterior to France's development. In 1962, French wine, like France itself, became more hexagonal than it had been for at least a century, even if, through a discourse of tradition, authenticity, and quality, France and its wines were presented as if they had always been hexagonal.[35] The sober revolution helped the state remap the economic, political, and gastronomic boundaries of France in ways that continue to shape its postcolonial identity and the world beyond.

1

UNDER THE INFLUENCE

The post-1945 sober revolution had its roots in the first half of the twentieth century in economic and social problems that undermined state authority. The economic problem was one of managing the quantity and quality of France's wine supply. French and Algerian vine growers were plagued by a series of surplus crises that limited the state's capacity to maintain stability in the countryside. While the Third Republic (1870–1940) faced a surplus problem, the Vichy regime (1940–1944) faced a scarcity and quality problem given tough wartime conditions and Nazi requisitioning and plundering. The social problem concerned high rates of alcoholism in the hard times of the 1930s and malnutrition during World War II. The success of the sober revolution would ultimately come from reformers' efforts to blame alcoholism not on individual moral weakness but on wine surpluses and the protectionist policies that led to them, thereby mobilizing consumers and a range of dynamic interest groups against the industrial wine system. No political leader risked making this connection prior to 1945 because of the power of the wine lobbies within French political institutions and culture. To gauge the challenges that sober revolutionaries faced in transforming the wine industry and the political order to which it belonged, this chapter outlines the emergence and development of the industrial wine system, its unforeseen problems, and the early efforts to regulate wine production.

Policymakers in the Third Republic and the Vichy regime struggled to tackle the problems besetting the wine industry given the political power of the producers, the economic value of wine to the state, and the symbolic value of agriculture and Algeria in French political culture. In a country with a population of 42 million in the 1930s, nearly 7 million were either directly or indirectly employed in the alcohol industry.[1] There were nearly 2 million vine growers in metropolitan France and another 20,000 in Algeria, not including their family members and other dependents who lived by the vine.[2] Approximately 450,000 indigenous subjects toiled in the Algerian vineyards.[3] More than 300,000 businesses—which included trades such as cooperage, glassblowing, and cork-making—depended on the wine industry.[4] The fate of other powerful groups—beet alcohol producers, cider producers, large commercial distillers, home distillers, merchants, and owners of wine shops and drinking establishments—was also tied to the wine industry. These groups' relations with the wine lobbies were tense yet overlapping, making the wine bloc all the more powerful.

These producers organized into various regional organizations—most prominently the General Confederation of Southern Vine Growers (CGVM) and the General Confederation of Algerian Vine Growers (CGVA). Such organizations had a strong presence in local political life and found effective allies in Parliament, thus giving the industrial wine system a profound influence on the levers of command. "It was . . . with glass in hand," one wine newspaper affirmed, "that the ideas from which our institutions sprung were first exchanged."[5] The largest proportion of parliamentary debates on agriculture during the Third Republic was devoted to the question of subsidizing and protecting the wine industry.[6] One liberal economist lamented that "few industries in France have obtained such considerable advantages and such persistent attention from Parliament" as the wine industry.[7] Two scholars would retrospectively call the industry the "spoiled child" of agricultural legislation.[8] In no other modern state, to be sure, did wine hold such sway.

The political power of wine was largely a product of its profit-ability. Metropolitan and Algerian wine yielded as much as 12 billion francs a year; only grain and steel were more lucrative, and only silk generated more income from exports.[9] Wine was an important source of tax revenue. The state earned 4 billion francs in wine taxes in the mid-1930s.[10] Wine was thus seen as a generator of wealth for the national economy, a fact that was frequently exploited by the opponents of wine reforms.

The wine industry obtained state protection not only because of its size and profitability but also because its lobbyists successfully tied their interests to the collective concerns of agriculture and French Algeria. The Third Republic has been characterized as both a peasants' republic and an imperial nation-state or empire-state.[11] Compared to Germany, Great Britain, and the United States, France industrialized cautiously. In 1870, over half of France's total active population was categorized as farmers.[12] Politicians across the political spectrum idealized small farmers as an anchor against the turbulence of fast-changing times. Because of the populous countryside, candidates to Parliament had to cater to rural voters to win elections. Jules Ferry, one of the leading politicians of the early Third Republic, famously declared that "the republic will be a peasants' republic or it will cease to exist."[13] Until 1931, the overall population was still considered rural, which the census defined as living in towns and villages of under two thousand persons.[14] During the Great Depression, many wine and alcohol lobbyists and their politicians perpetuated the myth that France was a "peasant nation" to be protected from the vagaries of the world economy.[15]

Along with metropolitan agriculture, the European settlers of Algeria added to wine's political power. European settlers of French, Italian, Maltese, and Spanish descent immigrated to Algeria in the nineteenth century and successfully lobbied to make Algeria an administrative part of France.[16] Many of these settlers dispossessed indigenous land and planted vines. By the early twentieth century, they had created the world's leading wine export industry. The colonial lobby, in which the settlers of Algeria had a strong presence, was among the most influential lobbies in the Third Republic.[17] The parliamentary representation of Algeria's settler population climbed in the 1930s.[18] The settlers also controlled the local administration of Algeria, formed a power base independent of Paris, and had the capacity to block metropolitan interference through the colonial assembly known as the financial delegations.[19] During the Great Depression, as world markets contracted and as colonial lobbyists touted the benefits of the French empire, known at the time as "Greater France," the settlers emphasized that France depended on trade with Algeria.[20] Although metropolitan and Algerian vine growers often saw their interests as competitive instead of as complementary, they agreed on persuading the state to support them during hard times. Rural and settler constituencies were thus a vital force in the political life of the Third Republic and helped create a favorable situation for the wine industry.

The economic crisis of the 1930s and World War II marked a turning point in the state's relationship to the wine industry, when forward-looking industry leaders, economists, intellectuals, and politicians advocated new forms of state management of the sector to address the industry's economic and social problems. For these groups, chronic wine crises caused by overproduction were symptomatic of a structural contradiction in French capitalism—namely, that the wine industry benefited from the Third Republic's protectionist policies that encouraged quantity over quality even though growers in the metropole and Algeria were obliged to compete within a limited metropolitan market. Significant portions of the regional economies of Algeria and the Languedoc depended almost entirely on the fortunes of the vine. For peasants in the Languedoc and indigenous Algerians, this often meant a life of poverty and misery. The state responded to their distress by protecting them from international competition, subsidizing surpluses, and pushing consumers to drink more. Out of this economic and imperial crisis emerged new ideas about how to regulate the industry, particularly through a regional appellation system. Yet the hardships of the economic depression and the war, combined with the political power of the industrial wine lobbies, compelled politicians to prioritize stability over structural reform. A broad alliance of wine and agricultural lobbies ensured that any attempt to overhaul the industry would be interpreted as a threat to the peasantry and French Algeria, hallowed yet unstable categories in the crisis years of the 1930s.

The Emergence and Development of
the Industrial Wine System

From the late nineteenth century to the post-1945 era, the bulk of French wine hardly conformed to romantic images of vine growing and winemaking; rather, it was the fruit of inequality and violence in the countryside and French Algeria. Prior to the imperial Third Republic, most French wine had been produced and consumed locally as part of subsistence agriculture. Market-oriented luxury wine producers certainly existed, scattered throughout Bordeaux, Burgundy, Champagne, and a few other areas, but even in these regions fine wine had been rare.[21] Starting in the middle decades of the nineteenth century, both non-market and luxury wine and brandy had to contend with an industrial wine system that centered on Algeria and the Languedoc and that delivered cheap, mass-produced, standardized wine to urban markets.[22]

The temptation to produce wine in bulk resulted from a confluence of factors: the development of a national mass market, the growth of a thirsty working class, a devastating wine blight caused by the phylloxera aphid, technological advances in the vineyard, and increased investment in Algerian vineyards.[23] Railways and roadways facilitated the expansion of industrialized viticulture by integrating the national market and by lowering transportation costs and shipping rates from Algeria to France. The introduction of tank cars in the late nineteenth century and tank trucks in the early twentieth concentrated vineyards in regions deemed appropriate for viticulture and helped the industrial producers of Algeria and the Languedoc gain a competitive edge over more localized producers working in other parts of France.[24] These industrial producers looked to satisfy the needs of workers in the bustling cities of northern France.

The phylloxera crisis of the late nineteenth century also contributed to the growth of the industrial wine system.[25] The aphid destroyed one-third of French vineyards and diminished wine production by about 70 percent. Their vines devastated, fifty thousand families consequently moved to Algeria and seized some 700,000 hectares of land from the indigenous population.[26] The decline in metropolitan production as a result of the crisis provided a large market for Algerian wines, thus accelerating the development of the Algerian wine industry along the northern coast near the urban centers of Algiers, Constantine, and Oran.[27]

New technologies were developed in response to the phylloxera crisis. While wealthy growers in famous regions like Burgundy had the financial means to graft French vines onto phylloxera-resistant American rootstock, many peasant producers and some large proprietors planted cheaper hybrids that required less care and fewer chemicals, could stand up to pests, and produced higher yields. These hybrid grapes produced wines with a lower alcohol content, which encouraged the merchants who bought them either to add sugar to them or to blend them with the more alcoholic wines of Algeria. The hybrids that were planted in the Languedoc and in some other regions thus necessitated the merchants' purchase of Algeria's blending wines.

Capital mobilization also fueled the growth of the industrial wine system. The Bank of Algeria provided easy credit for investment in agriculture. Metropolitan bankers and industrialists rushed to invest money in vine plantations with the hope of high profits.[28] "The vine grower is a *business man*," a geographer observed of the Algerian scene, "an American businessman who has the mentality of a gambler. . . . The settler . . . borrows especially in good times: his confidence in the future knows no limits and throws caution to the wind; he manages his business, buys land, develops a taste for luxury, and spends without counting his money."[29] In contrast to the general trend of fragmented plots in the metropole, Algeria's concentrated vineyards provided the opportunity to experiment with new machines and technologies that could bring down production costs. Threatened by Algeria's competitive advantage, metropolitan growers liked to portray Algerian growers as money-hungry capitalists, the "moguls" or "nabobs" of the wine trade.[30] While only 6 percent of Algerian growers held properties larger than 50 hectares, this minority produced 56 percent of the harvest.[31] In 1935, the average vineyard plot was about 20 hectares in Algeria compared to under 1 hectare in mainland France.[32]

While the Algerian wine industry threatened the metropolitan wine industry, the Algerian wine industry enriched certain other metropolitan sectors, giving added weight to the argument that "Algeria is France." Metropolitan bankers, barrel-makers, dockworkers, and shippers all profited from the Algerian wine industry.[33] Furthermore, as long as the metropole continued to buy Algerian wine, Algeria was more willing to purchase metropolitan industrial goods. Although Algeria produced other cash crops, wine constituted 60 percent of Algeria's total exports and about 50 percent of Algeria's export earnings. Algeria sold 98 percent of its harvest on the metropolitan market.[34] Vine growing was the most profitable sector of the Algerian economy. To the metropolitan and Algerian interests that depended on the success of the wine industry, wine was the "common soul" between France and Algeria.[35]

The successful development of the Algerian wine industry hinged on land expropriation, social inequality, racism, and the genocidal massacre of indigenous Algerians who resisted French rule.[36] Settlers owned 93 percent of the Algerian vineyards.[37] The wealth taken from Algerian vineyards by the European settlers contributed to social and racial tension. Like many businesses in today's globalized world, the industrial wine system thrived on cheap indigenous labor and low transport costs. Although some intellectuals pointed out that wine production increased the locals' purchasing power, others perhaps put it more aptly: "the culture of the vine has, above all, the most considerable colonizing power."[38] The colonizing power of wine created social tensions between indigenous Algerians and European settlers.

While one side of the industrial wine system was located in Algeria, the other rapidly grew in the Languedoc. When Languedoc growers recovered from the phylloxera's ravages, they converted their low-yield vineyards into vineyards of mass production in the hope of quickly recovering years of lost income. These growers abandoned the hillsides and planted in the plains and the sands of the Mediterranean littoral. In place of the centuries-long practice of disheveled growth came orderly rows of vines lined in rank and file. Rational rows made it easier to plow, prune, and wage chemical warfare on pests.

Intensive monoculture thus also prevailed in the Languedoc.[39] Growers in the Languedoc cultivated especially the Aramon, a grape variety that yielded an abundant amount of wine—up to 400 hectoliters per hectare—but often lacked color and alcoholic strength.[40] Between 1880 and 1920, the average yield per hectare for France as a whole jumped from about 14 hectoliters to about 39 hectoliters.[41] In 1850, the region's four departments—the Aude, Gard, Hérault, and Pyrénées-Orientales—had made up 10 percent of France's vineyard area; by 1897, however, that proportion had climbed to 25 percent.[42] These departments now accounted for 42 percent of the country's total production.[43] Wine experts deemed, as they still do now, that high-yielding vines usually produced low-quality wines and, conversely, that low-yielding vines produced high-quality wines. Over the next half century, then, the large quantity of industrial wine produced in France and Algeria would come at the expense of quality.

Although industrial monocropping replaced small-scale production in the Languedoc, the vineyards were not consolidated to any great degree. Instead, small, fragmented properties predominated, a legacy of breaking up the aristocratic estates during the French Revolution.[44] In 1892, for example, about 82 percent of the region's wine producers owned between 1 and 10 hectares.[45] In the Aude department specifically, about half of the proprietors possessed less than one hectare.[46] Parliamentarians needed to protect these small proprietors in order to get their votes at election time.

The Languedoc also had large properties. In the Aude, proprietors of over 10 hectares owned 59 percent of the land while those with under 1 hectare controlled just 8 percent.[47] On the big estates, yields reached 105 hectoliters per hectare before World War I, while the national average was only 33.5 hectoliters.[48] Big estates had large amounts of capital, access to transportation, and thus a larger customer base, whereas smaller growers in the region depended on the willingness of merchants to pay a fair price for their grapes.[49]

A powerful merchant class bound the industrial wine system together and controlled the wine market.[50] As urbanization widened the distance between producers and consumers in the late nineteenth and early twentieth centuries, new distribution channels occupied the growing gap between producers in southern France and Algeria and consumers in northern France. To increase profits, merchants looked for the cheapest grapes around, further driving vine growers into mass production.[51]

With few regulations in place, the industrial wine system unavoidably damaged the reputation of France's luxury wine districts. Merchants often bought the cheaper wines of Algeria and the Languedoc, blended them to make their own cuvées, and then sold them under a prestigious place-based label. In theory, merchants blended only one type of wine: for example, a wine from the Anjou region with another wine from the Anjou region. In years when the grape harvest was of a lower quality, however, merchants were often compelled to purchase stronger or sweeter wines from elsewhere; in this way, they kept their beverage consistent and their customers satisfied. Bordeaux merchants often improved wines of poor vintages with the stronger wines of Algeria and other Mediterranean countries.[52] In the Chablis region of Burgundy, merchants bought cheap white wine from Spain and blended it with the more expensive wines of their home region, bottling it under the prestigious Chablis label.[53] Other Burgundy merchants blended wines from the Châteauneuf-du-Pape area, not yet organized and still largely unknown, into their Pommards and Volnays. Merchants also dominated the market because vine growers often lacked the money to invest in the equipment to make, bottle, cellar, and market their own wines. In 1903, 90 percent of wines on the French market were reportedly blended.[54]

If merchants had more power than vine growers, the numerous owners of drinking establishments could also hurt the vine grower's reputation by adding water, grape must, or chemicals to the wines they were serving.[55] By adding cheap ingredients, they aimed to evade taxation, increase their profits, and circumvent the long arm of the state. The taxes on wine were higher than those on grape must and other ingredients, thus encouraging many merchants and drinking establishments to introduce the latter to the small amounts of wine that they had purchased. Apparently some city dwellers used raisins to make wines in their own bathtubs that they then sold as luxury wines.[56]

Even growers were known to add all sorts of ingredients to their wine. During the phylloxera crisis, the aphid weakened some vines and destroyed many others, forcing growers to plant new vines and over-fertilize in order to accelerate ripening and boost yields. These practices caused the wine to be thin, low in sugar, and highly acidic. Growers therefore added calcium carbonate, other chemicals, or sugar to remedy these defective wines.[57] Sugar, in a process called chaptalization, increases the alcoholic strength of a wine, but many growers added sugar and hot water to the fermenting residue to increase their output. In 1903, for example, thirty-five communities in the Hérault department declared an official harvest of about 1 million hectoliters in all, but over 2 million hectoliters left these communities for northern France.[58] The story was the same in the Gironde region of Bordeaux: 2 to 3 million hectoliters of wine were produced and 6 to 7 million hectoliters were sold.[59] That some growers added foreign ingredients to the wine encouraged other growers to follow suit in order to remain competitive.

France's economic orientation around its empire solidified the industrial wine system and Algeria's status as an administrative part of France. In theory the Third Republic embraced economic liberalism, but in practice it raised tariffs to protect all sorts of groups, including industrial wine producers.[60] In 1867, France and Algeria had formed a customs union. Algerian wine thus entered France duty-free and became almost entirely dependent on the metropolitan market. One observer would later claim that "as much as the 1889 naturalization law," which granted citizenship to non-French European emigrants, "the culture of the vine contributed to Frenchifying European Algeria."[61] With a series of tariffs on wine imports in the 1880s, culminating in the Méline tariff of 1892, the government protected the Franco-Algerian wine industry from major competitor countries such as Greece, Italy, and Spain.[62] Although tariff protection demonstrated the ability of peasants and settlers to organize and persuade the government to protect their way of life, liberal-minded economists argued that it made producers inefficient and unwilling to change. A parliamentary commission in 1930 accurately summed up this latter attitude: "everybody is convinced of the necessity of exporting wine, but nobody wants to make a move towards abandoning [the privileges of the home market] that would permit the exportation of his wine."[63] Tariff protection thus fused Algeria to mainland France, defended the vine growers' livelihoods, and minimized the risks involved in becoming competitive on world markets. The industrial wine system was thus part of a political and imperial order in which powerful interests had a stake.

Industrial Wine's Allies

It is worth mentioning four other agricultural groups whose interests would become intertwined with the industrial wine system, making that system all the more powerful and therefore difficult for post-1945 sober revolutionaries to reform: beet alcohol producers, cider producers, home distillers, and commercial distillers. Since Napoleon's reign in the early nineteenth century, the state had encouraged beet production to make France independent of imperial and world sugar markets and to meet the domestic demand for sugar. Napoleon had also intended to use beet alcohol in industry, especially to make gunpowder. Until the phylloxera crisis, wine had been the main form of alcohol used in distillation, but as wine production plummeted during the blight, beet growers sold their juice to distillers who then sold distilled alcohol to the spirits industry. At the same time, a commercial distilling industry developed in northern France near the beet fields.[64] Modern techniques of distillation had made beet and grain alcohol cheaper than wine alcohol.[65] With little wine available, consumers purchased cheaper beet-derived spirits. Once wine production recovered from the phylloxera crisis, wine producers faced new competition in the beverage market from beet producers, a problem, as we will see, that would require government attention in the first decades of the twentieth century. Although the beet growers and distillers were more concentrated and less numerous than the vine growers, the former equaled and perhaps exceeded the latter in power.

Cider production was centered in Brittany and Normandy. Like wine and beets, its production increased during the Third Republic, from an average of about 10 million hectoliters in the 1860s to 20 million hectoliters in the 1930s.[66] As with wine, experts complained about the low quality of most of this cider. Little of it could be exported outside of its region of production. Most cider was produced and consumed in the informal economy or distilled tax-free within the home. In 1929 in Brittany, only about 39 percent of the cider produced went to market.[67] Cider production, like beet alcohol production, limited the wine industry's ability to win over consumers in northern France.

The home distillers were the third group that had a direct relationship with the wine industry. Home distillers were scattered throughout France. They made brandy from apples, grapes, and other fruits and could legally produce 10 liters of pure alcohol a year without being monitored by state agents as long as their product was consumed within the household.[68] Anyone who owned a few rows of vines or an apple tree could ask their commune for a certificate that allowed them to benefit from the statute. The home distillers' ability—they called it a right, their opponents called it a privilege—to produce untaxed alcohol had its origins in the French Revolution. For this reason, they argued that any attack on their craft was a violation of private property and individual rights. The home distillers developed a reputation for evading the state's rudimentary surveillance of production, occasionally chasing away tax collectors with pitchforks. Their newspapers reported that tax inspectors paid the distillers a visit when only their wives were at home.[69] On several occasions, the state tried but failed to remove the practice.

Home distillation was not simply a hobby; it was also a calculated attempt by vine growers and cider producers to deal with surpluses and find a use for their lowest-quality fruit. Given the frequency of surplus harvests in the early twentieth century and favorable laws permitting home distillation, the number of home distillers jumped from half a million at the beginning of the Third Republic to about a million at the turn of the twentieth century. In the early 1900s, it was said that one farm out of every four had at least a portion of its harvest distilled.[70] Home distillation risked turning consumers away from commercial wine and brandy.

Finally, the commercial distillers purchased alcohol to make spirits and industrial products, thus further legitimating the industrial wine producers' existence.[71] Immediately after World War II, some sober revolutionaries would go so far as to suggest that the real power in the industrial wine system lay with these distillers and that "the myth of the small" merely served to prop up the distillers' interests.[72] The industrial wine system and its allies were thus a dynamic complex composed of vine growers, beet and apple farmers, merchants, distillers, and owners of drinking establishments. In the next section, we will see how in the early twentieth century wine lobbyists and their allies succeeded in building a structure of power that subordinated the state to their needs.

Early Efforts to Regulate Wine Production

From its inception, the industrial wine system was highly unstable as a result of its tendency to generate surpluses. Between 1900 and 1907 and again between 1928 and 1936, an oversupply of wine saturated the French market. Prices, property values, and incomes plummeted. Several factors caused these wine surpluses and thus the producer's plight: the new habit of selecting grape varietals that ensured higher yields; the expansion of industrialized viticulture in Algeria; new kinds of alcohol that entered the market to fill the void left by the phylloxera crisis; the emergence of wine industries in the Americas that threatened previously secure French export markets; the Third Republic's tariff policy, which often led to retaliatory measures in importing countries; and the growth of temperance movements in Canada, Sweden, and the United States that dried up markets.

The vine growers' efforts to assert control over the domestic market took place in this competitive imperial and international environment.[73] Desperate for state succor in resolving their economic problems, vine growers threatened public order. In 1907, over five hundred thousand inhabitants of the Languedoc demonstrated in the streets of Montpellier, the region's capital. Many residents participated in tax strikes. Businesses closed their doors. Local politicians resigned. In serious clashes with the army, troops fired on angry crowds of growers; several were killed and many more were wounded. The crisis of 1907 set the trend for subsequent revolts in the Languedoc, including some that crippled the region in the early 1930s.[74] These uprisings challenged state authority to such an extent that officials chose to protect producers instead of demand painful reforms.

To defend themselves from the flood of industrial wine on the market, and from the merchants who sold cheap wine under expensive labels, luxury wine producers also demanded that the state protect their interests. State officials half-heartedly aided them in the controversial work of vineyard delimitation with the creation of a series of laws, most notably those enacted in 1905, 1919, and 1927. A law against fraud in 1905 obligated producers to abide by practices that were "local, loyal to, and consistent with tradition," among them a measure requiring wine labels to indicate the wines' place of origin. Yet the law failed to specify the definition of best practices, nor did it allow for state surveillance of production. In consequence, the law did little to discipline the wine market. The 1919 law tried to go further in protecting fine wines, but the courts refused to include any mention of the most appropriate grape varietals that growers were supposed to use, or the most suitable soils in which growers were to plant their vines, or what was specifically meant by the expression "local, loyal to, and consistent with tradition." As a result, just about any grower on any piece of land could grow grapes however they wished. To increase profits, many turned to high-yielding hybrid vines. The law of 1927 thus discouraged the use of hybrids and underlined the importance of the grape varietal and the "traditional zones of production." Yet abiding by the law was optional, did not apply to all of the existing appellations, and failed to establish a minimum alcohol content and maximum yield, which led to the production of wine with an alcohol content of 7 percent by volume and yields four times larger than what was expected of luxury wine.[75]

Although the laws of 1905, 1919, and 1927 marked the state's first attempts to regulate the place and conditions of production, they also demonstrated the difficulties of establishing centralized norms. First, economic liberalism prevailed in the corridors of power, at least in theory. Second, many vine growers and merchants clung to their fierce individualism, especially when state-imposed norms threatened their autonomy. Third, when the economic depression struck France in the early 1930s, the government was reluctant to force peasant producers to carry out risky reforms. Nearly a seventh of French vineyards were planted with cheap hybrids at that time, a figure that would continue to rise through the 1950s.[76] Fourth, the local courts that presided over the appellations tended to side with existing economic interests, which favored the merchants.[77] Fifth, many industrial vine growers with the means to do so fled to the self-regulating appellation system and exploited loopholes in the law, which degraded the quality and reputation of the fine wine that the appellation system was intended to protect. They did this because strict regulations were concurrently being established for industrial wine, because appellation producers could continue to add sugar to the fermentation process to boost the alcoholic content (industrial producers could not) and because the development of appellations had the effect of branding all other wines as "ordinary." The production of wines declared with an appellation of origin thus jumped from 5 million hectoliters in 1923 to nearly 16 million hectoliters in 1934, the year before industry leaders and the government intervened and instituted the National Committee of Appellations of Origin (CNAO) to address this new problem.[78] The CNAO would become the National Institute of Appellations of Origin (INAO) in 1947. Two months before the government decreed the creation of the CNAO, a senator from Bordeaux expressed his regret that "the law against fraud had become a law that favored fraud."[79]

The onset of the Great Depression, which coincided with another surplus crisis, marked a turning point in the state's attitude toward intervention in the wine industry and the economy more generally. The chronic surplus problem and the diminishing global competitiveness of French wine incited a group of wine leaders to draw up plans to reorganize the industry. Wine was the very first sector to undergo the statist experiment of the 1930s, an unmistakable sign of its economic, political, and cultural significance.[80] Even though vine growers claimed that they were preserving traditional practices, doing so required a restructuring of the wine industry, the creation of standardized norms, and the construction of a new administration to investigate and organize knowledge about production. By bringing the state into the vineyards, producers in reputable districts hoped to protect their wines from imposters, and officials sought to police and tax production, stabilize the market, and reinforce state authority over regional economies.

Reform-minded wine leaders—notably Joseph Capus, an agronomist and senator from Bordeaux; Édouard Barthe, a Socialist deputy from the Hérault; and Pierre Le Roy de Boiseaumarié, a lawyer and vine grower who was trying to build the reputation of the wines of Châteauneuf-du-Pape—persuaded the state to classify and control wine production by segmenting the market: ordinary wine, what is here called "industrial" wine (*vins de consommation courante*), would come mostly from Algeria and the Languedoc, and luxury wine would come from the new regional appellations that were being delineated. The state would continue to orient ordinary wine around an insulated imperial market while tailoring luxury wine to global markets. The work of mapping and ordering wine into "ordinary" and "appellation" systems reinforced the boundary between quantity, which was largely merchant-controlled wine from Algeria and the Languedoc, and quality, which was largely grower-controlled wine in the metropole.

Industrial wine regulations consisted of a series of laws known as the wine statute, enacted between 1931 and 1935, that aimed to stabilize prices for growers in the short term and limit and improve production in the long term. Given that France was already in the throes of a glut, the government attempted to block wine from the market and prevent further vine plantings. The statute thus obliged growers to store part of their surpluses, imposed extra taxes on high yields, prohibited new vine plantings on vineyards of more than 10 hectares or on vine growers who produced more than 500 hectoliters of wine, subsidized the grubbing up of high-yielding vines, and required the distillation of surpluses when yields in France and Algeria exceeded a total of 65 million hectoliters. Growers whose average yield over the three previous harvests was more

than 500 hectoliters or whose production averaged more than 80 hectoliters of wine per hectare had to distill the excess.

These measures discriminated against the largest proprietors, located
mostly in Algeria, at the same time that they ossified the power structure
of the industrial wine system. Prohibitions on planting new vines made
it much more difficult for new players to enter the wine industry. At the
same time, distilling surpluses helped the state shore up the industry. A
consumer organization during the 1950s persuasively argued that the statute of the 1930s "crystallized overproduction but didn't combat it."[81] In
Algeria, outlawing new vine plantings forced a growing indigenous population into city slums, where it struggled to find work, a trend that would
have major consequences for the stability of French Algeria after World
War II.

To appease the industrial vine growers of Algeria and the Languedoc
and their agricultural and distilling allies, a state agency (Service des
alcools) purchased wine surpluses, distilled the product for use in industrial goods, and found resale outlets. This state alcohol agency had been
created in World War I to purchase beets for making industrial products.
After the war, the powerful beet lobby came to an agreement with the
wine lobby about maintaining the industrial market for beet alcohol and
giving wine alcohol free rein over the consumer market. But during the
crisis of the 1930s, the state alcohol agency also began purchasing surplus wine and cider. Wine subsequently became an ingredient in all sorts
of industrial products: perfume, rubber, even a "national gasoline" that
was supposed to curb France's dependency on the Anglo-American oil
companies.

Barthe successfully framed the 1930s wine statute as serving the general interests of agriculture. Other raucous and powerful agricultural
interests who received advantages through the state alcohol agency or
who hoped to obtain similar protection now threw their support behind
the legislation. Since the 1920s, Barthe had claimed that the state alcohol
agency would help France "escape the hegemony of the great worldwide
trusts" and "increase the financial and economic strength of the nation
by the limitless development of the richness of its soil."[82] A deputy from
the northern beet-growing region thanked Barthe for "the fine fight he
had waged for twenty years on behalf of industrial alcohol."[83] Grain producers joined the chorus when they were reminded that the "increased

cultivation of the beet meant a better cultivation of wheat."[84] The numerous home distillers also backed the wine statute in exchange for wine
industry support in extending their tax-free production privileges.[85] The
Society of French Farmers called the wine statute an "enormous advance
for all French agriculture."[86] Finally, the minister of finance claimed that
the agency boosted "France's domestic finances and her foreign-exchange
balance."[87] The state alcohol agency supported not just vine growers but
also fruit growers, beet alcohol producers, and grain farmers.

Consumer organizations, although much weaker than the wine lobbies
in influencing state policy in the 1930s, backed the state alcohol agency,
which gave it further democratic legitimacy. Consumers supported the
agency even though they had to underwrite it through taxes on wine and
gasoline.[88] The state alcohol agency created a budgetary deficit of 300 million francs in 1935, but this expense was tolerated as a political expedient
during the hard times of the economic depression.[89] One observer noted
that the alcohol-based gas "demands sacrifices and contributions from
the entire collectivity," and consumers were apparently willing to pay the
price.[90]

The wine statute fell short of its aim of limiting and improving wine
production: smallholders were mostly exempted, and the larger proprietors often evaded the law.[91] Each year, officials had to determine how
much wine was to be blocked and distilled, thus giving the wine lobbies
ample opportunity to influence the decision-making process. Further, state
inspection of production was rare. Jean Hennessy, of the famous cognac
family and a former minister of agriculture, suggested that "the situation
of the winegrowers is simply a boil to be lanced—that's to say this is a
means of treatment entirely exceptional and temporary . . . an exceptional
remedy for an exceptional situation."[92] That other powerful agricultural
interests had a vested interest in the state alcohol agency meant that a
complete restructuring of the wine industry would prove even more difficult. The state tried to keep depression-hit peasants on the land as the
bulwark of a teetering social order. Thus the wine statute of the 1930s
ended up being not a program of progressive reform but one that sought
to preserve the status quo.

Barthe's painstaking work in organizing the industrial wine market
helped Le Roy de Boiseaumarié, Capus, and luxury wine leaders give
greater definition to the appellation laws. How could a luxury be a luxury

if no "inferior" products existed on the domestic market to contrast it with? A decree of 30 July 1935 both regularized the state alcohol agency and established the CNAO. The CNAO, which Capus called "eminently corporative," represented a new alliance between luxury wine producers and the state that sought to stabilize wine markets by limiting production, improving quality, and rooting out imitators at home and abroad.[93] The CNAO replaced the local courts in standardizing procedures and enforcing the law on what became known as "controlled appellations," the cream of the crop in the luxury wine world. To obtain this new status, producers had "to discipline themselves, eliminate the high-yielding land for viticulture that was unfit for the production of fine wines, and replace crude grape varietals with noble grape varietals."[94] By "crude" varietals, the CNAO meant hybrids that churned out plonk and supposedly drove its drinkers insane.[95] Earlier appellation laws had focused solely on delimiting vineyards; now, the CNAO added production methods to its vision of tradition, authenticity, and quality.

The state's wine regulations of the early 1930s were a response to instability in regions with strong local identities. Politics had been radicalized in the hard times of the Depression. In the Languedoc, vine growers and their Socialist and Communist allies took to the streets and invoked the memory of 1907 in order to receive state aid. Representatives of Algeria in Parliament warned the government of a fratricide if it discriminated against Algerian wine.[96] At the same time, a growing indigenous population in Algeria, increasingly discontented with their living standards under French rule, began to organize various nationalist movements. In the cider country of Brittany and Normandy, militant home distillers, under the leadership of right-wing populist Henry Dorgères, violently protested the state's encroachment on their production.[97] Vine growers pressured the government for assistance, and home distillers agitated to be left alone; either way, both groups challenged the state's legitimacy. These economic and political problems, which would continue well into the postwar period, spurred the development of the appellation system.

These wine regulations must be situated in the broader political and cultural movements of the 1930s. During the economic crisis, figures like Alfred Sauvy, groups like X-Crise, and newspapers like *L'État moderne* championed more centralized political control, economic management, and greater commercial cooperation among European countries. Although these reformers had a range of views on how to reform France's political economy, most could agree that some form of corporatist or technocratic order was preferable to liberalism. Parliament, in their view, had become a useless talking shop. Economic plans were in vogue in the early 1930s among intellectuals and politicians from across the political spectrum.

For some of these reformers, wine exemplified the economic and political problems of the day. The government's inability to resolve the chronic wine crises underscored state impotence and economic sluggishness.[98] In 1932, the minister of the interior told André Tardieu, then prime minister and a darling of the technocrats, that Parliament would never work in the long-term interests of the country because "they are obliged to show the greatest caution towards the winegrowers of their respective regions." Tardieu doubted that "our legislative efforts can lead to a durable solution."[99] Even Barthe and Capus, parliamentarians from vine-growing regions, upbraided Parliament for watering down their original vision of the wine statute.[100]

The creation of the CNAO benefited from these corporatist and technocratic ideas. In the final years of the Third Republic, expertise in the administration gained ground on the politicians in Parliament. For thirty-two months between March 1934 and July 1940, the administration issued decrees instead of Parliament passing laws.[101] The laws against fraud in the first decades of the twentieth century, and especially the law establishing the CNAO, foreshadowed the growing diffusion of expertise into political and economic life after the war. Key reformers of both the post-1945 state and the wine industry—Michel Debré, René Dumont, Philippe Lamour, Pierre Mendès France, and Alfred Sauvy—came of age during this first struggle to regulate the wine industry.

Metropolitan vine growers also took advantage of public debates about the nature of authentic France.[102] Intellectuals, business leaders, politicians, and state officials expressed an interest in preserving or reviving "authentic" regional cultures at a time of heightened anxiety about hybridity, rootlessness, and Americanization. In the wine industry, "authenticity" almost invariably referred to the European metropole, not Algeria. In Burgundy, for example, vine growers, folklorists, the food industry, and politicians marketed quaint images of the peasantry and the land.[103] This served to empower vine growers against the merchants of the industrial wine system. Local elites commodified their

local wine industry through folklore, gastronomic fairs, and wine festivals.[104] The CNAO's corporative structure, emphasizing quality over
quantity and incorporating local versions of folklore and tradition,
helped distance appellation wine from the social crises of the 1930s—in
particular, the socioeconomic problems that agonized regions like Algeria and the Languedoc. Appellation-based production gave a timeless
quality to France's luxury wine districts, even though the CNAO was
in fact an active bureaucratic construct used to reinforce control over
production and revenue.

Amid the debates over authentic regional cultures, some metropolitan
wine lobbies and economists questioned the links between France and
Algeria, deploying a discourse that remained marginal in the 1930s but
would have greater resonance in the 1950s. The CGVM claimed that
Algerian wine was foreign and thus fraudulent, thereby denaturalizing
the metropole's link to Algeria. One of its leaders echoed a common sentiment in the Languedoc in the widely read *Revue des deux mondes* when
he bluntly asserted that "to consider Algeria as a strict extension of France
would be a mistake; it's too different from the mother country because of
its race, religion, and morals thus to be a part of the latter."[105] Another
observer reasoned that to cultivate a hectare of vines in the metropole
required 1,200 hours of work, 1,000 of which were carried out by French
workers and 200 by foreigners. The situation was nearly the inverse in
Algeria, where indigenous people carried out 70 percent of the labor. Thus
"a hectoliter of Algerian wine is . . . less French than a hectoliter of metropolitan wine."[106] For metropolitan wine interests, Algeria lacked a tradition of wine production, had been colonized by money-hungry capitalists,
exploited the indigenous population, and therefore lacked authenticity
and quality.

The CGVM's rhetoric resonated with those who observed structural
problems in French capitalism and who took stock of the specter of mass
insurrection in Algeria.[107] Metropolitan vine growers argued that Algerian farmers needed to convert their vineyards to the production of other
foodstuffs.[108] The National Economic Council, a corporative assembly
of the country's economic interests, warned that "there are products
that must be firmly discouraged or forbidden in the colonies . . . above
all wheat . . . and wines. If the growth of the Algerian vineyard is not
halted both the French and Algerian vine growers will be ruined."[109]

Furthermore, indigenous peoples grew increasingly disgruntled as they faced unemployment and hunger. The *Annales coloniales* anxiously asked: "Will Algeria remain French?"[110]

Despite metropolitan attacks on Algerian wine, few politicians dared upset the industrial wine system, or France's relationship to Algeria, during the Depression. While luxury vine growers in Burgundy worked to connect consumers to the producers and advertised a bucolic, European image of France, Édouard Kruger, an important Algerian wine lobbyist, invoked France's imperial identity through Greater France.[111] With limited markets during the Depression, Algeria became one of France's most important trading partners.[112] A metropolitan financial analyst advised the vine growers of the Languedoc to show more gratitude toward Algeria given their dependence on its blending wines.[113] If some observers criticized the lack of complementarity between the metropole and Algeria, the government in Paris chose to ignore this problem in the 1930s for fear of raising the fury of two wayward regions. The result was a divided market that defined and defended luxury wine against a sea of cheap industrial wine at the same time that this market was solidifying the structure of power in the industrial wine system. Regulations in the 1930s ultimately preserved the interests of the regulated instead of forcing producers to undertake structural reform.

Engineering Consent for the Industrial Wine System

The inability of state officials to tackle wine surpluses through structural reform led these officials to cajole metropolitan consumers to drink more wine, thus engineering consent for the industrial wine system and the political and imperial order that sustained it. As sober revolutionaries would later claim, the political problem of regulating the quantity and quality of the wine supply was responsible for a rapidly rising rate of wine drinking. Wine consumption, like wine production, rose vertiginously during the Third Republic. In the 1850s, before the industrial wine system and the Third Republic had emerged, each French adult drank approximately 120 liters per year, already a prodigious amount; between the 1920s and 1940s, when industrial wine production reached its high-water mark, that level had increased to about 240 liters.[114] Drinking establishments catered to the new drinking culture, rising from 464,000 liters in 1901 to a high of 509,000 in 1937.[115]

Many factors drive a person to drink, but sober revolutionaries would later reduce heavy drinking to the wine lobbies' ability to influence policymaking in the Third Republic. In 1931, Barthe, Le Roy de Boiseaumarié, Capus, Kruger and other industry leaders convinced the government to create a National Committee for Wine Promotion (CNPFV) and help finance its operations.[116] At the same time in Bordeaux, respectable doctors created the French Society of Pro-Wine Doctors (SFMAV), which received financial support from the CNPFV and which lauded the healthful benefits of wine drinking. The CNPFV and the SFMAV took advantage of modern advertising to convince the population to drink more wine.

World War I set a precedent for state-sponsored wine propaganda when the state allocated large quantities of wine to drain the surpluses and fortify soldiers on the front. Rations increased throughout the war, up to three-quarters of a liter of wine a day by war's end.[117] A professor of viticulture claimed that "soldiers who drank wine were less fatigued, had more energy, and were able to carry out more sustained military activity."[118] A parliamentarian averred that "a glass of wine . . . is a glass of morale."[119] Some observers went so far as to credit the military victory to wine. Soldiers from across France picked up the wine habit, one that would stick with them after the war.

State policy in the 1930s naturalized wine in everyday life to an extent unseen in French history by assuring the public that wine was a dietary staple, not a luxury. To promote wine consumption, the state made use of the agents and objects of the republican civilizing mission: schools, the army, and the empire. Wine was presented as a pillar of French civilization. The CNPFV suggested that "wine propaganda must start at primary school . . . it's at this stage of life that the child is the most malleable and receptive and this is when he should be told about wine."[120] Developing the wine habit in children, before they could know any alternative, was an effective way of ensuring lifelong consumption. The government also continued to target the army, noting that "the soldier must be accustomed to wine drinking. It would be useful to serve a half liter of wine per person with every meal in barracks."[121] Finally, wine propaganda was aimed at the sixty million subjects of the French empire who could be "civilized" by learning to drink wine.[122] The prime minister derided the existence of "the millions of Mohammedans and Buddhists who abstain from wine."[123]

To ensure that wine was viewed as a food, both doctors and politicians advocated its nutritional qualities.[124] At school, math problems were based on the idea that "1 liter of wine with an alcohol content of 10 percent by volume corresponds as a foodstuff to 900 grams of milk, 370 grams of bread, 585 grams of meat, or 5 eggs" (figure 7).[125] While the British government enacted a school meal service, the French Ministry of Education allocated wine to its hungry schoolchildren.[126] Postcards and stamps in the 1930s endorsed Louis Pasteur's dictum that "Wine Is the Healthiest and Most Hygienic of Beverages" (figure 8); others warned that "A Meal without Wine is a Day without Sunshine."

Consumers happily agreed. Who could say no to sunshine? During the entire interwar period, the prestigious Academy of Medicine maintained a longstanding distinction between wine and "unnatural" spirits, as if the former were a food and the latter were a drug. Moreover, between 1919

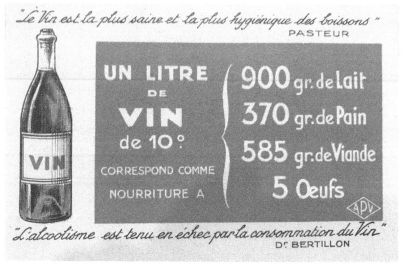

Figure 7. Promotional material from the Association of Pro-Wine Propaganda, c. 1930s. The text reads: "1 liter of wine with an alcohol content of 10 percent by volume corresponds as a foodstuff to 900 grams of milk, 370 grams of bread, 585 grams of meat, or 5 eggs." The quote at the top is from Louis Pasteur: "Wine is the healthiest and most hygienic of beverages." The quote at the bottom is from a Dr. Bertillon: "Alcoholism is kept in check by wine consumption." Courtesy of the National Archives of France, Pierrefitte-sur-Seine.

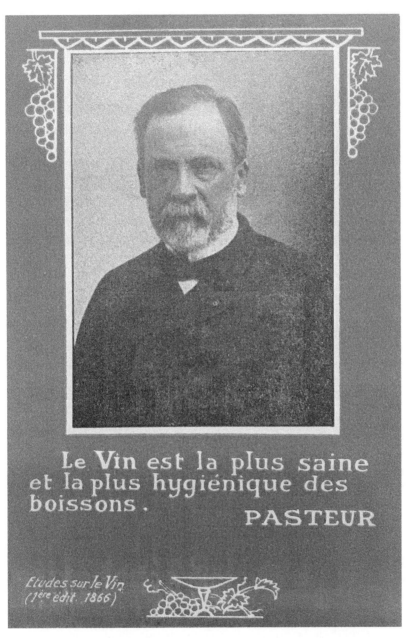

Le Vin est la plus saine et la plus hygiénique des boissons.

PASTEUR

Etudes sur le Vin
(1ère édit. 1866)

Figure 8. Promotional material from the Association of Pro-Wine Propaganda, c. 1930s. The material features a picture of Louis Pasteur and his famous dictum, "Wine is the healthiest and most hygienic of beverages." Courtesy of the National Archives of France, Pierrefitte-sur-Seine.

and 1939, the Academy engaged in but one big debate on alcoholism. Nor did the Ministry of Public Health want to make alcoholism into a public problem.[127] In the 1930s, then, at a time of economic crisis and debates about the nature of true France, wine's grip on state and society grew tighter.

Wine surely meant different things to different people, but scholars have shown how it was invariably linked to republican values including individual liberty, solidarity, the political parties, and a public sphere founded in part on France's numerous drinking establishments.[128] By lifting taxes on wine, the French revolutionaries of the 1790s had given the people the right to drink.[129] By the 1890s, some observers referred to wine as a right specifically of workers.[130] To keep workers happy and perhaps even stupefied, leaders of the Third Republic wished to protect that right. Drinking establishments sheltered clubs and labor unions. Victor Hugo had called cafés the "Parliaments of the People," a description even more apt in the 1930s than in the nineteenth century.[131] Wine and drinking establishments were both materially and symbolically tied to republican and working-class politics from the beginning of the Third Republic to its end in 1940. The link that the wine lobbies had made between wine and nutrition and wine and republican values made wine all the more difficult to decenter from daily life. In this way, wine drinking helped sustain both French Algeria and the parliamentary system. But when the authoritarian Vichy regime came to power under Nazi tutelage in 1940, its leaders used the humiliation of defeat as an opportunity to tighten regulations on the wine industry at the same time that wartime conditions shook the commonsense nature of wine in French life.

Vichy's Regulatory Environment

In June 1940, France fell to Nazi Germany, marking the end of the parliamentary Third Republic. The elderly and paternalistic Marshal Philippe Pétain, the hero of Verdun in World War I, was called on to establish an authoritarian government at the spa town of Vichy, where he governed most of southern France and the colonies and set about cleansing France of its republican past. Meanwhile, the Nazis occupied northern France and the Atlantic coast, and Italy controlled a part of the southeast. The defeat of 1940 and the subsequent Vichy regime was important to the post-1945 sober revolution for two reasons: it furthered the movement to regulate and improve wine production, and it raised awareness about the public health consequences of vineyard monoculture and the political system that enabled it.

It used to be the norm to treat the Vichy regime as an aberration in French history given its authoritarianism and its collaboration with Nazi Germany, but now we know that many of the political and cultural movements that began in the 1930s received Vichy's sponsorship.[132] The regime simultaneously promoted earlier ideas about economic modernization and essentialist images of rural France. Technocracy and nostalgic traditionalism went hand in hand. Pétain emphasized a conservative moral order in the hopes of ridding France of the selfish individualism, class antagonisms, and power of big business that he saw develop under the Third Republic. "Liberty, Equality, Fraternity" was replaced with the more dutiful motto "Work, Family, Fatherland." France, wrote Pétain, "will recover all its ancient strength through contact with the soil."[133] While Pétain preached the return to a moral order, the collapse of parliamentary institutions provided new opportunities for the reformers of the 1930s to overhaul the economy, even if difficult wartime conditions limited their ability to implement their visions.

The important question here is how the wine industry fits into the debate about continuity and rupture from the Third Republic to the Vichy Regime and how the Vichy experience contributed to laying the foundations for the post-1945 sober revolution. Despite certain continuities in efforts to regulate the wine industry, Vichy administrators created a symbolic break with the Third Republic by discrediting the parliamentary regime for its failure to resolve the wine surplus crises. The industrial wine system and the policies that supported it were seen as an unfortunate product of the Third Republic's liberal values. For this reason, Barthe came under fire as an example of parliamentary inefficiency. *Au Pilori*, a collaborationist newspaper, "blamed him for being 'against the Marshal': 'Barthe throws a wrench in the wheels of the new government. . . . He incites protest, alerts shadow syndicates, he is against the laws that the government passes. . . . He pushes the vine growers to refuse the state its wine tankers and Paris is deprived of wine.'"[134] Barthe was jailed between October 1941 and February 1942 for having advised the vine growers in southern France to resist German requisitions. He was subsequently released, placed under house arrest, and banned from any travel in the vine-growing regions.[135]

While industrial wine leaders like Barthe suffered under the new regime, appellation leaders such as Capus and Léon Douarche joined Vichy administrators in pillorying Parliament for having inadequately managed the wine crisis of the 1930s. Douarche asserted that "if, from a political perspective, the parliamentary solution is of a debatable efficiency, from an economic perspective, its interventions are necessarily harmful. . . . The insufficiency of the measures taken resulted from the French political regime."[136] From his perspective, Vichy's authoritarianism provided the CNAO with a chance to pursue further reforms. Douarche participated in the discussions about France's place as a junior partner in a German-led Europe. International demand for luxury wine made France "the most interested country in this new European economic order."[137] The CNAO supported the creation of a European economic sphere, even if it was to be under Nazi dominion.

Vichy officials hoped to improve the wines of the Languedoc in order to make them less dependent on Algeria. Pétain inveighed against the producers of the Languedoc for their commitment to vine monoculture. An August law obliged growers who owned vineyards of more than 5 hectares to plant 10 percent of their land in other crops.[138] The law was motivated by the pressing needs of food supply but also by the desire to transfer viticulture from the plains to the more suitable slopes. Wine experts in the Languedoc joined the movement to improve wine production. Jean Branas, a professor in Montpellier, promoted the improvement of vine-growing and winemaking techniques.[139] Lamour, already an ardent supporter of technocratic ideas in the 1930s, began championing the creation of a Delimited Wines of Superior Quality (VDQS) label, a halfway house between AOC and industrial wine. The VDQS aimed to determine the best grape varietals for a given soil and set yield limits and alcohol volumes that would guarantee the wine's quality. To encourage vine growers to adopt the VDQS, tax advantages were given to the VDQS at the expense of ordinary wines.[140] Branas and Lamour would advocate for the expansion of the VDQS label after the war.

That Algerian imports came to a halt further encouraged growers in the Languedoc to improve their production. A lack of labor and materials led to the deterioration of Algerian vineyards. Production reached a wartime low of 6.6 million hectoliters in 1943 (the high had reached 22 million hectoliters in 1934).[141] The Vichy regime furthered the Third Republic's exclusionary measures against Algeria. A decree of 1942 forbade Algerian producers from using quality designations like *cuvée réserve*, *réserve*, and *grande réserve*.[142] The experience of war and occupation thus advanced the movement against the industrial wine system.

The Vichy regime sought to continue the process not only of restructuring production but also of disciplining the industry by developing tighter relations among vine growers, merchants, and the state. Merchants, so vital to the industrial wine system but also to the sale of appellation wines, were associated with the rampant greed that had existed under the capitalist Third Republic.[143] Vichy administrators embraced the corporatist creed that gained traction in the 1930s.[144] Appellation leaders joined them in calling for a wine corporation "composed exclusively of technicians and practitioners, to the exclusion of all politicians."[145] In Champagne, growers, merchants, and the state came together to defend their common interests in the first Interprofessional Committee, a pattern that would expand to other regions after 1945.[146] In the interests of promoting quality production, the Vichy regime worked with the growers and merchants who showed a willingness to respect the rules of the CNAO and to expand appellations, even if the conditions of the occupation complicated these efforts. New appellations were created in Bordeaux and Burgundy, and new vine-growing regulations were imposed.[147]

While wine industry leaders and Vichy administrators continued the Third Republic's efforts to educate vine growers and enforce regulations on production, doctors and demographers initiated a separate movement to edify consumers about the dangers of daily wine drinking. The combination of state-sponsored wine propaganda in the 1930s, reports of a drunken army, anxieties over population decline, and a swelling Nazi army prompted some doctors to rethink the relationship between wine and health.[148] The wine that had been celebrated for inspiring victory in World War I was now condemned for sapping the army's strength. Alarmed that the state had returned to its World War I policy of procuring large quantities of wine for its soldiers, a doctor at the Academy of Medicine argued that the medical profession's "prolonged silence has contributed to consolidating in the people the opinion that wine does no harm and has no relationship to alcoholism."[149] On 28 May 1940, a wine commission at the Academy blamed the wine industry and the state for cultivating a belief about the benefits of wine drinking: "there is in our country an old tradition of wine, salutary drink, legend that, for already numerous years, has been confirmed, developed, and dare I say exploited by an extremely powerful political and commercial association."[150] In this view, consumers had become the victims of the wine lobbies and their political allies. While some blamed the Third Republic for the repeated surplus crises, others blamed it for causing alcoholism.

Vichy administrators enacted legislation that prohibited the production and sale of spirits, reduced the number of drinking establishments, and limited the activities of the home distillers.[151] Vichy's policy on alcoholism did not greatly differ from the Third Republic's during World War I; in both cases, the state most obviously targeted spirits, never openly attacking wine. The wine lobbies continued to be active during the occupation. Georges Portmann, a Bordeaux doctor and senator, had strong connections at Vichy.[152] Other wine-friendly doctors continued to promote the idea that wine was a food and a necessary source of calories, an idea that especially resonated during a time of shortages. The medical schools in Bordeaux and Paris offered courses on "The Vine as a Medicinal Plant" and "Wine in the Diet."[153]

Although the Vichy regime did not prohibit wine drinking for fear of losing its legitimacy, it could and did ration and requisition wine. The frequent oversupply that had beleaguered politicians in the 1930s turned into scarcity in the early 1940s. Given poor weather and a lack of labor and material, the declared national harvest fell during the war, from about 49,000 hectoliters in 1940 to about 29,000 in 1945.[154] Interestingly, wine production did not drop as dramatically during the occupation as during World War I.[155] Yet unlike in the first war, officials rationed wine to 2 liters per adult per week in 1940, a ration that would later be restricted to men.

Perhaps out of necessity, perhaps out of a concern for public health, or perhaps for both reasons, Vichy leaders gave the Germans access to the country's wine stock. In 1940, the Germans began requisitioning wine, about 2 to 3 million hectoliters per year during the war.[156] Although Hitler apparently showed little interest in wine, calling it "nothing but vulgar vinegar," much of the Nazi elite—Joseph Goebbels, Hermann Göring, and Joachim von Ribbentrop—did have a taste for France's luxury wines.[157] Nazi agents exported luxury wines from France to Germany, where they were then resold to help pay for the war. The equivalent of 320 million bottles were annually sent to Germany, the majority of which had not been requisitioned but were sold by vine growers and merchants.[158] The above quantities are surely the minimum taken by the Germans; much more was likely never declared. Wine rations, requisitions, and exports reduced the amount of wine available to the French population, thereby bolstering Vichy's collaboration with Germany and Vichy's moral crusade.

Wartime strains undercut the ongoing efforts at quality control. The wartime situation encouraged many people—for political reasons or survival or some combination of the two—to defy Vichy's authority by producing and consuming wine and brandy in the informal economy. The declared national harvest plummeted, doubtless as a result of shortages in labor and material, but likely as well because producers refused to declare much of their wine as an act of resistance to the new regime. More was to be earned on the black market. Because of state-directed rationing and requisitioning, and because the state was Vichy, black markets and fraud flourished.[159]

In regions without access to wine, peasants planted vines and made their own wine and brandy to be drunk by family and friends. As the Languedoc wine economist Jules Milhau remembered, "undeclared harvests coming from undeclared vines competed disloyally and mortally with wine from 'traditional vine growers,'" a problem that would continue to grow in the postwar years.[160] Moreover, inspectors in the Repression of Fraud agency lacked the resources to enforce quality production. Vine growers often exaggerated how much land they owned so that they could justify their high yields, and many declared the wines that they made from hybrid vines as appellation wines to increase profits.[161] Finally, despite laws against home distillation, the number of home distillers reportedly grew from about one million in 1941 to about three million in 1944.[162]

Given its need to supply the population with wine, the Vichy regime often did not enforce its own laws or relaxed them by allowing for more blending, watering, the use of hybrid vines, and lower minimum alcohol levels for industrial wine. Those parts of the 1930s wine statute that limited production—uprooting vines, restrictions on new plantings, irrigation, tax on yields, compulsory distillation—were suspended.[163] The CNAO quickly grew frustrated with the situation: "All the regulation on provisioning is conducted as much against the elite as against quality. It rewards high yields, penalizes the selection of grape varieties, prevents initiatives at improvement, kills the superior product by refusing to recognize its cost of production."[164]

Wartime supply problems seemed to provide evidence of the relationship between vine monoculture and alcoholism. In occupied Brittany and Normandy, where food had remained plentiful but alcohol was scarce because of poor harvests and restrictions, the mortality rate for alcoholism and cirrhosis among men aged thirty-five to sixty-four declined more dramatically than at the national level. Conversely, in the Languedoc, where wine drinking stayed relatively steady but food consumption diminished, rates of alcoholism and cirrhosis remained high. Whether or not such statistics were accurate, they provided weight to the scientific argument that wine was not a food and that restricted supplies would lead to reduced rates of consumption and thus a healthier population.[165]

Pediatrician Robert Debré and statistician Alfred Sauvy, both of whom had worked on population policy since the late Third Republic, were responsible for this new evidence and called on the state to intervene at the Liberation. Debré argued that the rare degenerate who ate away at French society was not at the root of French alcoholism; rather, alcoholism was a social habit caused primarily by wine.[166] For Debré and Sauvy, reforming wine production and consumption was part of a broader vision of reforming political institutions and remaking economic and social life. Even though one of Europe's most notorious dictators had just fallen when they made their view known in 1945, they still advocated for a "dictator of anti-alcoholism" who would restructure the wine industry.[167]

Yet at war's end, many vine growers fought to restore their liberties and interpreted the state's intervention in the wine industry as draconian and synonymous with the discredited Vichy regime. Growers in the Languedoc, tired of heavy taxes on their wines, demanded more favorable treatment.[168] Many growers anticipated a postwar spike in demand and thus planted high-yielding, low-quality vines, despite Milhau's dire warning that "this outlook is full of danger for the French economy in general and even more for the wine industry. . . . We have now reached the threshold of a catastrophe."[169] This tension between technocrats looking to resolve the repeated wine gluts, improve production through regulations, and adjust the economy to international competition, on the one hand, and peasant and settler vine growers struggling to maintain their way of life, on the other, would take center stage in the post-1945 sober revolution.

Conclusion

In trying to remedy the wine surplus problem with subsidies and advertising that extolled the virtues of wine drinking, the Third Republic served the interests of powerful agricultural lobbies and the settlers of French Algeria. Metropolitan wine drinkers were complicit—often unknowingly—in protecting the peasantry and the French presence in Algeria. Despite conflicting interests between the vine growers of Algeria and the Languedoc, this system helped bind Algeria to France and wine to power. The political necessity of "Algeria is France" was in direct contradiction to the economic reality of France and Algeria's competing wine industries. When the wine industry confronted a series of crises that threatened the livelihoods of several million people, the industry came together to solicit state support. Because producers were organized and had a tradition of protest, and because politicians depended on rural votes, the state opted to subsidize wine surpluses, find new outlets for them, maintain price levels, and raise tariffs against foreign competitors. Through advertising, the state inspired consumption. Drinking wine became so routine that it was taken for granted, helping naturalize the peasantry and French Algeria at the same moment that broad economic forces were starting to challenge their existence.

The crisis years of the 1930s and early 1940s laid the foundations for the sober revolution by introducing new ideas about the state's management of the wine industry. Although both Barthe and Capus would die just after the war, other able leaders would take up the torch. Many of the key post-1945 reformers of the wine industry began their ascent in the late Third Republic and the Vichy regime. Wine leaders like Le Roy de Boiseaumarié who were committed to addressing the wine problem ultimately turned toward the larger project of state reform as a way to restructure the industry. State reformers like Lamour, Michel Debré, Mendès France, and Sauvy subscribed to the new ideas about state and economic modernization and would turn to the wine and alcoholism problems as a way to implement their larger ideas. For post-1945 sober revolutionaries, overcoming the economic inefficiencies of the wine industry depended on overhauling the political institutions that shaped French capitalism, sustained vine monoculture in the Languedoc and Algeria, and kept people drinking daily plonk.

Yet these new ideas failed to materialize into an effective movement against the wine industry in the 1930s and 1940s, for several reasons. First, politicians in Parliament had to protect their constituencies if they wished to win reelection; political expediency outweighed a long-term plan. The state thus in some cases failed to enforce the new regulations and in others watered those regulations down. Second, wine lobbyists were successful in convincing politicians that protecting the industry was in the general interest of agriculture, a powerful political and cultural force in the Third Republic. Third, numerous economic and political actors viewed Algeria as an indissoluble part of France. During the Great Depression, the metropole depended heavily on trade with Algeria: the metropole bought Algerian wine as long as Algeria purchased the metropole's industrial products. Fourth, although the Vichy regime dissolved Parliament and continued earlier efforts to restructure the wine industry and promote quality wine, the hardships of the war and occupation thwarted thoroughgoing change. The problem of surpluses turned into a problem of scarcity and how to allocate supplies. In the 1930s and 1940s, opposition to the industrial wine system had not yet adequately organized.

The state's legitimacy hinged on appeasing agricultural and Algerian settler interests. The search for stability overshadowed the call for change. Even as a fringe of reformers came to the belief that the wine statute coddled inefficient producers, penalized the taxpayer, and sapped the national economy, the state kept growers on the land. For both the Third Republic and the Vichy regime, too much was at stake. For France's numerous producers and those who did business with them, wine was a way of life to be protected; for consumers, wine was a dietary staple and a source of conviviality; and thus for France's leaders, wine was a ticket to legitimacy. "The social order," one observer reductively claimed, "rests on a bottle of alcohol."[170] Formidable obstacles stood in the way of any fundamental transformation of the industry. And yet after World War II, that transformation, despite many twists and turns, would finally occur.

2

The Imperative of Intervention

While most French revolutions were fought over the barricades, one was fought over the bottle. In the wake of World War II, newspapers sounded the alarm about France's allegedly rising alcoholism. Between 1945 and 1952, the number of alcoholics reportedly tripled, from 1,420 for every 100,000 adults to 4,260.[1] Statistics from the newly established World Health Organization (WHO) were severe: with 30.5 liters of pure alcohol consumed per year per average adult, the French were easily the world's heaviest drinkers of alcohol.[2] In one year, the total number of workdays lost to alcoholism was estimated at 6.25 million; alcoholism caused 33 percent of work accidents and 40 percent of driving accidents.[3] Wine—Rabelais' muse, the source of the foot soldier's strength, the nation's ancestral drink—was reportedly causing a national scourge.

From the ruins of France's economic collapse in the 1930s and the war-time occupation, new forms of expertise turned wine from a virtue into a vice. Powerful groups with a stake in reconstructing France wielded this expertise to challenge the wine industry and the institutions and myths that protected it. Between the war and 1954, two popular but separate reform movements converged, one to combat surpluses and the other to curb alcoholism. On one side were technocrats hankering to resolve France's surplus problem; peasants and settlers became tropes of backwardness. On the other were public health activists intent on curbing alcoholism, working to eradicate the popular yet old-fashioned belief that wine was a dietary staple.

The technocrats—reform-minded agronomists, notably René Dumont and Philippe Lamour, and economists, statisticians, and demographers like Alfred Sauvy and Jules Milhau—lent their expertise to a network of state institutions that were charged with designing a plan for the modernization of the wine industry in particular and the French economy more generally: the planning commissions, the Economic Council, the National Institute of Demographic Studies (INED), and the Ministries of Agriculture and of Finance. These experts and institutions were supported by dynamic lobbies representing a range of industries—automobiles, trucking, tires, restaurants and tourism, health spas, chemicals, and oil—and consumer activists in trying to convince the government to regulate wine and cut subsidies as part of a general program of expanding the economy and driving down the price of consumer goods.[4] With Marshall Plan aid set to end in the early 1950s, the state faced an urgent need to rationalize the budget and find ways to finance economic development. Yet efforts to make the wine industry more efficient were stymied by the return of Parliament in the new Fourth Republic (1946–1958).[5] Wine and alcohol lobbies—the General Confederation of Southern Vine Growers (CGVM), the General Confederation of Algerian Vine Growers (CGVA), the General Confederation of Beet Growers (CGB), the National Federation of Cider Producers (FNPFC), the National Syndicate of Home Distillers (SNBC), and the large distillers grouped in the French Institute of Alcohol (IFA)—immediately reasserted their influence over parliamentary politics and sought to ensure the continuation of the state alcohol agency (Service des alcools) that defended their interests.

At the same time, however, public health activists—doctors like Robert Debré, Léon Dérobert, and Étienne May—were redefining alcoholism not only as a moral or medical issue, as they had since the nineteenth century, but more controversially as a problem of state institutions that subsidized wine and alcohol surpluses. French anti-alcoholism advocates were active internationally, particularly at the WHO, but they frequently pointed out that French alcoholism resulted from the country's wine tradition and social habits and less from psychopathy found in other industrialized countries.[6] The drinking norm was the problem, not deviations from the norm. Their views were adopted by another network of state and non-state institutions: the Academy of Medicine, the National Institute of Hygiene, the Ministry of Public Health, and the National Committee for the Defense Against Alcoholism (CNDCA), the country's main temperance organization. In making alcoholism a problem of French political institutions and economic arrangements, public health activists attracted the technocrats' interest. This unlikely coalition set about upending the myth that industrial wine was central to the country's economic and social wellbeing, casting it as a cause of France's economic backwardness, as unhealthy, and as an instrument of political oppression. Such a dire assessment might make the population amenable to new modes of expert intervention in the wine industry and help the technocrats achieve supremacy over the alcohol lobbies and parliamentarians who obstructed their vision of French renewal.

The struggle that sparked the sober revolution centered on the state alcohol agency that purchased alcohol surpluses in order to prop up powerful yet inefficient agricultural interests in mainland France and Algeria. The alcohol agency thus became a key site of contestation between the forces of freer trade and modernization that favored the localization of wine through the appellation system, on the one hand, and the forces of protectionism and the status quo that sided with the industrial wine system, on the other. In the heat of a surplus crisis in the summer of 1953, the statistician Sauvy wrote in *La Journée vinicole*, a major wine newspaper, that "the defense of vested interests pushed to the extreme will lead France to decadence" and that "the problem of alcohol and winegrowing is one of the most striking examples of this degeneration."[7] In the same newspaper the following summer, Pierre Le Roy de Boiseaumarié, the leader of the National Institute of Appellations of Origin (INAO), criticized French vine growers for stagnating behind protective walls and for "falling asleep with a false sense of security resulting from the certitude that never, and nowhere, will other countries reach the perfection of our noblest wines."[8] Defenders of the state alcohol agency in the IFA attacked officials for granting Sauvy the power "to supply through statistics . . . a sophisticated form of lying . . . the facts of French political economy."[9] The CGVA censured Le Roy de Boiseaumarié for calling on the government to uproot vines in Algeria and thus unfairly discriminating against a French region.[10] This first postwar struggle to transform wine offers a window onto a broader debate over the direction of France's political economy, as it pitted a parliamentary and imperial republic that needed to maintain the privileges of peasant and settler agriculture against a more technocratic republic that looked to centralize state power, liberalize the economy, and protect public health.

The Movement to Rationalize Wine Production

The agents of the industrial wine system, weakened by unfavorable wartime conditions, quickly restored their authority in the first years after World War II. Taking advantage of high prices resulting from years of lean supply, growers expanded their vineyard areas and increased yields. Algerian production doubled from 9 million hectoliters in 1945 to 18 million in 1953. Metropolitan yields jumped from 40 million hectoliters in 1943–1944 to around 60 million hectoliters in 1953–1954.[11] By the early 1950s, the wine industry had a surplus of approximately 20 million hectoliters.[12] As in the past, the oversupply led to falling prices, poverty, and misery in Algeria and the Languedoc. The wine lobbies mobilized their parliamentarians to protect their interests through the state alcohol agency, much as they had in the 1930s.

Unlike before the war, young finance inspectors indicted the state alcohol agency for its economic inefficiency. In 1953, a surplus year that saw protest movements in the Languedoc, the state purchased over 4 million hectoliters of alcohol, more than twice as much as the market could absorb. The state had three possible outlets for this alcohol. First, it could export the alcohol, but its world price was lower than its domestic price. Second, it could use the alcohol for industrial purposes such as the "national gasoline," but by the early 1950s scientists and economists were demonstrating the costliness of this product compared to foreign oil.[13] Third, it could sell the alcohol to consumers, but the size of the consumer market was estimated to absorb only half the amount the state alcohol agency was purchasing. The state, as a result, profited from none of these outlets; in fact, the agency cost the Treasury about 20 billion francs a year.[14] Yet the alcohol lobbies and pro-alcohol politicians persuaded the agency to revert to its 1930s practice of buying the surpluses instead of demanding structural reforms.

The state alcohol agency faced new international constraints, however. The post-1945 world was very different from the 1930s world in which the agency had been created. The instability caused by the economic depression and war had put new pressures on policymakers to open the economy. With the United States in a position of international leadership and advocating freer markets as a way to ensure peace and prosperity, some French agricultural and economic experts wished to integrate France into an American-backed West European common market. The immediate post–World War II years marked the era of the "green pool," when experts devised plans to integrate the agricultural economies of Western Europe.[15] Yet the industrial wine producers, along with other agricultural interests, opposed the prospect of a Franco-Italian customs union in 1949 given Italy's competitive wine industry.[16] Although the green pool failed, the technocratic dream of an open market for Western Europe persisted.[17] The state alcohol agency stood in the way of preparing the wine industry for such competition.

Desperate to rebuild after years of depression and war and preparing for heightened international competition, state institutions like the planning commissions and the INED had increased legitimacy to advise politicians on how to manage, renovate, and "free up" economic and social life. This expertise was putatively apolitical, but in fact it served the interests of those who would gain the most from economic liberalization: the technocrats themselves, who developed the economic expertise and who wished to assert their authority against the parliamentarians, along with key industrial and agricultural sectors. The planning commissions, Ministry of Finance inspectors, the Ministry of Agriculture, the Economic Council, and the INED all engaged with the problem of restructuring the wine industry as a way to legitimate their authority over the political process. Key technocrats who provided expertise to these institutions had witnessed the problems confronting the wine industry in the 1930s, including Sauvy, Dumont, Lamour, and Milhau. Although these technocrats claimed to serve the general interest, they were all driven by the ideology of maximizing economic growth even if it meant obliterating the local ways of knowing and doing that blocked reforms.

At least rhetorically, technocrats and vine growers were worlds apart.[18] While technocrats resided in Paris and spoke the language of rationalism, functionalism, and profit, vine growers lived in the provinces and largely considered their craft a labor of love. Technocrats applied science and data to solve economic and social problems; vine growers adhered to local know-how. "Today," one agricultural newspaper observed, "we have to deal with bureaucrats, whose youth makes them presumptuous and who are all the more contemptuous of the realities of peasant life since they are often of rural stock. They no longer want to have any contact with the countryside except for during vacation."[19] In the first post–World War II years, the wine lobbies and other agricultural groups would sense a gulf between their way of life and the interests of technocrats in far-off Paris.

Alfred Sauvy, a well-connected economist and statistician and key expert in the state institutions charged with modernizing the economy, was among the most influential Paris-based critics of the wine industry and the archetypal technocrat who had abandoned the land. Most famous for coining the term "Third World," Sauvy compared the rural under-development of mainland France to the underdevelopment of the colonial world. The corollary was that if the French state did not take action in the countryside and in the colonies, these regions would revolt against the state, much as the revolutionaries of 1789 had revolted against the king. As a child, Sauvy had participated in the violent wine protests in his native Languedoc, including the revolt of 1907 that had demonstrated for the first time the political might of the region's vine growers. In this sense, Sauvy was a critic from the inside, and yet still an "unrepentant technocrat."[20] Sauvy and his colleagues drew comparisons between the Languedoc and Algeria; in both regions, vine monoculture led to wasteful surpluses, deprived the local populations of other foodstuffs, and created the conditions for alcoholism throughout the French Union, the euphe-mistic label given to the French empire after 1945.[21] Through his political connections, Sauvy extended his influence to the various branches of gov-ernment and tried to serve as a bridge between Paris-centered technocrats and province-based wine producers.

French wine policy seemed to exemplify the "Malthusianism" that technocrats so loathed.[22] Sauvy defined Malthusianism as a state of mind

that showed satisfaction with the status quo, a "French disease . . . resulting
from the secular aging of the population, which atrophies the creative
spirit and puts in its place the fear and anxiety of protection."[23] For modernization to succeed, French mentalities needed to change, and the state
was responsible for changing them. In a paternalistic tone, René Dumont,
a colleague of Sauvy's who had begun his career studying agricultural
practices in the French colonies, observed that "the technical training and
even more the economic orientation of our peasantry is truly in its infancy
since we've let it commit such crude errors. *All together, these errors will
lead to the ruin of our economy.*"[24] Dumont assumed that new forms of
agricultural science were better than the peasants' tried and tested ways
of farming. Peasants, in his view, had to be taught that viticulture was a
business and that economic rationalization would be good for them.

The wine industry represented economic wastefulness akin to that
found in the peasant societies of the Third World, a comparison that resonated in a period of heightened anxieties over the colonial war in Indochina, Americanization, and the decline of France as a world power.[25]
Dumont highlighted similarities between the inefficiencies of the French
wine industry and the Vietnamese economy: "three hours of work for
the vine grower on the slopes per liter of alcohol allows an automobile to
travel about ten kilometers. In the Far East, a hardworking coolie could
cover the same distance with two men in a rickshaw in an hour and a half.
Wouldn't it make more sense to allocate our 'surplus' vine growers to
this type of towing?"[26] Official statistics showed that 1.5 million growers
planted vines on 1.5 million hectares of land.[27] Technocrats argued that
this labor force could serve more productive purposes.[28] Moreover, the
weak wines of the Languedoc depended on the stronger blending wines
of Algeria. For this reason, the metropole was both the world's largest
producer and importer of wine.[29]

The comparison between rural France and the Third World was one
recurring theme in the technocrats' discourse; another was the "feudalism," as some critics termed it, of the industrial wine system that made
it seem antiquated and undemocratic.[30] In this account, instead of protecting the peasants' way of life, the industrial wine system propped up
feudal privileges, mired the peasantry in poverty, and prevented general
prosperity. References to feudalism suggested that the technocrats of the
post-1945 period had something in common with the revolutionaries of

1789. These technocrats, if given the authority to do their work, would emancipate producers and build a modern republic based on peace and prosperity for all.

To drive home their case about the pitfalls of economic stagnation, political inequality, and social injustice, technocrats marshaled statistics to demonstrate that the place of wine in French society was diminishing in importance, thus implying that a protective wine and alcohol policy served only the producers, not the national economy. These statistics led Dumont to believe that wine surpluses were no longer episodic but permanent. France and North Africa simply produced more than consumers could drink.[31] The economist Jules Milhau agreed, showing that wine's value in agricultural production was in constant decline. Milhau anticipated "inevitable and painful socio-economic transformations" in the French wine industry. In 1948–1949, viticulture made up nearly 13 percent of the value of agricultural production; in 1951–1952, it dropped to 9 percent.[32] The decline of viticulture resulted from a permanent reduction in wine consumption, which he linked to a demographic revolution that had been underway since the war. As before the war, France had 42 million inhabitants, but 1.5 million more children than adults. This transformation affected demand: as family expenses surpassed individual expenses, Milhau predicted that milk consumption would surpass wine consumption.[33]

Dumont and Sauvy complained that while politicians subsidized frequent wine gluts that could not be exported, the country produced an insufficient amount of perceived dietary necessities such as milk, meat, and sugar. Given that a hectare of vines required four times the workforce of a hectare of grain, wine production took time, space, and energy away from the production of other crops and livestock.[34] Despite France's rich agricultural potential, the country depended on agricultural imports, which adversely affected the balance of payments at a time when the government was trying to finance economic modernization. Dumont believed that France could either produce alcohol and watch as the country degenerated or produce milk and meat and watch as the country grew.[35]

To reorient and diversify production and make the Languedoc less dependent on Algeria's blending wines, technocrat Philippe Lamour continued his wartime work of convincing the vine growers of the Languedoc to irrigate in order to compensate for the region's arid climate and convert to other crops.[36] Lamour, who had helped develop the Delimited Wines of Superior Quality (VDQS) label during the war and who was inspired by the work of the Tennessee Valley Authority (TVA) in the United States, devised a plan to build Europe's biggest canal in the Rhône and Languedoc regions.[37] Producing a wider range of foodstuffs could help resolve the surplus problem, render France more self-sufficient, relieve labor-intensive wine production, and move people off the land and into industry. In the technocrat's mind, a wine revolution could support a dietary revolution; combined, these revolutions could stimulate economic growth.

While plans were being hatched to restructure the Languedoc economy, technocrats in Paris hesitated to impose the same kind of restructuring on Algeria. It was not yet clear, in the first years after World War II, that power was shifting from the settlers to the indigenous population. True, after the war, the Economic Council called for a reduction in the size of the Algerian vineyard and the planning commissions expressed concern that the industrial wine system caused malnutrition in Algeria and alcoholism in the metropole.[38] Yet criticisms of the Algerian wine industry were more forthcoming than were realistic reform programs, especially when the new expertise conflicted with vested interests. Dumont complained that in North Africa "the transition to irrigation is still very slow."[39] The settlers primarily and the metropolitan consumers of Algerian wine indirectly were major obstacles to reform. The local government in Algeria supposedly lacked the funds to carry out agricultural reforms, and state officials in Paris hesitated to use tax money to subsidize such reforms.[40] Despite competition between the Algerian and metropolitan wine industries, the settlers were insistent on maintaining the status quo, even if some of them publicly expressed interest in improving their production and competing internationally.[41] A few Algerian vineyards obtained VDQS status in the early 1950s, making up 6 percent of the Algerian wine harvest in 1954.[42] Finally, reports indicated that metropolitan drinkers were ever more drawn to Algerian wines.[43] For these reasons and others, policymakers in Paris maintained their claim that "Algeria is France."

The aim of ensuring a diversified food supply and enhancing France's economic performance was doubtless sincere, but by doing so state officials could also break up the political power of the industrial wine system and reinforce state authority over underdeveloped and subversive regions. As we saw in chapter 1, the settlers of Algeria and the peasants of the Languedoc, along with their cider-producing and home-distilling allies in Brittany and Normandy, were notorious for their strong local identities and for defying centralized power. The early 1950s marked the most crippling crisis that the wine industry had undergone since 1907 and the early 1930s. Left-wing parties had a preponderant influence in the Languedoc, a cause for concern in the context of American aid and the Cold War. In Algeria, economic and social unrest racked the diverse populations: the settlers demanded a more supportive wine policy at the same time that indigenous elites blamed vine monoculture for the problem of hunger.[44] In northwestern France, rabble-rousers like Henry Dorgères and Pierre Poujade, both of whom also had supporters among the settlers of Algeria, mobilized peasants against centralized authority. If technocrats could succeed in ending monocultural practices, the people of Algeria, Brittany, and the Languedoc might share fewer common interests and become easier to govern.

Contrary to technocrats' claims about being above politics and ideology, their interests aligned with those of powerful economic interests that wished to reform the state alcohol agency and free up and expand the economy. "Freeing" up the economy, in France or elsewhere, is always deeply political and divisive, reflecting the interests of the powerholders even if it is couched in terms of the general welfare. In both 1950 and 1953, the Economic Council, in opposition to its agricultural groups, voted in favor of reforming the state alcohol agency.[45] The automobile industry, the main drivers' lobby, the oil industry, the tire industry, the tourism industry, and the trucking lobby also came out against it.[46] French drivers were unanimously against the alcohol-based "national gasoline," deploring its low quality and high cost and complaining that it would hurt French tourism because foreign automobiles were not designed for it.[47] Consumer activists, who had supported the state alcohol agency in the 1930s, had a change of heart in the early 1950s. The Federal Union of Consumption (UFC), a consumer activist group that began its work after the war, blamed the state alcohol agency for making wine prices artificially high.[48] The UFC encouraged the state to reverse its 1930s policy of prioritizing the welfare of producers over that of consumers at a time when technocrats saw consumer behavior as the key to economic growth. Some of France's most dynamic, export-oriented sectors and consumer activists joined the campaign to limit and improve production for export markets.

At first glance, it would seem likelier that the industrial wine system, with its emphasis on monoculture and product standardization, was more in tune with the technocrats' rationalist discourse than the artisanal appellation system. Yet the industrial wine system included many peasants who, from an economic standpoint, worked land in the plains and whose labor could be more useful to the national economy if moved into other sectors; in Algeria, indigenous vineyard workers were increasingly unhappy with French rule. Industrial wine was difficult to sell to anyone other than metropolitan—and often poor—drinkers. Although the AOC and VDQS classifications tended to cultivate on small plots on the slopes, which limited mechanization, their growers jibed with the logic of economic rationalization because they produced on officially classified land, their harvests were closely monitored and taxed, their yields were often lower, and their wines commanded a high price on global markets.[49] Appellation wines accounted for a small portion of the overall wine harvest. In 1954, for example, producers declared just under 13 million hectoliters of appellation wine compared to over 46 million hectoliters of industrial wine.[50] The state had more control over appellation wine than it did over the numerous peasants, settlers, and indigenous laborers who produced for the industrial wine system and who faced a deteriorating socioeconomic situation in the early 1950s.

The appellation system's claims to authenticity, quality, and tradition made its wines more exportable than industrial wine. Most consumers within the French Union could not afford luxury wines, so AOC producers looked to sell on more lucrative world markets.[51] An estimated 623,000 hectoliters of the 707,000 hectoliters of wine that France exported were appellation wines, while four-fifths of the wines sold *within* the French Union were industrial wines.[52] Mis de Lur-Saluces, a producer of luxury bordeaux wine and president of the National Committee for Wine Promotion (CNPFV), informed the public that exports of appellation wine generated over 17 billion francs in revenue. Unlike other sectors like industrial wine, textiles, or metallurgy that required raw materials from the colonies or beyond, AOC wine was a net profit for the Treasury because it was produced entirely within metropolitan France.[53] AOC wine was not only exportable; it also helped render France self-sufficient and held the potential to stimulate France's regional economies, a concern of the postwar state.[54]

Although the appellation system had emerged as a way to delimit and protect luxury wine, it became a strategy deployed by the INAO to transform the industry as a whole, save the smallholder, and bring peace and prosperity to the wine regions as the state prepared the economy for international competition after 1945. For this reason, and because the surpluses of the industrial wine system hurt the appellation business, Le Roy de Boiseaumarié and other industry leaders sought to impose the regulations of the appellation system on all of French wine production.[55] Yet they continued to face resistance from the peasants in the Languedoc, the settlers in Algeria, and these groups' agricultural and distilling allies who guarded their privileges, as well as from the many consumers who still saw industrial wine as a staple and a right.

The Movement to Rationalize Consumption

As technocrats worked to "emancipate" peasants from poverty by rationalizing agriculture and opening the economy to international competition, another group with a different agenda echoed the call for less wine and more milk, meat, and sugar in the interest of setting consumers free from the chains of tradition and habit. At the end of the 1930s and during the war, members of the Academy of Medicine had come to a new understanding of French alcoholism, now seeing wine as a primary cause.[56] Moral arguments against habitual drinking did not disappear, but they faded into the background of a new public health campaign to limit wine production by reforming France's political and imperial order. Immediately after the war, public health activists rarely drew the same 1930s distinction that the state had made between appellation and industrial or ordinary wine. From the medical perspective, *all* wine posed a public health risk: quantity, not quality, mattered. While public health activists could find common ground with the technocrats who were looking to modernize wine and agriculture, a public health campaign that blamed alcoholism on wine threatened to alienate the growing appellation system. The wine industry usually united when confronted with the anti-alcoholism message.

To economic and public health experts, freeing citizens from the unhealthy habits created by the industrial wine system ironically required weakening parliamentary power and imposing authoritarian measures. For this reason, public health activists did not contribute to the collective amnesia over the Vichy regime; they underlined how the authoritarian Vichy government, with no Parliament to impede action, had enacted a series of decrees that regulated the drink trade and rationed and requisitioned wine.[57] Public health activists assumed that state policy, as much as wartime shortages, explained falling consumption; these activists failed to acknowledge that the official statistics did not take into account the thriving black market during the war. Yet the policy argument became the basis of a claim that the postwar state, despite a return to parliamentary democracy, needed to continue its efforts to regulate wine production in order to curb drinking.

The postwar economic and political climate—one where state officials intensified efforts begun in the late Third Republic and the Vichy regime to coordinate the economy and promote the population's welfare—informed the new understanding of alcoholism. Public health activists took as fact what was instead a claim: that a correlation existed between surpluses and the rate of alcoholism. In asserting this connection, they sought to demonize Parliament as undemocratic and as serving the vested interests of the wine industry to the detriment of the general population. French democracy, they lamented, had been turned into a *bistrocratie*.[58] The argument that surpluses necessarily led to heavier consumption had important implications: it suggested that citizens were powerless to act in an environment where wine was readily available. The corollary was that the state should intervene to save consumers from the wine industry's greed.

Public health activists fused anxieties over alcoholism to the state's concern over agricultural modernization. In this way, the wine industry was called on to consider consumer interests, not just producer interests. Instead of converting wine production into more nourishing foodstuffs, public health activists feared that the state would, as in the 1930s, preserve the status quo by protecting the producer, burdening the national budget, and pushing the consumer to drink more wine. Dumont countered conventional wisdom that "the economy has always been organized for the profit of the producer, and not for the benefit of the consumer, and therefore the general interest: this is a dangerous deviation."[59] From his perspective, in protecting wine, the state was tampering with the laws of the market, which prevented farmers from growing healthier, more profitable products.[60] Dumont neglected to admit that altering production would require reforming consumption; the state would thus have to intervene in the market to create new norms.

The supposed link between wine surpluses and alcoholism raised questions about state responsibility, both in the metropole and in the colonies. If wine production resembled Third World agriculture, then wine drinkers took on the supposed irrational attributes of non-European peoples. Public health activists claimed that the political institutions of the Fourth Republic, like those of the Third Republic, stupefied its citizens and colonial subjects. In this view, citizens and subjects could not know what was best for them. Instead of genuinely seeking out wine because they found pleasure in it, consumers had been duped into thinking it was necessary. Such a portrayal helped justify statist intervention in the wine economy in the name of consumer welfare.

Public health activists also worried that the subtle persuasion of alcohol advertising made citizens into victims. To them, the state's behavior in the 1930s had confirmed this point. In 1948, the state reconstituted the CNPFV, which, backed once again by influential doctors, claimed that consuming luxury wine "remains the best way to fight against alcoholism."[61] Public health activists lamented the amount of alcohol advertisements found in the newspapers, on the streets, and on the highways. In 1950–1951, Sauvy gave a series of lectures at Sciences Po on alcohol advertising and its insidious intent.[62] Alcohol companies sponsored sporting events. Children reportedly wore paper hats that familiarized them with the various alcohol brands, conditioning them to drinking before they were old enough to make their own choices about it. France's main temperance lobby complained that the Ministry of Agriculture had granted the CNPFV 50 million francs to advertise wine, whereas the Ministry of Public Health could only give France's main temperance lobby 500,000 francs.[63] In this way, public health activists supported the technocratic effort to demonize Parliament for irresponsibly governing the country and failing to serve the general interest. This legitimated their own expertise and authority over policymaking.

Demographers juxtaposed the vice of wine to the virtues of milk. Wine became an icon of old and feeble France, an obstacle to increasing milk consumption, which symbolized young and vigorous France. At a time when the birthrate was rising, demographers showed concern for France's high infant mortality rate, especially in the towns of the Languedoc.[64] Doctors noted that children usually took wine to school for lunch; if they had to travel far, they brought spirits to provide them with energy. One observer reported that in western France the "teachers have failed to have wine replaced with milk."[65] Doctors and demographers with an interest in reforming the wine industry called on the planning commissions to link economic modernization to the "human factor," which meant that France should produce goods that benefited the population. In other words, more milk and less wine. The planning commissions hoped to elevate French milk consumption from 99 liters per person in the 1930s to 127 liters, the same level as in England, Germany, the Netherlands, and Denmark before the war.[66]

The debate about the proper governance of wine was magnified in the colonial context. At a time when a population boom, unemployment, and hunger were driving colonial independence movements to organize and revolt against French imperial rule, dumping wine surpluses on undernourished colonial peoples drove home the contradictions of the civilizing mission.[67] The combination of wine surpluses and limited export potential in the 1930s had led the state to push wine onto its colonies. Between 1939 and 1951, France's alcohol exports to its colonies increased by 37 percent.[68] In 1954 and 1955, about one-half of France's exports went to its colonies.[69] Public health activists upbraided France's governing institutions.[70] One doctor confessed that "if we've brought to the colonies a lot of the benefits of civilization, we've alas also introduced a growing quantity of alcoholic beverages."[71] Another observer noted that "it seems paradoxical, if not shocking, to observe that alcohol consumption in black Africa increases at a dizzying speed whereas sugar consumption develops only gradually."[72] In 1953, René Dumont observed that "the Algerian vineyard, in contributing to French alcoholism, has compromised the dietary balance of this country [Algeria]."[73] Sauvy warned that vineyard monoculture and the lack of food in Algeria would cause problems for France "at the United Nations or elsewhere."[74] Wine, icon of French civilization, was becoming the source of discontent among independence movements and metropolitan reformers who looked either to overthrow or reform the empire.

Liberating the colonies from the industrial wine system was not the same thing as emancipating the colonies from French rule. Reformers hoped that the temperance message would deliver a more just form of governance in the colonies and the metropole. One critic of the state's submission to the wine lobbies argued that addressing the wine problem was synonymous with preserving European civilization in the colonies.[75] If underdevelopment existed in the colonies, wine policy was partially to blame. Public health activists had faith that less alcohol would lead to economic growth, thereby re-legitimating the French presence in the colonies.

Not only did the wine lobbies and their parliamentary allies supposedly victimize consumers in metropolitan and colonial France, but the costs of habitual wine drinking to the state were also becoming clearer. After World War II, social security began to cover alcohol-related illnesses, which forced policymakers to reconsider the economic value of wine.[76] The more the state paid for treatment, the more citizens were likely to seek treatment. Alcohol-related illnesses became more visible. Both the INED and the Ministry of Finance showed that, although in the short term the state generated revenue through wine taxes, the public health consequences of wine saddled the national economy in the long term. One INED researcher observed that "the illusion created by the monetary revenues is deep-seated and the particular interests in question are devoted to maintaining it. The best way to destroy this illusion would be to assess, in as exact and complete a way as possible, the economic loss that alcoholism makes the nation undergo in human life and in wasting productive power."[77] A bureaucrat at the Ministry of Finance demonstrated that the direct cost of alcoholism for the state came to approximately 132 billion francs in 1950 and reached 152 billion in 1952. The Treasury only received a fraction of the returns it was owed. The state allegedly lost 80 billion alone in 1950.[78] Through statistical assessments, experts hoped to challenge dearly held beliefs about wine as a source of health, wealth, and power.

Public health activists expressed their anxiety about alcoholism in economic terms, seeing a correlation among French drinking habits, France's excessive mortality rate compared to other industrialized countries, and poor economic performance. Doctor Étienne May calculated that by reducing alcohol consumption "we could thus increase our lifespan by 4 percent which . . . would represent a gain of 2.5 percent of work hours. Related to a gross production of 13 billion in 1952 and in assuming that the production is exactly proportional to the hours of work, this loss of activity of 2.5 percent corresponds to a material loss of 323 billion francs."[79] As this passage suggests, public health activists connected drinking to broader concerns over productivity. This was a language that technocrats could understand. Life, in this passage, boiled down to hours worked and profits made. The state could profit from neither a drunkard nor a dead man.

Statistics offered a seemingly objective argument for public action. With this approach to alcoholism, public health activists sought to make the campaign seem natural and necessary, a prerequisite to larger economic reforms. The INED, along with a new generation of technocrats at the Finance and Public Health Ministries, monopolized the production of knowledge on alcoholism.[80] Any knowledge or opinion produced without the state's endorsement was deemed less rigorous, reflecting the state's ability to discredit other perspectives. Because the state's interest lay in productivity and economic growth, these technocrats placed the issue of alcoholism within the framework of the general interest, making the state's intervention in the industrial wine system an economic and public health imperative.

By rendering alcoholism not only a problem of moral degeneration but especially one of economic torpor, public health activists sought to advance their agenda by collaborating with the technocrats who saw the state alcohol agency as a major obstacle to restructuring the wine industry, promoting exports, and achieving economic growth. In their attempt to reform France's political institutions, technocrats and public health activists would gain more legitimacy by working together. Yet no natural alliance existed between them. Doctors hoped to protect public health, which could drive down consumption and torpedo the technocrats' goal of generating revenue. Sauvy and the INED became an important interlocutor between these two groups. Not only did Sauvy have close ties to eminent doctors like Robert Debré, but he also had connections to agronomists like Dumont who were key players in the planning commissions responsible for making wine and agriculture more competitive.

Although technocrats no doubt increasingly expressed concern about the costs of alcoholism, they would have attacked wine surpluses and subsidies whether or not there had been a public health campaign to reduce wine drinking. In the early 1950s, like in the 1930s, reform-minded agronomists, economists, and wine industry leaders all proposed to scale back wine production and improve quality without invoking alcoholism. As the director of a medical school put it, "up to the present we have always established and changed the wine statute without ever consulting those who are responsible for public health."[81] That would change. Concerns about alcoholism gave the technocrats' cause additional ammunition: it brought public health activists who blamed alcoholism on surpluses into the fray.

It is significant that public health activists focused much less of their attention on the INAO, the industrial wine companies like Postillon, or the large spirits manufacturers such as Pernod or Ricard. They saw these entities as a potential danger, but because they were efficient, powerful, and, excepting the merchants in industrial wine, globally competitive, they would have had trouble persuading technocrats to target them. Without riding the wave of the state's modernizing project, public health activists could not have advanced their agenda. By focusing on consumer welfare, they helped technocrats mobilize public opinion against the industrial wine system.

After the war, then, two different fields of expertise converged: political economy and public health.[82] This alignment of the two began with Sauvy and Debré's collaboration on *Des Français pour la France*, a book that linked alcohol surpluses to alcoholism. Doctors had railed against the wine industry and proposed measures to regulate it more effectively.[83] At the Economic Council, for example, May, Robert Debré's colleague from the Academy of Medicine, called on the state to attack alcoholism by attacking the alcohol supply: "It's vain to search to limit consumption if the mass of alcoholic drinks is not also diminished."[84] Technocrats offered remedies to alcoholism.[85] One of the economists at the INED, for example, having blamed state institutions for alcoholism, astutely observed that "behind this praise of flavor and quality is concealed—barely—an advertising that is meant to encourage quantity-driven consumption, less poetic but more real."[86] The political economy problem and the alcoholism problem became one and the same. The state adopted a kind of "technopolitics"—based on supposedly neutral scientific research—to regulate the wine industry. To give their movement a democratic air and to impel politicians to reform the state alcohol agency, this new anti–industrial wine coalition of technocrats and public health activists set out to convince consumers of the dangers of daily wine drinking, what many still considered as "the most hygienic beverage."

Mobilizing Public Opinion: A Drink or a House?

An energetic campaign against alcoholism was a fortuitous development for the technocrats, who were struggling to gain the democratic legitimacy they needed to reform the state alcohol agency. In the early 1950s, technocrats tried to rally public opinion to their cause by launching a press campaign that showed how the agency burdened the consumer through taxation, alcoholism, and a low standard of living. The Paris-based press—*La Croix*, *L'Express*, *Le Figaro*, *Le Monde*, and *Réforme*—was especially sympathetic to their cause.[87] The business press, *La Vie française*, for example, also expressed concerns about the economic consequences of alcoholism.[88] In order to mobilize public opinion, the coalition went so far as to blame France's housing shortage and a low standard of living on the state alcohol agency. Sauvy demonstrated that the alcohol-based gasoline cost the state 15 billion francs, "the equivalent of ten thousand new homes every year, or rather a city the size of Cherbourg."[89] A member of the Family, Population, and Public Health Commission in the National Assembly, upon hearing that the alcohol agency would cost the country 15 billion francs for the year, asserted that "it would be better to build houses and not reduce the money devoted to construction."[90] *Le Monde* censured the government for wasting money on alcohol when new homes needed building. "If the government hesitates to protect interests that have between them no common interest, if it does not choose for the good of the country, we demand a referendum: 'A roof for each family or a drink for each French person?'"[91] According to these portrayals, alcohol undermined the "general interest" and deprived citizens of basic needs and services.

The rhetorical linking of alcoholism to housing shortages fed into the debates about how to adapt French society to the baby boom and about how to raise the standard of living. After a century-long stagnation, France's population was growing. Although resistance to credit and consumerism could still be found in the countryside in the 1950s, workers around Paris increasingly aspired to owning their own homes.[92] Houses began to compete with cafés as a symbol of the good life. Yesterday's sociable, radicalized worker was to become tomorrow's domesticated, satisfied consumer. By turning the choice between a drink and a house into a choice between poverty and prosperity, technocrats tried to build mass opposition to the industrial wine system.

As tropes, the significance of choosing between a drink and a house went even deeper. Referendums were an exercise in direct democracy, thus undermining parliamentary power. The Paris-based media presented the state alcohol agency as a corruptor of citizenship and democracy. In the early 1950s, several observers writing in *Le Monde* blamed the industrial wine system for causing social troubles in Algeria and for turning citizens into alcoholics.[93] The journalist Alfred Fabre-Luce censured the "feudal lords" of Algeria for "reinvesting all their profits in sectors that already had surpluses" and thus for slowing Algeria's industrialization.[94] Fabre-Luce implied that the social structure of Algeria resembled feudalism and that local elites in Algeria, not the French state, should fund Algeria's development. *Réforme* excoriated the mainstream press for being the puppets of the alcohol lobbies and for providing the population with misinformation: "problem of the formation of public opinion in a democratic regime, therefore a problem of financial or political means, alcoholism is maintained by the powers of money that make a living on it."[95] *L'Aurore* ran an article whose very title bluntly asserted that the people responsible for alcoholism were the parliamentarians.[96] Technocrats, public health activists, and progressive newspapers therefore condemned the alcohol lobbies and their political allies for indoctrinating public opinion and for hurting the country's wellbeing.

In trying to overcome the wine and agricultural lobbies with a stake in the state alcohol agency, reformers looked to a potentially progressive political force that had finally received the vote in 1945: women. Since at least the late nineteenth century, women had been called on to teach rational consumption to their children and to provide moral guidance in the home.[97] In pursuing the female vote, which represented over half of the population, reformers hoped to overcome the wine industry's parliamentary defenders. Sauvy noted that "the parliamentarians haven't yet really seen all the consequences of the female vote instituted in 1945 that doubled the electorate. Women are the biggest victims of alcoholism and can one day defend themselves if we give them the means."[98] Women, who were represented as guardians of the family and the home, which reinforced their place in the domestic sphere, were potential allies in the campaign to reform drinking habits and the industrial wine system that they underpinned.

The postwar press campaign that blamed alcohol for the low standard of living had reportedly begun to influence public opinion. An INED poll in 1948 showed that 61 percent of men and 71 percent of women believed that alcoholism threatened the future of France.[99] Popular attitudes had not much changed when the INED conducted another survey in December 1953.[100] Conversely, the public did not see harm in the wine habit. In 1948, 92 percent of men and 77 percent of women believed wine to be good for health, against 88 percent of men and 72 percent of women in 1953.[101] Since the war's end, then, public opinion had become more aware of the dangers of drink, even if it continued to believe in the benefits of wine.

The campaign against alcoholism intensified from 1950, just as another round of surpluses sparked yet another protest movement among vine growers and alcohol producers to force the state to come to their rescue, and as a series of debates inflamed Parliament on the future of the state alcohol agency. Jean-Raymond Guyon, a Socialist deputy from wine-producing Bordeaux and the president of the National Assembly's finance commission, scoffed at his critics who linked alcoholism to the state alcohol agency. In defending the agency, he resurrected the rhetoric of his 1930s predecessors: "the essential and primordial problem of alcohol, it's the problem of French agriculture. When, for various reasons, the state alcohol agency is called into question, it's the entirety of the balance of our agriculture that's at stake."[102] Such arguments could elicit the sympathy of the entire rural population. Defenders of the agency emphasized that harvests varied from year to year, and therefore farmers needed guaranteed outlets and price supports.[103] In addition, alcohol-producing crops were a raw material that could be used for industrial purposes and make France less dependent on imports. Guyon pointed out that most of the alcohol purchased by the state went to industry, not drinkers.[104] In invoking the collective interests of agriculture and industry, Guyon hoped that the wine lobbies would continue to forge a wider alliance to defend their cause against the technocrats' new economic imperatives. Parliament thus put up stout resistance to the technocratic efforts to reform the state alcohol agency. One ally of the agency, referring to the links that technocrats were making between the agency and parliamentary paralysis, lamented that "the alcohol producer has become the scapegoat who is responsible for all the wounds of the Fourth Republic!"[105]

The advantage tilted in favor of the anti–industrial wine coalition during the geopolitical and economic crisis of 1953. Faced with the imminent conclusion of Marshall Plan aid, a budgetary deficit caused by the war in Indochina, and a desire to modernize the country, two premiers persuaded Parliament to grant them emergency powers to rule by decree in 1953. In a similar vein to 1935 and during the Vichy regime, technocrats were now empowered to carry out wine reforms without the usual parliamentary obstacles. State officials used this opportunity to reform the alcohol agency and raise alcohol taxes. First in May and then in August and September 1953, two different premiers—René Mayer and Joseph Laniel—placed the reform of the state alcohol agency into their larger plan to redress the economy.

La Journée vinicole immediately condemned this "dictatorship of the decree-laws."[106] After the May decree limiting state alcohol purchases, the lobbies with a vested interest in the alcohol agency quickly mobilized their political allies, branded the premier the "murderer of French agriculture," and had a powerful hand in the fall of the Mayer government in May 1953.[107] Supporters of the state alcohol agency brazenly took credit for the ministerial crisis of May 1953.[108] Laniel, the next premier, appeared unmoved, also obtaining special powers from Parliament and issuing a decree in August 1953 that provided for the gradual reduction of alcohol quotas. The quota price of wine alcohol fell below cost.[109] The reformed alcohol agency did not satisfy the anti–industrial wine coalition. A statistician at the INED, fearing that the lobbies would find a way to suspend the decrees, criticized the government for not having gone far enough, noting that in five years the state would still subsidize the distillation of more than 7 million hectoliters of alcohol that it could instead have invested in thirty thousand new houses.[110] This statistician concluded that "an outdated agricultural structure will thus be artificially maintained thanks to a protection that's accorded to no other agricultural product."[111]

During the crisis, policymakers also seized the opportunity to move the wine industry further down the path of quality through classified and controlled production. In September 1953, the government enacted decrees that reinforced the wine statute of the early 1930s by taxing high yields, controlling the type of grape varietals planted, forbidding new plantings, limiting production, creating a vineyard cadaster in order to secure a clearer understanding of where and how much wine was being produced, and determining which regions had the aptitude to produce quality wines. The Institute of Industrial Wines (IVCC) was established, modeled on the INAO, to regulate grape-growing and winemaking practices and to improve the quality of industrial wines. The updated statute of 1953 went further than that of the early 1930s in emphasizing quality production over quantity by subsidizing vine uprooting and converting less favored land to other crops. The statute of 1953, like the earlier one, discriminated especially against the large proprietors in Algeria and the Languedoc.

Neither Mayer nor Laniel linked alcohol surpluses to alcoholism like the anti–industrial wine coalition had wanted, finding it politically safer to separate the two issues. Yet January 1954 marked a turning point when members of the Economic Council, which had been studying the problems emanating from the alcohol agency since the late 1940s, switched the discussion from the problem of alcohol surpluses to the problem of alcoholism. Doctor Étienne May delivered a report to the Council on French alcoholism, calling on the state to attack alcoholism by attacking agriculture and concluding that "the war on alcoholism will therefore be accompanied by important changes in the agricultural orientation of France."[112] The campaign to reform agriculture in the name of public health continued. In July, just after reform-minded premier Pierre Mendès France took power, the Family, Population, and Public Health Commission of the National Assembly examined the links between alcohol production and alcoholism.[113] The following month, while Mendès France pleaded with Parliament to permit his government to rule by decree in order to renovate the economy, the commission released its report, arguing that to reduce alcoholism, the country needed to rationalize agriculture.[114] To the extent that the interest groups participating in the Economic Council represented the economic and social concerns of the nation, the country saw in alcoholism a way to combat the outdated structure of alcohol production.

In August 1954, when the National Assembly finally granted Mendès France special powers to rule by decree in order to reform the economy, a broad-based movement—including newspapers that advocated economic expansion, some prefects, the general representative councils for each department, town councils, the INED, the Christian Labor Union (CFTC), the Academy of Medicine, professors, as well as representatives of the automobile, oil, steel, and chemical industries who opposed the "national gasoline"—called on the government to connect alcoholism to surpluses and the policies of the state alcohol agency.[115] These latter groups had no direct interest in alcoholism, but they wanted to undercut the tariffs, subsidies, and price supports that reduced their profit margins. On the same day that Parliament granted the government the power to rule by decree, the Family, Population, and Public Health Commission delivered a final plea to Mendès France to work up the courage to act.[116] After all, a house and a higher standard of living were at stake.

Let Them Drink Milk

The controversial connection between alcohol surpluses and alcoholism was made at the state level for the first time when Pierre Mendès France came to power in June 1954. Mendès France, who had begun to develop a reputation in technocratic circles in the 1930s, was the consummate modernizer of the immediate postwar years. Since the war, French leaders had called on his economic expertise, his youthful dynamism, and his tough-minded approach to reconstructing the economy. Not only did he have a broad coalition pressuring him to reform the state alcohol agency when he became premier, but the country was also in a state of emergency because of the costly war in Indochina and economic stagnation and governmental instability at home. These circumstances were what ultimately prompted the National Assembly, with the exception of its Communist members, to grant him decree power.[117] Consequently free of parliamentary waffling, Mendès France set about regulating alcohol production and consumption.

Mendès France took advantage of the technocratic and public health campaigns of the immediate postwar period to justify controversial reforms that he claimed would rejuvenate France during a time of national crisis. He staffed his administration with some of France's leading modernizers, men like François Bloch-Lainé, Georges Boris, Claude Gruson, Étienne Hirsch, Simon Nora, and Jean Saint-Geours. Immediately upon assuming office, Mendès France and his team acknowledged that wine surpluses and the state alcohol agency were a major cause of France's economic inefficiency and political impotence.[118] While previous French leaders had often publicly glorified wine, Mendès France condemned it for causing immobility and backwardness.

Between September and January, his government thus carried out further reforms to the state alcohol agency and to the tax-dodging home distillers. Taking up Lamour's advice, the government planned to install an irrigation canal in the Languedoc, subsidize the uprooting of vines, convert vines to other crops, and develop regional tourism.[119] Mendès France also ordered beets to be turned into sugar and promised to indemnify those distillers who would lose business to the sugar refineries. Beet farmers would apparently lose no income, as prices for beet sugar would equal those for beet alcohol. "For the producer nothing has changed," guaranteed Mendès France. "For the nation, there's an immense difference: more sugar and less alcohol."[120] Mendès France envisioned subsidizing sugar exports and distributing sugar to the people of the French Union, especially to children. The government decreed that as of 1 January 1955, sweetened milk would be distributed in both public and private schools.[121] Mendès France even tried to get soldiers and workers to drink sweetened milk, a new manhood and nationhood in the making in the months following the army's surrender at Dien Bien Phu.

Mendès France scandalized a good part of the French population by drinking milk at public functions. But by doing so, he was taking a symbolic stand against past policy and charting a new path for the state, one that could help modernize the economy, make the French more responsible rulers, and improve France's international image at a time when France's peasant- and imperial-friendly policies were making the country look backward. Mendès France worked closely with the big, commercial agricultural producers in the metropole while ignoring the lobbies that defended the vine-growing and cider-producing peasants and home distillers. Because beet producers and dairy farmers were well represented in the National Federation of Farmers' Unions (FNSEA), France's most powerful farm organization that supported large-scale capitalist agriculture, this lobby pressured Mendès France to enact the decree establishing free milk distributions. Industrial vine growers, organized in the CGVM and the CGVA, had less representation in the FNSEA and appeared to have less contact with Mendès France. Significantly, Jacques Lepicard, who had been president of the CGB, became president of the FNSEA in 1954. This connection ensured support for Mendès France's sweetened milk policy. As the FNSEA had already stated in August:

> These distributions will be salutary for the health of our children, they'll help to circulate a part of our milk and sugar production; and they'll set off a progressive alteration in the consumer habits of our country where rich and energetic foods like milk and sugar aren't consumed as much as the health and vigor of the race would like, whereas, in other neighboring countries, which are similar to ours, these foods contribute more importantly to the average intake of the population.[122]

The FNSEA encouraged free milk distributions as a new outlet for over-produced milk. In the 1930s, dairy producers had emerged as a highly organized political force, expanding beyond a local clientele and producing milk for the national market. Between 1946 and 1954 the agitation of dairy producers reached a new level, as they sought to maintain a high price for their product.[123] Days after Mendès France gave official support to the cause of milk drinking,[124] Lepicard spoke on a radio program in order to encourage milk distributions.[125] The FNSEA publicly defended Mendès France's milk drinking. Another leader of the FNSEA reminded his followers that "he [the President of the Council] drinks milk, and one mustn't welcome this fact with jokes, for it constitutes an excellent propaganda for increasing the consumption of this product."[126]

Mendès France, who continued to hold his seat in Parliament while heading the government, also needed to defend his dairy-producing constituency in the Eure department. Since the 1930s, he had pursued similar reforms in that part of Normandy.[127] In order to help peasants survive the economic depression, he had launched a project of milk distribution in schools, first in Louviers in 1935, then in the rest of France in 1937. In support of his decision to distribute milk, he had advanced two main arguments: the financial assistance that it would bring to the numerous dairy farmers of Normandy and the nutrition that it would give to the many undernourished children of the poor and the unemployed.[128]

By drinking sweetened milk, Mendès France was setting an example for France's growing population of young people and promising a future of improved nutrition in the overseas territories. In targeting children, he could counter the wine propaganda of the 1930s in the schools and show that there was an alternative to daily wine. In targeting colonial people, another population perceived to be helpless, Mendès France hoped to re-legitimize the imperial state. In September 1954, in the French Union section of the planning commission, it was declared that "overseas alcoholism is the gravest social problem which we face at the present hour. . . . It'd be better to import into Africa butter and cheese than alcohol."[129] France's global mission was on the line. Thus, by drinking sweetened milk, Mendès France isolated the critics of wine and alcohol reform: it would be bad press to thwart a campaign to protect and promote health. Mendès France sought to appease the powerful beet and dairy lobbies that suffered from an oversupply of their respective products, limit state alcohol purchases, make French agriculture more competitive, and turn consumers in the French Union away from wine and alcohol, a product that threatened their health and supported underdevelopment in Algeria and several metropolitan regions.

Mendès France directed his attention away from the problem of the state alcohol agency and toward the problem of alcoholism in November 1954, immediately following insurrections in the Aurès Mountains that ignited Algeria's fight for independence and just as Pierre Poujade and his followers mounted their tax protests across the countryside. Poujade was a virulent nationalist and supporter of the peasantry and French Algeria. By shifting from the behind-the-scenes production reforms to alcoholism, Mendès France could politicize the public and mobilize it against the producers during a time of crisis. Mendès France never publicly strayed from the belief that "Algeria is France," but his anti-alcoholism decrees fell on precisely those groups that had an interest in the industrial wine system and that, through the state alcohol agency, were seen to impede economic growth, endanger public health, and subvert state authority: beet alcohol producers, cider producers, vine growers in Algeria and the Languedoc, and home distillers. These decrees, which extended to Algeria, limited the privileges of the home distillers to only those who were employed as farmers; regulated more closely the use of stills; reduced the opening hours of drinking establishments; raised alcohol taxes; and, perhaps most importantly, established the High Commission for Studies and Information on Alcoholism (HCEIA), which would coordinate government activity and educate the public about "proper" drinking behavior until its demise in 1991. Mendès France's decrees targeted the state alcohol agency and tax evaders instead of the drinker suffering from alcoholism, thereby squarely situating his campaign against alcoholism in his broader program of ensuring public order and economic growth and demonstrating to the world that the French were fit to rule themselves and those in their colonies.

Those producers that technocrats deemed unfit for world markets refused to be sacrificed on the altar of economic growth. By December 1954, peasants in Normandy showed hostility toward the government. Officials observed that at a local rally right-wing agitator Henry Dorgères had said that "President Mendès France is the most anti-peasant head of government that we have had in France up to this point."[130] By late January 1955, the agitation became more feverish. At one demonstration in Normandy, a local firebrand launched into a stinging diatribe against the premier, declaring that "there were home distillers before the family of Pierre Mendès France came from Portugal and there will be some after."[131] Mendès France's Jewish and Portuguese origins were used against him, as his reputed rootlessness was exactly what the far right opposed. Home distillers presented themselves as defenders of the national interest against the supposed statelessness of technocrats like Mendès France.

Producers who had a vested interest in the state alcohol agency also protested and blamed other groups. A senator from the plonk-producing Languedoc claimed to see through Mendès France's program, arguing that the government's milk policy imposed great sacrifices on the wine regions to the benefit of the dairy regions and that this policy had less to do with the protection of children than with the protection of dairy producers.[132] Producers who depended on the state alcohol agency asserted that an increase in the alcohol taxes would only lead to further acts of informal production and tax evasion. The more consumers looked for alcohol in the informal economy, the more that surpluses would plague the state alcohol agency. The alcohol lobbies used the rhetoric of the country's main temperance organization to discourage tax increases, arguing that the problem lay with the home distillers, whose production was "hardly controlled or controllable" and "represents for the Treasury at least an annual loss of 43 billion francs without including fraud."[133] Industrial vine growers thus saw the war on alcoholism as an opportunity to attack their non-market rivals.

The home distillers, grouped in the SNBC, did not necessarily oppose modernization, only Mendès France's version of it.[134] Yet unlike industrial wine producers, they did not have the financial resources to influence public opinion or policymaking. Their newspapers often solicited financial support from their readers. They tried to work through the channels of Parliament,[135] where André Liautey, their loudmouthed leader, was a member of the Finance Commission, and they pressured key figures at the Ministry of Finance.[136] The home distillers sent letters to their deputies and senators warning them that they needed to support home distillation or else lose votes at election time.[137] An inter-parliamentary commission in support of the home distillers was even established to study the causes of alcoholism, but Mendès France did not grant its representatives a hearing.[138] Although home distillers had support in Parliament, they lacked influence in the national press and therefore had little power to alter how the alcohol problem was being framed.

Alcohol became a symbolic battleground for Poujadists, Dorgèrists, and Communists, all dissident groups that opposed global capitalism and considered Mendès France an anti-peasant, anti-empire, and anti-French politician who conspired with international trusts, stateless technocrats, and American agents.[139] "If you had a drop of Gallic blood in your veins," Poujade berated Mendès France, "you would have never dared, as a representative of France, world wine and champagne producer, to be served a glass of milk at an international reception!"[140] Dorgères claimed that "the anti-alcohol campaigns that are based on lies and calumny threaten the entire production of alcohol"[141] and that the "technocrats and bureaucrats have no expertise in agricultural matters."[142] One of Poujade's comrades weighed in by saying that the "average French person, portrayed as a drunk, drinks a liter and a half of (pure) alcohol per year, whereas their ancestors, those who experienced Verdun, drank four and a half liters."[143] Clearly some in France still associated alcohol with vigor, not vice.

To a large extent, the right-wing, Communist, and provincial press shared the view that the Mendès France government was seeking to

Americanize France. Conservative cartoonists such as Sennep, a reputed wine enthusiast, portrayed Mendès France derogatively as an American cowboy. The Communist newspaper *L'Humanité* chose Tarzan or a Superman-like figure as its American reference (see figures 9 and 10). Although the typical Marxist viewed the peasantry as backward and as an obstacle to proletarian revolution, the French Communist Party defended peasants against industrial capitalism. Foreign journalists were also shocked by Mendès France's milk drinking. The *New Yorker* correspondent Janet Flanner remarked that Mendès France's "announcement that . . . France's surplus milk will be distributed to school children and to the boys in the French army has caused consternation among French mothers, for the French think that no drink is as bad for the liver as milk."[144] Either genuinely or sarcastically, observers viewed Mendès France as alien to a characteristically French way of living.

Thus, in connecting alcoholism to the uncompetitive segments of the alcohol trade, Mendès France could also attack his main ideological

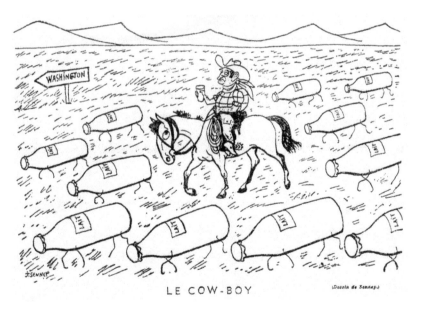

LE COW-BOY

Figure 9. "Le Cow-Boy." Depiction of Pierre Mendès France's trip to the United States. Cartoon by Sennep. *Le Figaro*, 17 November 1954. Reprinted by permission of *Le Figaro*.

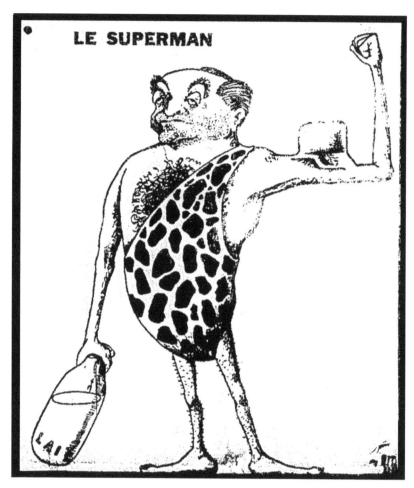

Figure 10. "Le Superman." Depiction of Pierre Mendès France as a superhero. *L'Humanité*, 20 November 1954. Reprinted by permission of *L'Humanité*.

opponents. Supporters of Mendès France associated the Communists and the far right with tradition, backwardness, and ignorance: "Politicians must understand that, if they continue to defend the cause of the alcohol lobbies, they will remain behind the times, even if they belong to 'advanced' parties."[145] They alluded undoubtedly to the Communist Party. Nor did representations in the progressive press favor the home distillers and their defenders. The home distillers represented everything that Mendès France hoped to upend: ignorance, poverty, and political corruption.

Mendès France used Franklin Delano Roosevelt's strategy of fireside chats to promote his campaign and to pressure the legislature to support his measures. His speeches on alcoholism placed the onus on producers: "It's of course not a question of imposing a type of prohibition on the French. It's a question of making men free and conscious of the dangers that threaten them and to help them avoid these dangers."[146] Hoping to avoid any moral insults on consumers, Mendès France borrowed the rhetoric of the anti–industrial wine coalition, making consumers into the victims of the country's producers. His appeal to the people made him popular among the public, but it increasingly galvanized Parliament.[147] Mendès France hoped to overcome demagogy and the paralysis of parliamentary politics in the name of the general interest. In the critical political context of 1954, one in which the French Union was destabilizing and the economy was stagnating, no political party could afford to oppose efforts to improve public health and stimulate economic growth.

The press's definition of alcoholism garnered public support for Mendès France's campaign. State agencies conducted polls that gave Mendès France's campaign legitimacy against parliamentary criticisms. One poll questioned the public about state subsidies to the beet, cider, and wine industries (table 1).[148] In December 1953 and again in January 1955, these institutes asked the public about the possibility of limiting the home distillers' privilege (table 2).[149]

TABLE 1. Public opinion of alcohol subsidies, 1955

	September 1954	January 1955
Opponents of subsidies	54%	81%
Supporters of subsidies	23	5
Other responses	—	2
Undeclared	23	12

Source: French Institute of Public Opinion (IFOP), "Public Opinion Poll on the Topic of Alcohol Subsidies," *Sondages* 1 (1955), 19.

TABLE 2. Public opinion of limits on tax-free home distillation, 1955

	December 1953	January 1955
Opponents of limits	24%	22%
Supporters of limits	54	61
Undeclared	22	17

Source: French Institute of Public Opinion (IFOP), "Public Opinion Poll on the Topic of Limits on Tax-Free Home Distillation," *Sondages* 1 (1955), 20.

In both 1953 and 1955, public opinion agreed to limiting the practice of home distillation. By January 1955, a large majority favored reforming the alcohol economy. Only one out of ten persons considered Mendès France's anti-alcoholism to be unimportant; 67 percent considered it "very important," though less important than other social problems.[150] Significantly, all the political parties—though the Communists the least—endorsed the campaign against alcoholism.[151] As evidenced by the polls, public sentiment about alcohol was clearly shifting, and the Mendès France government exploited this new trend, but perhaps this fact is not too surprising given that the media had framed alcohol subsidies and tax-free home distillation as obstructing a higher standard of living.

How the Communists changed their position on alcoholism illustrates the effectiveness of Mendès France's political strategy. In Parliament in late November, a Communist deputy tried to repeal the decrees against the home distillers, but the Senate blocked the attempt. The press immediately vilified the Communist Party for its attempts to repeal an important public health measure. As a result, the French Politburo suggested that the Communist Party take a more pragmatic approach to the problem. It called for a "note on the problems of alcohol and the government's measures on this subject";[152] at the end of the month, however, the leader of the Communist Party suggested that its members modify their wording to "a note defining the position of the Communist Party on the ravages of alcoholism and the means to combat it, and the latest governmental measures."[153] In early January 1955, Waldeck Rochet, an agricultural syndicalist and member of the Communist Party, presented a long report to the members of the Politburo that sought to incite the Communist Party to take action against the problem, for the popular press portrayed the Party as the "defenders of alcoholism."[154] Communists recognized the need to jump onto the anti-alcoholism bandwagon. The Mendès France government made Communists toe the line.

Despite the consensus in favor of reform, a wave of demonstrations rocked the French countryside. Between mid-December and mid-January, protest reached a fever pitch in the beet-producing departments. In nearly one month, 42,150 demonstrators took to the streets. The rage against the government's agricultural policy culminated in Lille on 1 February 1955, just days before Mendès France was forced to leave office. The beet producers' newspaper detailed the events, showed photographs of the violence, and ran as a headline "President Leclercq Seriously Wounded by Riot Police after a Meeting of 15,000 Peasants."[155]

In February 1955, the Mendès France government fell, not directly because of the ire raised by its alcohol reforms but because of its inability to cope with the crisis in Algeria. Yet the defenders of alcohol and Algeria were allied and strong.[156] Supporters of the industrial wine system were frequently supporters of French Algeria. It should come as no surprise, then, that those with a stake in agriculture and Algeria voted against the government.[157]

The alcohol lobbies may have used the crisis in Algeria to air their grievances. One author speculated shortly after Mendès France's dismissal that "the alcohol bloc . . . gave the word to 'its' parliamentarians: overthrow the government. Little did it matter that the pretext was the debate on North Africa."[158] During the Fourth Republic, the status of the wine industry, the peasantry, and French Algeria were being called into question by a wide alliance but were still sufficiently entrenched in French institutions and political culture.

Mendès France's removal from office permitted the wine and alcohol lobbies to reverse many of his government's reforms. In 1955, the home distillers delayed the termination of their tax-free distillation privileges; deputies repealed the higher license fees for drinking establishments; beet growers reestablished some of their privileges; and some distilleries reopened for business.[159] The influence of the peasant groups and their allies in the subsequent government helped in rescinding the Mendès France decrees.[160] Because of the industrial wine system's continued hold on Parliament, the Fourth Republic, like the Third, failed to rationalize the wine economy.

Concerns over the beet alcohol producers subsided in public debate about the wine industry after the Pierre Mendès France government collapsed. It is difficult to know exactly why. It is likely that the beet lobby and the commercial distillers convinced state officials that they had little to do with wine surpluses and alcoholism, and thus the state distanced these wealthy and concentrated sectors from controversial public debates concerning wine, the peasantry, and French Algeria. Moreover, based on the beet lobby's newspaper, beet producers became more interested in the sugar market and were less implicated in the problem of alcohol surpluses after 1955.[161] In the years after the Mendès France government, the industrial vine growers of Algeria and the Languedoc lost a powerful ally in blocking reforms to the industrial wine system.

Conclusion

Looking back on the immediate postwar years, Sauvy remembered, perhaps hyperbolically, that France "was under the domination of the most powerful lobby that it had ever known," referring to the apple-beet-vine bloc that had had a vested interest in maintaining the state alcohol agency.[162] Sauvy and like-minded technocrats believed that it was their duty to emancipate the population from the industrial wine system's grasp. They wrongly assumed that their movement was above political and class interests. Between the 1930s and the Pierre Mendès France government of 1954–1955, the wine industry became a site of contention over the orientation of France's political economy, whether reinforced around a protected empire that sustained peasants and settlers or around an empire rebuilt and industrialized to face international competition. New economic and public health expertise that linked wine surpluses to alcoholism became a source of debate, but the notion struggled to gain political legitimacy.

Why the resistance to the sober revolution? Why the return to previous policies that were now said to encourage alcohol surpluses and alcoholism? First, the Fourth Republic preferred accommodating the wine industry to the political risks of demanding painful reforms. For vine growers, wine was a way of life that would not be robbed by the prophets of modernization. Worried about its legitimacy, the state appeased vine growers in the Languedoc and Algeria and their alcohol-producing allies in the state alcohol agency. Second, when technocrats attacked the state alcohol agency, they attacked not just the industrial wine lobbies but also other powerful agricultural interests. In response, the apple-beet-vine bloc united to defend the agency. Third, even if public opinion approved of tackling alcoholism, it still viewed wine as a source of nutrition, not as a public health problem.[163] In this way, consumers consented to the industrial wine system. Finally, the new expertise struggled to overcome a parliamentary system that continued to see wine, agriculture, and Algeria as central not just to France's political and economic arrangements but to national identity as well. Pierre Mendès France's brief stay in office spotlights the obstacles to reforming the industrial wine system in a parliamentary and imperial republic.

The industrial wine lobbies and their allies thus stood firm as a united bloc in this first postwar battle to transform wine and France. Despite Mendès France's failure to carry out thoroughgoing reforms, the anti–industrial wine coalition had begun to represent their adversaries as backward and as an impediment to economic expansion and consumer wellbeing. Public opinion was generally susceptible to combating an alcoholism that was believed to deter improved living conditions. After foreign occupation and dietary deprivation in World War II, as families grew and as people longed for stability and prosperity, surplus alcohol was blamed for burning the national budget. To reformers, the alcohol lobbies and their parliamentary allies obstructed a higher standard of living by wasting tax money on subsidies. Unlike nineteenth-century critics who feared that drink politicized workers in subversive ways, postwar technocrats viewed drinking as a habit that bred passivism.[164] The status quo, in this view, had to go. Give up the daily drink, technocrats promised, and a sober and stronger France would be born.

3

QUANTITY OR QUALITY?

After the fall of the Pierre Mendès France government in 1955, the sober revolution took an unexpected turn. Desperate to gain any advantage they could over "the monarchy of alcohol" that had just helped bring Mendès France to his knees, the technocrats and public health activists who had so courageously campaigned against the industrial wine system and its protectionist policies now started defending the regulatory National Institute of Appellations of Origin (INAO) in its bid to expand its norms and prepare the industry for international competition.[1] Working together, this coalition for quality wine and brandy sought to drive a wedge through the industrial wine system by targeting the settlers of Algeria and the home distillers, two groups toward which public opinion was becoming increasingly indignant. In 1959 and 1960, as the war in Algeria and unrest in the metropolitan countryside challenged the legitimacy of the newly established Fifth Republic, the quality coalition supported the state in promoting economic development, protecting public health, and removing vine-growing settlers and home distillers from the national wine heritage that the INAO was trying to (re-)create through reform and new norms.

The continued presence of an estimated several million vine growers and home distillers in France and Algeria in the late 1950s—and the continued centrality of agriculture and Algeria to national identity— suggests that the sober revolution could have quickly lost its momentum or turned out differently.[2] Its advance was neither inevitable nor easy. Rather, it depended on a specific set of circumstances: the need of the newly created High Commission for Studies and Information on Alcoholism (HCEIA) to find common ground with the modernist wing of the wine industry—the INAO and the National Confederation of Wine and Spirits (CNVS) that defended producers and distributors, respectively; the ability of this alliance to influence how the media framed the problem and turn an increasingly urban and affluent population against settlers and home distillers; and last but not least, the transformation in French democracy from the parliamentary Fourth Republic into the authoritarian Fifth Republic in 1958, which gave technocrats in the administration more ability to overcome Parliament and to impose centralized norms.

In the late 1950s, policymakers confronted two concurrent and intertwined events that would have profound implications for the French wine industry and its representations of wine and nation. On the one hand, an unpopular war in Algeria raised the controversial question of whether or not Algeria was in fact France. On the other, France's entry into the European Economic Community (EEC) threatened the state's authority in controlling national culture and forced a consideration of whether or not France was more continental than colonial. This uncertain context served as an impetus to centralize state power over the wine industry and rebrand French wine in a way that rooted it in the metropolitan regions. This rebranding was intended to improve the socioeconomic conditions of the countryside and Algeria and fight alcoholism. Concerns over alcoholism and the INAO's discourse of tradition, authenticity, and quality became increasingly useful as the fledgling Fifth Republic set about consolidating new nationwide norms of wine production and preparing for competition in the European common market. "Quality," as defined by the Ministry of Agriculture, "is a consequence of respecting old practices."[3] Yet the home distillers' and the settlers' brandy and winemaking practices—in some cases over a century old—were deemed unfit for the INAO's classifications.

New regimes need founding myths to gain popular support and consolidate their authority. The Fifth Republic under Charles de Gaulle, a man obsessed with maintaining the country's independence and restoring French grandeur, could draw on the INAO's narrative of metropolitan France's excellence in the world of wine to launch a project of redefining the nation as historically hexagonal. Although several important figures in the Ministries of Agriculture and Finance and the intellectual world called the future of the Algerian wine industry into question, a reformed Algeria was not excluded from the Fifth Republic's vision of nation and tradition until it achieved independence. Algeria's gaining AOC status and remaining a part of France were still possibilities until the ink dried on the Evian Accords in 1962. Retrospectively, however, it is clear that the problems of the industrial wine system initiated a process of modernizing the wine industry and airbrushing the narrative about the place of wine in the French nation, a process that became linked to modernizing and sanitizing France under the Fifth Republic. The INAO not only supported the new republic in promoting economic growth and protecting public health; its invocations of tradition, authenticity, and quality gave the state greater legitimacy in marginalizing alternative visions of production that would have otherwise tried to prevent the increased power of technocrats over policymaking, the expansion of the appellation system, and European economic integration.

The State's Anti-Alcoholism

Thanks to Mendès France, the industrial wine system in the late 1950s faced a new state agency whose purpose was to limit its influence over consumers. Established in November 1954, the HCEIA gathered information on alcoholism, proposed measures to reduce it, and undertook an ongoing campaign to educate the public about the dangers of habitual drinking. Most importantly, the HCEIA would check the wine industry's ability to shape consumer behavior. Older, carefree wine slogans like "A Meal without Wine is a Day without Sunshine" would now have to compete with new, more cautious ones such as "The Pleasure of Drinking

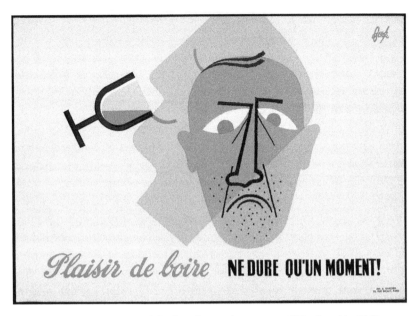

Plaisir de boire **NE DURE QU'UN MOMENT!**

Figure 11. "The pleasure of drinking lasts only a moment!" Designed by Philippe Foré, HCEIA propaganda, c. 1957. Courtesy of the National Archives of France, Pierrefitte-sur-Seine.

Lasts Only a Moment!" (figure 11). Based on this new message, one might conclude that an ethos of living in the moment was losing ground to hopes of a more prosperous future that lay ahead if consumers disciplined their drinking.

The HCEIA fused the new economic and public health expertise that treated alcoholism as a problem caused by unregulated production. Framing alcoholism as an economic problem mobilized a wider range of stakeholders than the depiction of alcoholism as solely a public health problem. At the outset, the HCEIA was composed of ten figures with an abiding interest in public health, economic modernization, and the centralization of state power.[4] The HCEIA's composition demonstrates that it reached beyond the public health domain and engaged with the bigger debate about economic and political reform.

Mendès France nominated Robert Debré as the HCEIA's first president, a position he would hold until the late 1970s. Debré was a man with excellent connections.[5] He brought to the HCEIA Marcel Bleustein-Blanchet, an advertising magnate; Christian Chavanon, one-time director-general of the state-run French Radio and Television Broadcasting (RTF) network, and Havas, a major advertising and public relations firm; Eugène Forget, a leader of the National Federation of Farmers' Unions (FNSEA), France's major farm lobby that represented the conservative large-scale agricultural interests of northern France against the left-wing smallholder associations of the Languedoc; Max Sorre, a geographer who had written on the history of the wine trade of the Languedoc; as well as other prominent doctors, bureaucrats, and metropolitan and overseas politicians. Then there were the HCEIA's experts: Alain Barjot, who helped develop the social security system and served as a councilor of state in France's highest court; Étienne Hirsch, head of the planning commissions; Alfred Sauvy, director of the National Institute of Demographic Studies (INED); and Jean Stoetzel, administrator of the French Institute of Public Opinion (IFOP).[6] Debré's broad connections facilitated the incorporation of a range of actors whose interests reached well beyond wine. In this way, the wine problem was linked to the broader project of state reform and economic modernization, thus ensuring that officials would take the HCEIA's advice into account when developing wine policy.

Moreover, the HCEIA resided in the office of the prime minister, above the ministerial and parliamentary fray that had destabilized the Fourth Republic and stalled reforms to the industrial wine system. When Mendès France created the HCEIA, he had hoped that it would overcome the political instability that had prevented governments from implementing lasting change: the "general interest" of economic growth was to overcome the "particular interests" of the status quo. Debré's status as a pediatrician obliged policymakers to take consumer health and safety into account when developing wine policy. It may be recalled that since the war, technocrats had complained that "the wine lobbies think about the wine problem solely from the vantage point of the vine grower."[7] Given the political power of wine producers, state officials often ignored the relationship between production and consumption. A bureaucrat in the Ministry of Finance pointed out that "the struggle against alcoholism could be the occasion for agriculture to free itself from a system of expedients and security."[8] By educating consumers, the HCEIA could raise awareness about the problems stemming from the industrial wine system and contribute to the modernizing impulse to cut subsidies, generate tax revenue, and make wine production more competitive on world markets.

The HCEIA was thus always more than a group with a mission to curb alcoholism; it also contributed to remaking the wine industry, reinforcing state power over refractory regions, transforming democratic institutions, and preparing the economy for international competition.

The Wine Lobbies Mobilize Science and Tradition

In response to the establishment of the HCEIA and the brake that it could put on the wine industry's ability to shape popular opinion, wine lobbyists in the influential National Committee for Wine Promotion (CNPFV) and the French Society of Pro-Wine Doctors (SFMAV), groups formed during the surplus crisis of the early 1930s, immediately defended wine in the political arena and contested the new expertise that linked wine to alcoholism. These lobbyists tried to maintain wine's legitimacy by appealing to both science and tradition, thus accommodating the new economic and public health imperatives to French culture, a culture that was metropolitan and elitist to be sure. The national wine lobbies hoped to create confusion about the etiology of alcoholism and extol the benefits of the "moderate" drinking of "natural," "authentic," "quality" wine, which nearly invariably meant the INAO's wines.[9] A public that supported these drinks could help fend off "fraudulent" competitors—which implicitly referred to Algerian wine, home-distilled brandy, and foreign drinks—and hamper the state's attack on the "honest producers" who had the means and the willingness to conform to the INAO's regulations.[10]

While Robert Debré headed the HCEIA and combated wine-related alcoholism, the Bordeaux doctor and politician Georges Portmann was one of the most outspoken defenders of wine in the CNPFV, in the SFMAV, and in the Senate.[11] Both Debré and Portmann were doctors, were members of the Academy of Medicine, and loved wine.[12] Each in his own way had an interest in reforming French drinkers. While Debré hoped to reduce overall alcohol consumption, Portmann hoped to educate French drinkers about how to taste wine.

Having been inactive during the war, the CNPFV was reorganized in 1948 "to develop the consumption and exportation of wine and grapes."[13] This gave appellation wine leverage over industrial wine, as the latter was difficult to export. Indeed, the Algerian wine lobbies complained about the CNPFV's elitism and its inattention to Algerian needs.[14] Subsidies granted by the Ministry of Finance to the CNPFV skyrocketed from 5 million francs in 1948 to over 69 million in 1954.[15] In 1957, the CNPFV was reorganized once again, this time in response to the creation of the HCEIA and the need to prepare the industry for competition in the EEC. It sought to counter the HCEIA's anti-wine propaganda by educating the consumer about how to drink, thus placing the onus on the individual instead of the product and emphasizing the values of quality over quantity. The CNPFV claimed that wine advertising appealed to reason and the cultivation of taste: "know how to drink, know how to taste wine" was its mantra.[16] While the HCEIA labored to reduce drinking, the CNPFV worked to refine drinking.

The SFMAV also continued its mission after the war of mobilizing doctors in France and abroad to praise the healthful benefits of wine drinking. In the 1920s, the League of Nations had created study groups to examine the condition of alcoholism; after World War II, the World Health Organization (WHO) took up the cause. In response, pro-wine doctors established their own international connections and conducted scientific research to defend wine drinking against what they perceived to be teetotalers. At a conference in Bordeaux in 1949, for example, Portmann commented that "we used to say never give pure lemon juice to children; now we give it to infants! Why not do the same with good wine? We must defend wine, but from a physiological basis that has been subjected to scientific research."[17] Thus the SFMAV aimed to continue to use scientific research to demonstrate the healthful benefits of moderate wine consumption, an approach that was in line with the rationalizing discourse of technocrats and public health activists.

While the wine lobbies relied on scientific research to prove the health benefits of wine, they also appealed to tradition. The CNPFV defended quality wine against the increasing industrialization and rampant consumerism of the postwar years. The president of the Drinks Commission in Parliament pursued the logic of the economists who argued that France's habitual wine drinking stood in the way of the development of a mass consumer society. He described the following scene: a father, a mother, and their children sit around the dining room table. An invisible hand replaces the liter of wine with one hundred francs. After a few months of this, the family is able to buy a refrigerator or a dining room, and it does so on credit. If the family replaces 2 liters of wine for 200 francs, it could afford a vacuum cleaner, a floor polisher, a washing machine, and other modern appliances. The president of the Drinks Commission concluded that "after having eliminated the liter of wine," the family "could also get rid of its daily bread . . . and then it would be the head of the family's turn to be replaced by a robot. Voilà the future appearance of French civilization."[18] Clearly, France had to achieve a balance between capitalism and humanity, between the industrial age and the civilization of wine.

The SFMAV emphasized that wine had longstanding legitimacy in French medicine. Portmann pointed out that "since earliest antiquity, way before the scientific era, when we still didn't know the chemical composition of wine, or how alcoholic fermentation worked . . . we acknowledged, based on our everyday experience . . . that natural wine, taken at a moderated dose, is a hygienic drink, useful to the individual."[19] For centuries, doctors had administered wine to patients for its positive therapeutic effects. Proverbs had supported the use of wine in popular medicine: "Good wine and a good woman put medicine in the air" or "a glass of wine is worth five francs spent at the doctor." Wine supposedly prevented colds, cured fevers, killed parasites, and, by drinking white wine with five small nanny goat turds, cured jaundice.[20] French scientists frequently cited Louis Pasteur's maxim: "wine is the most hygienic beverage." When, in 1960, Jean-Max Eylaud, general secretary of the SFMAV, published his book *Vin et santé: vertus hygièniques et thérapeutiques du vin*, he was writing in the medical tradition of showing the links between moderate wine drinking and good health.[21] For Eylaud, wine was healthy and downright fun. "Austerity does not prolong life," his doctor friend Portmann warned, trying to encourage his readers to follow the doctor's orders.[22]

The established place of wine in French medicine allowed doctors and wine lobbyists to challenge and nuance the new understanding of alcoholism being promoted by the technocrats in Paris. The wine lobbies contested Sully Ledermann's seminal study on French alcoholism, which was shaping the way government officials viewed the problem. This INED statistician showed that habitual wine drinking was at the root of French alcoholism. His illustration of "the Ledermann curve" claimed that the number of alcoholics in a given society could be determined by the total consumption of the population. "If such is really the case," Ledermann argued, "it would appear vain to hope for a reduction of alcoholism in France without diminishing, in a noticeable way, the average consumption per individual, that is to say the overall consumption and, finally, the French production of wine and alcohol."[23] This meant that in order to reduce alcoholism, state policy would have to be directed at "normal" drinkers and the products that they consumed. An attack on the drinking norm assumed an attack on the foundations of French culture, which was also assumed to play a crucial part in transforming the political economy that supported the industrial wine system.

Roger Andrieu, a professor at the Scientific Foundation of Anthropological Research and the French Institute for the Study of Human Problems, exposed Ledermann's tenuous link between overall consumption and the number of alcoholics in a given society. He argued that "human biology is quite simply the Science of Good Sense" and that "it finds few skilled people among the Technocrats."[24] Andrieu suggested that alcoholism should be treated on a case-by-case basis, not in terms of raw numbers. In this view, one person's physiological response to alcohol was surely not the same as another's: "The mathematical abstractions of the polytechnician Ledermann join the astronomical calculations of the polytechnician Paul Choisnard in an imaginative cloud of the same order."[25] Andrieu's comparison of Ledermann to Choisnard, an odd figure who sought to demonstrate the validity of astrology through statistics, was no accident.

Pro-wine doctors marshaled statistics to make their case about the benefits of moderate wine drinking. Both they and the wine lobbies consistently and persistently posed the question: if wine endangered health, then why did the wine-drinking departments of the south suffer much less from alcohol-related conditions than the spirits-drinking departments of the north? Statistics showed that alcohol-related deaths were far more common in Brittany and Normandy than in, say, Bordeaux or the Languedoc.[26] Medical insouciance about alcoholism in the south no doubt had an impact on the statistics for alcoholism in that region, as doctors likely declared a lower rate of deaths as being directly related to the alcoholic condition. Polls showed that doctors in the winegrowing Languedoc were less concerned about alcoholism than their counterparts in Brittany or in Paris.[27] Portmann noted with much pride that, because of its wine-drinking tradition, the Gironde had the most nonagenarians and centenarians.[28] With this evidence, the wine lobbies pointed out that the wine-drinking Latin regions had much to teach the spirits- and binge-drinking north.

For Portmann and like-minded doctors, it was a crime to reduce wine to its alcoholic properties. They believed that for technocrats, wine was wine, without nuance and without distinction from alcohol. Portmann agreed that "wine contains alcohol." But he hastened to add that "the alcohol is part of a complex where one finds glycerine, tartrates, tannins, and vitamins; it's such a particular complex that it's the only product from the soil of France that continues to live when it leaves the soil."[29] The agronomist Michel Cépède demonstrated that research conducted on rats had shown that they reacted differently to wine than to alcohol. Unlike wine, spirits stunted the rats' growth and induced liver maladies.[30] The wine lobbies associated wine with "knowing how to drink" (*savoir-boire*) and alcohol with "excessive drinking" (*trop-boire*).[31]

Pro-wine doctors drew on a nineteenth-century rhetorical distinction between wine and industrial alcohol. Authentic wine was natural and rooted in the land, apparently unlike other forms of "industrial" alcohol that had to go through a distillation or blending process. Paul Pagès, a member of the medical faculty of Montpellier, agreed with the official statistics concerning the links between wine, alcoholism, and cirrhosis of the liver but claimed that the industrial wines were to blame.[32] When doctors and the wine lobbies agreed on a link between wine and alcoholism, mass-produced, blended wine, which was more difficult for the state to regulate, was at fault. One wine lobbyist lamented that "wine, yesterday a loyal friend to mankind, is no longer thus because of its industrialization!"[33]

From 1955, the wine lobbies mobilized counter-expertise based on both science and elitist French traditions to influence public opinion and state officials about the virtuous qualities of wine, and they largely succeeded. Fully 79 percent of people polled in 1948, 70 percent in 1953, and 65 percent in 1955 agreed that wine was healthy.[34] Only 7 percent in one poll believed that wine could be harmful to health.[35] To be fair, the belief that wine was healthy was not altogether unsound. As late as 1957, approximately ten million inhabitants of metropolitan France were still without piped water.[36] French people usually added wine to their drinking water to disinfect it or in some cases perhaps simply replaced wine with water. If Winston Churchill is to be believed, "ordinary wine is the drinking water of the French."[37] In an age when hygiene was not guaranteed, wine continued to be perceived as the safest and most hygienic drink. This caused trouble for the technocrats and public health activists in the HCEIA who were looking to regulate wine more effectively and raise its price. Although the HCEIA surely meant well, its movement, unlike that of the INAO and its allies, was largely devoid of culture. To gain legitimacy in reforming wine, technocrats would have to win over the hearts and minds of consumers. As we will see, they would attempt to do so by exploiting the legal distinction between luxury and ordinary wine and by trying to convince consumers to choose the former. The state's aim with promoting appellation wine—with its appeals to tradition and authenticity and its place-based image—was to endow drinking with richer historical meaning. Wine was to become increasingly a symbol of hexagonal France that could draw people together, just as broad economic forces were threatening to tear them apart.

The Quality Coalition

Medical disputes about the extent to which wine was culpable for causing alcoholism and the public's insistence on the virtues of wine bolstered the wine lobbies in the political arena and blocked the reforms that the HCEIA hoped to accomplish. From its inception, the HCEIA had to contend with parliamentary skepticism about waging war on alcoholism in a country where alcohol was a source of political power and at the center of economic and social life. In the months following the collapse of the Mendès France government, the alcohol lobbies tried to derail the HCEIA's mission. The Drinks Commission in the National Assembly[38] opposed Mendès France's December 1954 decree—which had dictated that taxes on café licenses would fund the HCEIA—as an unfair measure against France's shopkeepers.[39]

Between 1955 and 1958, Parliament reduced the HCEIA's budget from 400 million francs to 200 million francs.[40] Robert Debré complained to the Finance Commission of the National Assembly that "these reductions have had some extra-financial reasons," implying that the political influence of the lobbies had been behind the budget cuts.[41] Another member of the HCEIA admitted pessimistically that "it's an almost daily fact of life that the evocation of the HCEIA brings to the lips of the parliamentarians or high functionaries a compassionate smile, but one that is disabused or ironic."[42] In its campaign to reduce alcoholism, the HCEIA struggled to achieve political and popular support.

Yet new opportunities came to the fore. Immediately after the HCEIA formed, the wine lobbies pressured the government to grant them representation at the HCEIA's meetings. Although Debré had originally refused their pleas, he reconsidered as the HCEIA's budget continued to diminish. Debré needed to find a way to work with the industry without compromising the HCEIA's mission. The HCEIA took two steps to adjust to the hostile political environment. First, its members deliberated on having a wine representative sit in on the HCEIA's meetings.[43] The HCEIA preferred conciliation to outright conflict with the wine lobbies. Second, Debré and his colleagues went before the powerful Drinks Commission to reassure its members that the HCEIA had never discouraged the moderate consumption of quality wines.[44] Debré was becoming aware of the importance of promising to maintain culture as he carried out reforms.

By supporting the modernizing impulse within the wine industry to promote quality production and its traditions, the HCEIA hoped to use the INAO's connections in the press, in Parliament, and in the administration to spread the temperance message. Quality wine would command a higher price and enrich those vine growers who planted state-approved vines on state-approved land at the expense of the merchants who dominated the industrial wine system and who indiscriminately looked for the cheapest grapes available, notably in Algeria. Given its cost, quality wine would also encourage consumers to think more about what they were consuming. This reformist impulse was in line with the HCEIA's aim of discouraging daily wine drinking, an aim that would affect the industrial system and its peasant and working-class consumers more than the growing middle classes of France and beyond. The HCEIA encouraged *La Journée vinicole*, one of the industry's leading newspapers, to pressure its allies in Parliament and to launch a press campaign against the home distillers, the group that had historically defied the state's intrusion in its affairs.[45] Debré asked Pierre Le Roy de Boiseaumarié, president of the INAO, and other appellation leaders to urge the Ministry of Finance to act against fraud.[46] By avoiding the wrath of INAO leaders who were trying to create new production and market norms, the HCEIA hoped to use the INAO's political influence in the Ministries of Agriculture and Finance to reduce an alcoholism that was blamed on industrial wine and home-distilled spirits.

At the same time that the HCEIA was struggling to stay afloat, INAO leaders were trying to consolidate their industry and win over those consumers who continued to show a preference for Algerian wine and homemade brandy. Campaigns against alcoholism clearly threatened the INAO's ambitions. Just under 15 percent of vine growers who declared their harvest had appellation status, even though it was these produc-ers who held the most promise and generated the most revenue in global markets.[47] Domestically, in 1954, the average wine consumption rate for each French citizen was around 140 liters a year, but only 10 percent of that came from appellation wines.[48] Even so, the consumption of appel-lation wines doubled between 1949 and 1955.[49] Appellation leaders had reason to be optimistic as long as temperance campaigners did not sully their good name publicly.

To distance themselves from alcoholism and safeguard their budding business, wine industry leaders thus attempted to corral the technocrat/public health coalition. To this end, they succeeded in persuading gov-ernment officials to force an HCEIA representative to participate in the meetings of the CNPFV.[50] The assumption was that the HCEIA's temper-ance propaganda and the CNPFV's pro-wine propaganda shared the same aim. Étienne May, Debré's colleague in the HCEIA and the Academy of Medicine, agreed to participate in the CNPFV. Both May and the minister of public health attended an international wine conference in Bordeaux in 1957. May told the doctors in the audience that "wine is an excellent drink" and that he condemned its abuse, not its use.[51] May wished that "wine and alcohol become one day for everyone . . . a reasonable pleasure of civilized peoples," suggesting that wine had a cultural, not a physi-ological, function.[52] At the state level, industry leaders tried to harness the campaign against alcoholism as a way to educate the public about how to discern and appreciate quality wine and blacken the reputation of their cheaper competitors.

Wine industry leaders tried to coopt the anti-alcoholism campaign as they faced the prospects of West European market integration. In March 1957, France and its Western European partners signed the Treaty of

Rome, which established the European Economic Community (EEC), predecessor of today's European Union. The Treaty of Rome called for the creation of a European common wine market over the course of the next decade, to begin in 1970. Yet the policymakers who participated in drafting the treaty tended not to be agricultural experts but instead generalists from the foreign affairs ministries.[53] The concerns of agriculture were pushed aside even though common markets for agriculture were included in the Treaty's provisions. Thus policymakers with broader concerns held influence over the future of the French wine industry.

The anti-alcoholism campaign became a way for wine industry leaders to reinforce their call for more stringent regulations at the very moment that international norms began to challenge national ones. In the months after the signing of the Treaty of Rome, national wine lobbyists and the HCEIA increasingly spoke the same language about the need to promote quality wine and brandy. Equating quality with certified origins was not inevitable but rather a political tactic to defend producer and state interests as they faced stiffer international competition. Regulating production would protect the French wine and spirits industry from cheaper domestic and foreign impostors, promote public health, and strengthen the state, whose sovereignty and economic interests were threatened by the incipient EEC.

Thus in 1957, the year that the EEC came into being, members of the HCEIA opened a dialogue with leaders of the INAO and the CNVS, producer and distributor groups, respectively, that had historically been opposed to one another but that had come together after the war to promote the appellation system. As the INAO started to gain prominence and shifted the balance of power from merchants to vine growers and as the appellation system's interests began to align with the state's anti-alcoholism, the CNVS chose to support the appellation movement in order to distance merchants from the problem of fraud and alcoholism. The CNVS argued that a close correlation existed between the rise in alcoholism and the increase of fraudulent wine and spirits on the market, calling on the state to strengthen the fraud police and to ensure that the HCEIA financed it.[54] Framing alcoholism as a problem of unregulated production and distribution placed the INAO and the CNVS in the vanguard of the campaign against alcoholism and provided further protections to the appellation system against the prospects of looser

European norms. In September 1958, the final month of the Fourth Republic's existence, the president of the CNVS told Debré that his "latest letters have sufficiently proven to us that you're really concerned about fighting alcoholism."[55] In the campaign against alcoholism, the tables had turned.

The HCEIA, the INAO, and the CNVS agreed on common messages: "Drink Well, Drink a Little, in order to Drink for a Long Time" (figure 12). While "well" meant appellation wine and brandy found in metropolitan France, "a little" meant no more than a liter of wine a day. Guy Mollet, head of the government in 1957, acknowledged that "the fact that the government's propaganda implies that a dose of a liter of French wine per day is not dangerous in itself appears to me . . . very favorable from the perspective of foreigners who generally consider that infinitely smaller doses are toxic."[56] In the early 1950s, Le Roy de Boiseaumarié had called on the wine industry to "Produce Better, but Less"; now, Robert Debré appealed to consumers to "Drink Better, but Less."[57] Refining wine production and consumption had become mutually reinforcing.

In the period between 1955 and 1958, the HCEIA and the INAO and its allies started to fuse their movements at strategic moments to defend quality. The HCEIA could not categorically attack wine if it was going to win popular support. In turn, the INAO had to change the way the average French producer and consumer conceived of wine if it was going to maintain and expand its rules and regulations in the new Europe. This quality coalition stigmatized the producers, distributors, and consumers who either defied or were excluded from the appellation system's norms. Working together, they sought to provide wine with deeper cultural meaning at a time when Algeria was challenging French self-definitions and the prospects of a European common wine market were threatening to homogenize goods, which would give added weight to France's industrial wine system. By negotiating the conflicting interests of technocrats, public health activists, and the INAO and using these interests to marginalize less favored producers in the countryside and Algeria, the state could centralize its power, promote regional economic growth, and rebrand wine in a way that concealed social conflict and conjured up quaint images of hexagonal France.

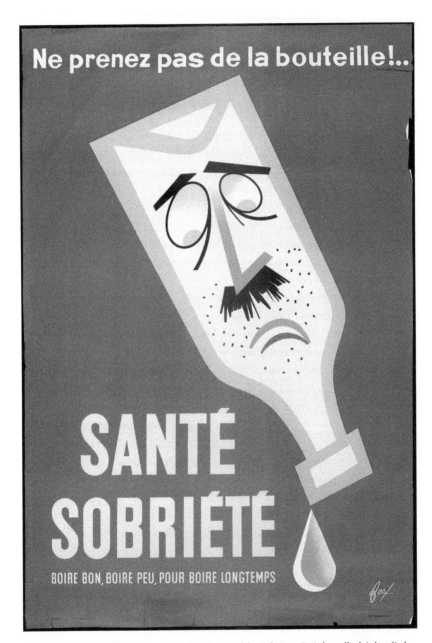

Figure 12. "Don't fall victim to the bottle. Health. Sobriety. Drink well, drink a little, in order to drink for a long time." Designed by Philippe Foré, HCEIA propaganda, c. 1957. Courtesy of the National Archives of France, Pierrefitte-sur-Seine.

Demonizing Home Distillers and Settlers

The quality coalition was injected with further momentum when intellectuals and Paris-based newspapers of various political opinions stigmatized the home distillers and settlers of Algeria in the late 1950s, alerting the public of the need to reform these two categories of French citizens. Reports linked them to alcoholism in France, malnutrition in Algeria, and economic backwardness in both. In contrast, the expanding appellation system was ignored in these reports, as if appellation wine had no potential for causing surpluses and alcoholism. This suggests that combating the industrial wine system was about much more than combating alcoholism; above all, it was about puncturing drinking myths that helped sustain a particular kind of political and imperial order that was impeding economic expansion and the ability of technocrats to oversee that expansion.

In metropolitan France, the home distiller became synonymous with the parliamentary power and perceived corruption that technocrats hoped to constrain. Novelist and journalist François Mauriac observed that "a right-dominated Assembly can follow a left-dominated Assembly; in order for the difference to be erased, all one has to do is utter the magic word: home distiller."[58] Not only did Parliament hold much power, but the home distillers had unqualified support across the political spectrum as well. Writer Robert Escarpit, frustrated with Parliament's continued extension of the home distillers' practice, censured "the politicians of the old stock, republicans through and through who have a tri-colored but patriotically cirrhotic liver."[59] The modernist periodical *L'Express* encouraged parliamentarians who voted to preserve home distillation to pin up or place in their wallets a photograph of "these dazed, disfigured children, who either come from a family of alcoholics or are alcoholics themselves . . . next to that of their own children" (figure 13).[60] Such representations suggest that the home distillers' 10 liters of tax-free brandy a year did more harm to the French population than large spirits firms or the commercial wine trade. In 1955, French television presented a program about alcoholism, inviting several public health activists and alcohol lobbyists to participate. When André Liautey, the raucous leader of the National Syndicate of Home Distillers (SNBC), took the floor, the cameraman stopped filming in order to change reels.[61] The claims of home distillers were falling on

Comment auraient-ils voté hier ?

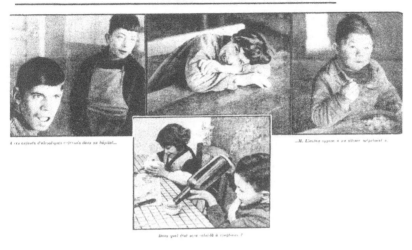

Figure 13. Children victimized by home-distilled brandy. The newspaper headline reads, "What did they [the parliamentarians] vote for yesterday?" *L'Express*, 9 November 1955.

deaf ears and blind eyes. Books made for a popular audience blamed the home distillers and working-class drinking establishments for maintaining the authority of French drinking habits and thus sustaining the country's economic backwardness and alcoholism.[62] These examples suggest that the Parisian cultural elite was turning against the home distillers and their parliamentary allies in order to centralize state power.

While the home distillers were associated with parliamentary power and corruption, the European settlers of Algeria were represented as greedy capitalists who exploited the indigenous population and who were uneasy about redistributing land and power to help pacify French Algeria. In 1955, the year that official reports started questioning the economic value of empire, several agronomists, economists, INAO leaders, Parisian newspapers, and the nationalist movement in Algeria raised public awareness about how the Algerian wine industry was causing economic inefficiency, malnutrition, and violence. This was not the first time that metropolitan elites had condemned the Algerian wine industry, but in the context of the war, criticisms of the industry and its consequences for the future of French Algeria reached a wider audience.

The war and the shifting balance of power in Algeria made people more attentive. In the late nineteenth and early twentieth centuries, the settlers in Algeria and state officials in Paris had largely divided power; the settlers had a large amount of freedom from distant Paris. The rise of the nationalist movements and the war of independence drove a wedge between settlers and state officials. Between 1936 and 1948, the size of the European population remained stationary; at the same time, the indigenous population rapidly grew. State officials in Paris had to negotiate between settler and indigenous demands. The significance of wine to the Algerian economy meant that the vineyard became a key site of state-directed reform, which further alienated the settlers from Paris. In trying to integrate the indigenous population more fully into French life through socioeconomic reform, officials in Paris showed how the settlers, through their defense of the vine and of the status quo, harmed not just indigenous living standards but metropolitan drinkers as well.

Early in the war, Pierre Fromont, an agronomist and supporter of the INAO, argued in *Le Figaro* that vine monoculture in Algeria was the cause of the region's malnourishment and bitterness.[63] It is true that the settlers had more incentive to grow vines than other food. In 1951, for every 100,000 to 150,000 francs that a hectare of vines brought in, a hectare planted with grain earned only 20,000 to 25,000 francs.[64] Wine production was thus more lucrative, but the indigenous population generally lacked the capital to participate in it. Indigenous Algerians were left in an autarkic situation, producing an insufficient amount of grain to feed a rapidly growing indigenous population.[65] The vineyard was thus the source of a severe dietary and socioeconomic imbalance in French Algeria.

Not only did the wine industry impede wellbeing in the present, but wine provided little hope for the future of the indigenous population. Hildebert Isnard, an historian of the Algerian wine industry, censured the settlers for lobbying to uphold the Franco-Algerian customs union that protected the wine industry and limited Algeria's ability to trade with other countries and expand.[66] This criticism came at a time when French policymakers had begun the negotiating process for the establishment of an integrated European market. "Algeria," he claimed, "no longer needs new growers in the fields; the Algeria of tomorrow needs technicians, specialists, engineers."[67] *Le Monde* published an article suggesting that Algeria was an economic burden on France and was turning metropolitan

Frenchmen into alcoholics. "France," the article dramatically concluded, must "leave Algeria to its fate."[68]

The INAO publicly distanced itself from the socioeconomic problems arising from the Algerian wine industry. Le Roy de Boiseaumarié, the INAO's head, blamed the "insane extension" of the Algerian vineyard for the wine industry's ills and reported that "there's no overproduction of good French wines, but there's about 12 million hectoliters that the consumer doesn't want and that poisons the market."[69] Le Roy de Boiseaumarié's reference to 12 million hectoliters, which was roughly the amount that flowed into the mainland from Algeria, was no doubt a jab at the Algerian wine industry; he was wrong, however, to assume that consumers disliked Algerian wines. In critiquing the Algerian wine industry, the INAO could conceal its interest in expansion behind a concern for the wellbeing of indigenous Algerians and mainland drinkers.

While various metropolitan interests voiced concern about the socioeconomic consequences of the Algerian wine industry, the National Liberation Front (FLN) saw wine as one of the most striking examples of imperialist oppression.[70] Between the late 1920s and the 1950s, the Algerian nationalist movement frequently confiscated large agricultural properties, which included the vineyards.[71] During the war of independence, the vineyard was a regular site of nationalist attacks on the settlers.[72] At the Evian peace negotiations, an FLN leader argued that Henri Borgeaud, one of the wealthiest settler vine growers, deserved "the title of national hero" because "without him and those like him, there would be no united Algeria."[73] Albert Camus, who grew up in Algeria and whose father had been a vineyard worker, noted that "one knows that the parliamentary majority has systematically intoxicated the French nation, generally for ignoble reasons."[74] In his critique of the death penalty, Camus linked the state's support of alcohol to France's rate of crime. Camus insinuated that the state had a hand in criminal behavior and perhaps as well in the acts of terrorism during the war. State subsidies to wine, as we have seen, not just encouraged drinking but also preserved the privileges of the industrial wine producers and reportedly led to a low standard of living in Algeria and certain metropolitan regions.

State officials responded to both Paris- and indigenous-based criticisms of the status quo with several reports on Algeria's potential for industrialization. It is significant that of the handful of reports that were released in the late 1950s that assessed the viability of French Algeria and that aimed to improve its socioeconomic situation, two were written by technocrats charged with the wine surplus problem. The influential Maspétiol Report, named after an agronomist who also headed the Institute of Industrial Wines (IVCC) that had been established in 1953 to discipline industrial wine production, revealed the costs to the Treasury of developing Algeria. In 1952–1953, 53 percent of Algeria's development funds had come from the mainland; in 1954–1955, that figure had increased to 81 percent.[75] Charles Frappart, who headed the state alcohol agency from 1956, also drew up a report on Algeria's socioeconomic development.[76] That the heads of the IVCC and the state alcohol agency, two state institutions that had direct relations with the Algerian wine industry, were also charged with thinking about the modernization of Algeria as a whole suggests the significance of wine to the Algerian economy.

It is unclear how inequality or the war affected the public's view of the settler vine growers specifically, but we do know that as the war dragged on public opinion became increasingly indifferent to the claim that "Algeria is France." Between the onset of the war in 1954 and early 1956, a majority wished to preserve Algeria's status as an administrative part of France. Starting in 1957, however, polls showed that metropolitan French people became detached from the settlers, had little interest in funding Algeria's industrialization, showed a lack of enthusiasm for the war, and were skeptical about France's long-term interests in Algeria. In 1958–1959, a majority of the public agreed that Algeria would eventually obtain independence.[77] The public's disaffection weakened the settlers' cause.

The public was also increasingly hostile toward the home distillers. In 1955, the main temperance lobby claimed to have obtained an astonishing eleven million signatures petitioning against the home distillers' practice.[78] In May 1960, a public opinion poll revealed that for every ten persons, five were in favor of abolishing the existing home distillers' practice, three were partisans of the status quo, and two were indifferent.[79] As France urbanized, as disposable income rose, and as the media stigmatized the home distillers as the source of alcoholism, consumers showed a preference for commercial drinks.

At the same time that public opinion turned against the settlers and the home distillers, a new generation of farmers in mainland France was coming of age that was more enterprising and ready for competition in the common market. Through Catholic Agricultural Youth Leagues (JAC), which since 1929 had sought to improve education and leisure in the countryside and had a strong presence in Brittany, young, forward-looking farmers came to accept the imperative of modernization. Medical students and young agricultural leaders spoke at a press conference about the dangers of drink.[80] The president of the distillers' union noted that the mentality of youth had changed and was less attached to the practice of home distillation.[81] Young farmers wanted to push for more fruit farming in place of alcohol production.[82] The CNDCA, the country's main temperance lobby, recognized "the indifference that the young peasant generation, in its entirety, manifests toward a 'privilege' that has become the least of its concerns. . . . The country must do its best to satisfy the young generation if it wants to conserve or give to the countryside the rural elite that will rejuvenate life in the 'French desert.'"[83] Notorious home-distilling departments in western France proved attentive to ways to combat alcoholism. Municipal councils gave substantial financial support to the local temperance committee in order to fight alcoholism.[84] Fighting alcoholism, modernizing the countryside and Algeria, and promoting appellations were different components of the same process.

Both the vine-growing settlers—grouped in the CGVA—and the home distillers—grouped in the SNBC and the National Syndicate of Ambulating Distillers (SNBA)—armed themselves with their own arguments about the causes and remedies of alcoholism and how to promote quality wine and brandy. *Le Tribune agricole* insisted that not all French Algerians were "feudal lords" or "reactionary settlers."[85] *La Journée vinicole* questioned Paris representations of the settler as alcoholic.[86] To be fair, some vine growers in Algeria worked diligently to improve production and prepare their industry for competition in the EEC just like metropolitan vine growers. They pointed out that French consumers preferred Algerian wine and that the vine growers of the Languedoc could not survive without Algeria's blending wines.[87] The viticultural specialist Jean Branas characterized all Algerian wine as "industrial" in order to legitimate the movement to localize wine production in metropolitan France through the appellation system, a characterization with which Algerian wine lobbyists took issue.[88]

Similarly, the SNBC and the SNBA supported public health measures by encouraging the production of quality brandy. *Le Figaro* could admit that the home distiller "doesn't intend to give up his natural product, which he knows is good, so as to resort to commercial alcohol that isn't all up to par."[89] The home distiller operated by a different logic than state officials; whereas the former found quality in the homemade, the latter found quality in regulated drinks. The home distillers claimed to protect national products against international trusts and foreign competition.[90] "Why this campaign against the home distillers?" asked one of the SNBC's leaders as he connected the home distillers' plight to the Suez Crisis of 1956, answering that "we must at any price reduce alcohol production in France . . . in order to import a little more oil."[91] One home distiller wondered how Parisian elites could castigate homemade wine or brandy for causing alcoholism while blithely imbibing scotch or whisky.[92] Responding to an article in the Paris-based *Femina-Illustration* that advised people suffering from a liver condition to drink whisky with water, a leader of the SNBC warned that "the liver knows how to recognize the nationality of alcohol."[93] Finally, the home distillers defended the inviolability of the home against the intrusion of the state and the right to family-based alcohol production and consumption. While Parisian intellectuals reported on the "complete jacquerie" found in regions like Brittany and Normandy, the home distillers claimed that by taking away their tax-free production, state officials were infringing on private property with "inquisitorial and abusive searches."[94]

Paris-based representations of settlers and home distillers as purveyors of political corruption, economic backwardness, and alcoholism pathologized the Fourth Republic for its inability or unwillingness to corral these groups. One temperance activist called home distillation "the typical problem, which puts in sharp conflict the national interest and the electoral interest."[95] Looking back on the fall of the Fourth Republic and no doubt intending to ensure that the new republic overcame localized power, *L'Express* blamed the lobbies for France's political paralysis: "the fact that the Fourth Republic . . . has always capitulated before the alcohol lobbies was proof of its weakness and one of the causes of its discredit."[96] As this quote illustrates, the Paris-based newspapers, along with the quality coalition discussed earlier, used the wine problem and the related Algerian War and European integration to call on officials to build a stronger state. The technocrats, long interested in boosting their power, now had their chance to carry out deep change.

The Political and Fiscal Revolution of 1958–1960

In 1958, the Fourth Republic, having failed to cope with the crisis in Algeria and address pressing socioeconomic problems, collapsed. Charles de Gaulle was summoned to draft a new constitution, develop a more effective Algerian policy, and promote economic and financial stabilization in preparation for the EEC.[97] The new constitution allowed de Gaulle and the executive branch to rule over Parliament. Technocrats could finally take their revenge on the parliamentarians who had blocked so many reforms.

The negative representations in the media of the home distillers and settlers helped discredit the Fourth Republic in the eyes of the public; in turn, these representations and the installation of the more authoritarian Fifth Republic abetted the appellation system in modernizing the drink trade.[98] In the Fifth Republic, where it was "better to know two well-placed civil servants than twenty deputies," the appellation system had friends in high places.[99] Michel Debré, son of Robert, had become de Gaulle's first prime minister and had versed himself in the technocratic school of the 1930s and 1940s.[100] Although a proponent of French Algeria, he had a keen awareness of the need to modernize wine and agriculture in the name of peace and prosperity. He was not alone. The Fifth Republic gave greater voice to other leading technocrats whom we have already encountered, figures like Étienne Hirsch and Alfred Sauvy. Sympathetic institutions and political actors, then, were in place at the beginning of the Fifth Republic to expand the appellation system in the interests of economic growth, public health, and cultural renewal. The Fifth Republic set about legitimating itself by marking a rupture with past institutions and policies, all the while drawing on the national traditions that the INAO was protecting and promoting—modernity, via nostalgic traditionalism.

At the beginning of the Fifth Republic, the government drew up plans to resolve the socioeconomic problems facing the country, quell unrest, and adjust to the new and potentially hostile economic environment created by the EEC. In October 1958, de Gaulle announced his Constantine Plan that would finance the industrialization of Algeria and increase the living standards of indigenous Algerians.[101] The plan's subcommission on viticulture called for the maintenance of the Algerian vineyard, arguing that it generated wealth for the entire Algerian economy, that metropolitan wines continued to depend on it, and that there were "financial problems" with vine reconstitution.[102] This conclusion likely reflected the settlers' refusal to reform the industry, the continued centrality of wine to the economy, and the difficulties that reducing the Algerian vineyard presented, especially during the war. Algerian wine exports made up 55 percent of the value of all exports in 1958 and a similar proportion in 1960. Wine was a key commodity in agricultural employment and income. In 1955, the wine industry received 25 percent of the gross investment in Algeria.[103] To be sure, the ripping out of vines had increased after the 1953 decree that revised the wine statute. Although yields remained high throughout the 1950s, Algeria's vineyard reached 371,000 hectares in 1954 and then fell to 344,000 in 1961.[104] Uprooting vines reportedly indicated a divestment in Algeria and "an intention of abandoning it."[105] To match the industrialization of Algeria, de Gaulle's government also created a committee under the leadership of the liberal economist Jacques Rueff to remove the obstacles to economic expansion and prepare France and Algeria for competition in the EEC. The committee included Alfred Sauvy, who had a long history of thinking about the wine problem and who had also participated in the HCEIA. The Rueff Committee called on the government to scale back wine production, improve the quality of wine, and limit the home distillers' practices.[106] For economic, social, and cultural reasons, wine attracted attention at the highest levels at the beginning of the Fifth Republic.

In this context, Robert Debré created a sub-commission with the CNVS, wine and spirits exporters, the aperitif firm Saint-Raphaël, and Nicolas, the largest merchant in appellation wines, to discuss ways to tighten the state's control over the wine industry and modernize production.[107] Significantly, the sub-commission excluded the voices of the settlers and smalltime producers who were grouped in the CGVA, CGVM, SBNC, and SNBA. A supporter of industrial wine production reacted by fulminating against the "partisan and totalitarian mindset" of the groups promoting appellation wine and "a harmful wine policy that aimed to asphyxiate the production of industrial wines in order to ensure their own survival."[108] The sub-commission encouraged the government to incentivize quality wine production by raising taxes on outputs, to police fraud more effectively, to restrict tax-free home distillation, to enforce the laws against prohibited vines, to more closely surveil the circulation of wines coming from non-market-oriented family vineyards, and to educate the public about how to appreciate quality appellation wine and spirits.[109] While seeking to reduce alcoholism, these measures especially reinforced state power over the wine industry and combated "unfair" competition from non-appellation producers. Interestingly, the HCEIA's funding, which earlier had been so hard to maintain, started to increase just as it began collaborating with the CNVS to promote quality wine.[110]

Newspapers in luxury wine regions expressed joy at the news of this quality coalition. *Le Bien public* of Dijon was happy to see that public health activists were "not against wine but against the abuse of wine . . . there's as much difference between a drunkard and a connoisseur of good wine as between a glass of water and a glass of Beaujolais."[111] A public health activist in Alsace noted that "a lot of wine producers deplore like us the miseries caused by the abuse of wine. . . . For helping the wine producers out, we'd really like to be able to say to the French: 'Drink wine, but observe temperance.'"[112] Another activist declared that "we're in favor of the reasonable consumption of natural wine. It's indispensable that consumers know that what we're fighting against . . . is above all adulterated, industrially produced wines, and, above all else, against fraud."[113] Quotes such as these reinforced a common distinction between use and abuse, on the one hand, and authenticity and fraud, on the other.

Some public health activists believed that their campaign to reduce drinking was being derailed. Public health activists in the Isère department protested against the possibility that the country's main temperance lobby would accept financial support from the wine lobbies.[114] They warned of the danger of making an official distinction between "good" and "bad" wine, as if the consumer could unrepentantly drink "good" wine. A psychiatrist noted that "the questions relative to the quality of wine, whether trafficked or adulterated with more or less dangerous chemical substances, constitutes a *trap*."[115] Some public health activists believed that their cause was being compromised by the CNVS's and the HCEIA's association of appellation wine production with temperance.

The month after formal collaboration began between the HCEIA and the CNVS to promote quality wine, the new government implemented major economic reforms. In December, de Gaulle valiantly devalued the franc. Also in December and then again in May 1959, de Gaulle's administration obtained special powers to raise the wine taxes. In devaluing the currency, the state could facilitate wine and other exports; in raising the wine taxes, the state could change the status of wine from a dietary necessity into a luxury and thus limit domestic demand. Both of these measures could help reduce alcoholism and generate more revenue to underwrite development projects. Antoine Pinay, the minister of finance, reasoned that the financial renewal desired by "the immense majority of the nation" would especially fall on "the consumers of alcoholic drinks," but he doubted that the higher taxes would discourage affluent consumers from purchasing appellation wines because they "appreciate the diverse qualities of these wines."[116]

Nevertheless, the currency devaluation and the tax hike galvanized both public opinion and the industrial vine growers. *Le Figaro* complained that the price of a liter of wine required thirty-five minutes of work in 1911, but now it required thirty-six minutes of work.[117] The Communist Waldeck Rochet argued that the tax was an attack on both the small vine grower and the average consumer, showing that wine drinking had declined 11 percent in France between September 1958 and April 1959 as a result of the decree.[118] The Federation of Vine Growing Associations (FAV) and stalwart defender of Algerian wine Édouard Kruger called the new tax a "wineocide" (*vinocide*).[119] The vine growers of the Languedoc, having a diminished ability to influence the policymaking process and reeling from the government's recent decrees, fell back on their tradition of direct action. In 1959, the Workers' Movement for the Defense of Family Businesses (MODEF) was created as a Communist alternative to the conservative FNSEA.[120] Languedoc vine growers joined its ranks and protested in the streets. *Le Monde* warned its readers that "soon it will no longer be possible to guarantee public order."[121]

The economic shakeup left broader peasant and Algerian interests feeling betrayed as well. In 1959, the government accepted the Rueff Committee's position that France's agricultural backwardness held back economic growth and that the price of agricultural goods tended to be inflationary. For this reason, price indexing came to an end in February 1959, a move that sparked violent demonstrations.[122] Also in 1959, de Gaulle called for Algerian self-determination, declaring that "the old Algeria is dead, and if you don't understand that, you'll die along with it."[123] In January 1960, militant settlers retaliated by clashing with the police, leaving 20 dead and 150 wounded. The week of the "barricades uprising" had begun.

Peasants on the mainland and settlers in Algeria were challenging the new republic's legitimacy.

The forward-looking media provided a moral justification for these economic reforms, suggesting that it was the state's responsibility to intervene in order to improve living conditions. *Le Monde* asked "how can we contest that there's a problem of state when there are regions . . . that we'll lose to the ravages of alcoholism?"[124] *L'Express* othered the metropolitan countryside just as it had othered Algeria, suggesting that both had fallen prey to "feudal interests" that blocked socioeconomic reforms. To liberate rural life from these feudal interests, *L'Express* demanded that the state foot the bill for the development of the countryside through equipment, electrification, water conveyance, garbage collection, land consolidation, agricultural education, and rural migration, "in short, the metropolitan equivalent of the Constantine Plan."[125] This bold comparison implied that the metropolitan countryside and Algeria had much in common; the state needed to fund development projects in order to pacify and preserve these regions.

Amid these disturbances and the obstacles of reforming alcohol, the countryside, and Algeria, Michel Debré, like Mendès France before him, abandoned the behind-the-scenes policy decisions that had excluded the public, such as the tax hike, and launched a public campaign against alcoholism to politicize consumers and turn them against the industrial wine system. The wine lobbies could see which way the wind was blowing. When Michel Debré went before Parliament to explain his reasons for combating alcoholism and to request the power to rule by decree, the Socialist Party dubbed him an anti-parliamentarian for attempting to circumvent the legislature's power.[126] One Socialist deputy saw the war on alcoholism as a way to discredit Parliament, noting that "the exploitation of anti-parliamentary propaganda is carried out shamelessly against these deputies who wish for . . . the rapid extension of alcoholism."[127] Socialists were put in a difficult position. As the traditional defenders of the industrial vine growers of the Languedoc, they had the tricky task of deflecting accusations that their constituency was responsible for widespread alcoholism; on the other hand, however, the Socialists were a major opposition party to de Gaulle's regime and wanted to defend Parliament against technocratic rule. As the reformers framed it, though, to defend Parliament was to defend alcoholism.

Aware that it would spell political suicide to directly attack the settlers who were desperately struggling to hold on to power in Algeria or upset the peasant vine growers whose living standards had not kept up with their urban counterparts, Michel Debré conceded to the wine supporters in Parliament. He accepted the demands of several metropolitan senators to uphold the wine statute of 1953 that set out to convert quantity production to either quality production or other foodstuffs.[128] To further appease the metropolitan wine industry, Michel Debré acknowledged in the Senate that the primary cause of alcoholism was not metropolitan wine but the cheap, highly alcoholic wines of Algeria.[129] But even with such an admission, the government took no decisive action against the Algerian wine industry except enforcing the 1953 statute, given the war, the challenges of industrializing Algeria, and the settlers' power.

While wine-loving parliamentarians fulminated against Michel Debré, parliamentarians from Brittany, a bastion of cider production and home distillation, supported the new government's campaign against alcoholism and the much-maligned home distillers.[130] The popularity of both cider and homemade brandy was waning in this region. Cider consumption fell from 18,203 hectoliters in 1953 to 12,353 hectoliters in 1957.[131] The number of home distillers dropped from 3,030,000 in 1952 to 2,118,000 in 1957, a decrease of 30 percent.[132] Still, a think tank reported that the home distillers' practice and tax fraud made the commercial wine business lose half of its business and the Treasury 18 billion francs.[133] The continued power of the industrial vine growers and the weakened position of the home distillers meant that industrialized viticulture faded into the background as the state pursued an easier target.

When a law of 30 July 1960 authorized Michel Debré, like his predecessor Pierre Mendès France, the power to rule by decree, the prime minister launched a campaign against the country's "social scourges": alcoholism, homosexuality, and prostitution. Home distillers were surprised to find themselves grouped with homosexuals and prostitutes.[134] Yet, at first, they did not display much hostility toward the movement against them.[135] In fact, the home distillers helped bring themselves down. Many of their parliamentarians voted in favor of the law against home distillation so as to prevent the harsher Mendès France decree from going into effect, which would have taken the privilege away from those who did not claim themselves as farmers. One senator who supported home distillation had encouraged his colleagues in the Senate to vote in favor of the law but now felt that Michel Debré had deceived them.[136] An ordinance of 30 August 1960 dictated that the home distiller's tax-free production would end with the person who currently practiced it. Home distillers could no longer transmit their privilege to their offspring. Those who abandoned the privilege would receive subsidies to produce fruit for non-alcoholic purposes.[137] In November, as part of the campaign to eliminate home distillation, the government also issued ordinances to continue the process begun in 1953 to improve and limit cider production. These measures were intended not only to combat alcoholism but also to aid the development of appellation brandies like armagnac, calvados, and cognac.

Terminating the home distillers' practice and rationalizing cider production supported the Fifth Republic's political and fiscal revolution. The home distillers' influence diminished with the power of their elected officials. The political tactics and raucous debate that had worked during the Fourth Republic simply failed to do so at the beginning of the Fifth. When, in a dramatic display, André Liautey, a former deputy and leader of the SNBC, was spotted giving advice to his political successor in the National Assembly, security guards immediately escorted him from the premises of the National Assembly.[138] What may have been tolerated just a few years earlier was no longer allowed. For the home distillers, Liautey's expulsion from Parliament was the beginning of the end. Liautey's political style belonged to a past that the new republic wished to forget, not resurrect. With the transition to the Fifth Republic, the SNBC lacked the necessary political connections and the financial means to influence policy. A journalist predicted that the abolition of the home distillers' practice would increase the state's tax revenue by 60 billion francs per year, a higher estimate than the think tank cited above, thus contributing to the new republic's fiscal revolution.[139]

France's drinking establishments, those "Parliaments of the People," also felt the effects of the Fifth Republic's stricter regulatory environment. The state decreased the number of establishments from one for every 180 French denizens to one for every 3,000 citizens, approximately one per village.[140] The new zoning laws prevented the installation of cafés near athletic fields, hospitals, new housing developments, and schools. As the power of the political parties and the industrial working classes gradually declined, these institutions were no longer economically viable. The bistro smacked of a working-class and revolutionary past that the rising new middle class hoped to forget. Proprietors of drinking establishments, like home distillers, merchants, and some vine growers, had also been accused of perpetrating fraud. Owners of drinking establishments were notorious for filling empty bottles of fine wine and spirits with cheaper concoctions.[141] Limiting the number of drinking establishments, like ending the home distillers' practice, helped prevent the circulation and sale of fraudulent beverages and control quality.

In 1958, the newly established Fifth Republic had begun to come down on the side of the INAO's definition of quality, and it justified the endorsement on the grounds of needing tax money for development projects and fighting alcoholism. "Quality," in this sense, meant a respect for old practices—metropolitan to be sure—that were invariably state-approved and state-regulated, which supported the new republic's bid to consolidate its technocratic authority by directing economic growth, protecting public health, and rethinking the nation in a period of imperial crisis and Europeanization. In 1960, Michel Debré, like Pierre Mendès France, used alcoholism as a way to mobilize the public against the industrial wine system and carry out reforms to the industry. These reforms were controversial because they raised larger concerns about the status of French democracy and the future of the peasantry and French Algeria. Unlike Mendès France, however, Debré benefited from a more favorable political context: not only did he have a larger segment of public opinion supporting his reforms, but also he led a more authoritarian state. Even so, the settlers' refusal to share power and the instability caused by the Algerian War limited the government's ability to enact thoroughgoing change to wine in 1960. Despite the limitations on reform, the vine growers of Algeria and the Languedoc, having lost their beet, cider, and home-distilling allies, were now more isolated than they had been before. As we will see, however, it would take more than de Gaulle's army of technocrats to push industrial vine growers to the margins of French life.

Conclusion

The period between 1955 and 1960—a period that witnessed the escalation of France's war in Algeria, the inauguration of the EEC, and the transition from a parliamentary to a technocratic republic—was an important turning point in the sober revolution that helped expand state power over the wine industry and localize production in metropolitan regions. Since war's end, technocrats had struggled to upend the industrial wine system because of the political power of the peasant vine growers of the Languedoc, the settlers of Algeria, and their agricultural and distiller allies. At the same time, public health activists were just beginning to raise public awareness about the dangers of wine-related alcoholism. Both technocrats and public health activists needed popular support to mobilize the state against the wine industry.

But how could this coalition win popular support against wine, a product that was seen as essential to French life? The coalition found an answer in borrowing the legal distinction between quantity and quality wine and favoring the latter. The late 1950s was a decisive period for the INAO as it struggled to cajole the rank and file of the vine growers and brandy makers to conform to its norms. Working together to achieve their particular ends, technocrats, public health activists, and the INAO—the quality coalition—attracted the new Fifth Republic at a moment of great economic, political, and cultural uncertainty. Given the urgency of managing the Algerian War and France's entry into the EEC, these groups, in demonizing the settlers and home distillers, helped the new Fifth Republic justify a more stringent regulatory environment. The quality coalition also took advantage of that environment. The first years of the Fifth Republic accelerated a process of rationalizing the drink trade, which meant showing a preference for quality wine that was rooted in regional appellations at the expense of quantity wine that had no specific homeland.

The quality coalition treated the transformation of wine and the transformation of state institutions as interlocking processes. The INAO, with its notions of tradition, authenticity, and quality, helped consumers think about the contours of the nation as hexagonal and mask the conflicts that controversial economic reforms entailed. Settlers and home distillers were blamed for a variety of ills that had beleaguered the Fourth Republic, such as parliamentary corruption, economic stagnation, undernourishment, and, finally, the "anachronistic scourge" of alcoholism.[142] By raising the wine taxes, ending the home distillers' practice, and treating wine as a luxury product, the Fifth Republic sought to create a symbolic rupture with the perceived failures of the Fourth Republic. By successfully laying claim to tradition, the INAO was intimating that settlers and home distillers—despite their own longstanding traditions—were fraudulent and foreign to the French heritage. The INAO stressed its continuity with the past even as it tried to impose new production norms on the country-side and marginalize those who could not live up to those norms. Today, few will remember the hand of the settlers and home distillers in making France's modern wine industry and legitimating the Fifth Republic.

4

DRINKING AND DRIVING

In May 1953, the *Touring Club de France*, the magazine of the automobile and tourism lobby of the same name, published the transcript of a recent radio broadcast by the minister of public works, transportation, and tourism. "French provinces," the minister told his listeners, "you must maintain your folklore, your costumes, your dances, and your songs. Become even more aware of them. Foreign tourists want to see the face of your history. They also want to taste the flavors of your cuisine and the aromas of your wine."[1] On the very next pages in the magazine, an automobile lobbyist, anticipating an influx of foreign tourists whom the French would need to impress, pleaded with his French readers to do something about "the procession of undisciplined, selfish, cynical, drunken, and boorish individuals who drive as if they were the only ones on French roads."[2] In his view, French drinking and driving habits threatened a vibrant tourism industry and the romantic images that it sold of the French heritage.

The juxtaposition of these two articles highlights a central tension in maintaining and expanding France's reputation as an international destination in the 1950s and 1960s: how to promote automobile-based foreign tourism in wine country while ensuring road safety and sobriety among French drivers.[3] To reconcile these seemingly contradictory imperatives, the doctors and technocrats in the High Commission for Studies and Information on Alcoholism (HCEIA) joined forces with the technocrats at "Ponts et Chaussées," France's most prestigious engineering school, and the automobile, insurance, and tourism industries. This coalition for road safety embarked on a campaign to establish a legal blood alcohol limit that would at once limit automobile accidents, reduce alcoholism, stimulate regional tourism, and curb the power of the industrial wine system.[4] As we have seen, the parliamentary Fourth Republic, as a guardian of individual rights and the industrial wine interests that economic expansion would have endangered, resisted the state's attempt to enforce thoroughgoing change to the industrial wine system. In the debate over drinking and driving, the industrial wine lobbies were joined by the local courts that wished to protect their right to determine the role of alcohol in automobile accidents. The coming of the expert-led Fifth Republic in 1958 and the development of international road safety research slowly cleared the path to more Paris-based regulation over drinking and driving in the name of safety and economic growth. Defining a threshold of responsible drinking and implementing a breath test device to enforce it became an instrument of state power in negotiating the tensions between wine tourism and automobile use.

The near-universal use of automobiles after World War II and the campaign against drinking and driving had two important consequences for the sober revolution and the related rise of the appellation system. First, automobile tourism and the revenue that it generated contributed to the impulse to link notions of authenticity and quality to the place of production and integrate French wine into global markets, thus helping the appellation system advance against its cheaper competitors. Second, the growing number of alcohol-related car accidents spurred state officials to engineer new nationwide drinking norms—deploying the quality coalition's slogan "drink better, but less"—as a way to modify consumer practices and regulate greater mobility. The automobile revolution and road safety campaigns thus coincided with and contributed to the sober revolution and the rise of the appellation system.

Looking to promote the ideals and values of the mass consumer society that was emerging in postwar France, sober revolutionaries invariably associated the automobile with progress, mobility, and modernity and wine with backwardness, roots, and tradition. The perceived necessity of the automobile revolution to economic growth was underlined by the fact that those with a stake in automobile tourism succeeded in implementing the state's drinking and driving policy at the expense of the protected and privileged industrial wine system. The imperative of limiting motor accidents in order to promote automobile use enabled doctors, technocrats, and the automobile-related lobbies to distance the industrial wine lobbies from the decision-making process. One wine lobbyist complained that "to attack the makers and distributors of national drinks doesn't resolve the problem of alcoholism, for it ignores the real causes of the condition. No one would think to render the builders and sellers of automobiles responsible for road accidents and prohibit the advertising of powerful, fast cars."[5]

The campaign against drinking and driving was international in scope, but its translation into French law should be understood in terms of the particularities of French political culture—namely, the ongoing effort to transform wine production and consumption and the institutions and protectionist policies that preserved the status quo.[6] Wine became a highly politicized issue, not only because France's high rates of road accidents and alcoholism threatened to impede economic growth and tarnish France's international image but also because technocrats aimed to overcome Parliament and rationalize wine production, eliminate the industry's least competitive producers, and make the industry more export-oriented. This reform proved especially difficult because, into the 1960s, wine continued to underpin the status of agriculture and France's relationship to Algeria, on the one hand, and the French consumer's understanding of wine as a dietary necessity, on the other. Widespread wine drinking and automobile use after World War II created new tensions that—given their economic, political, and social weight—sober revolutionaries would have to reconcile and regulate by mobilizing international road safety expertise against Parliament and French drinking myths.

Automobile Tourism and the Appellation System

The automobile revolution and the appellation revolution—two seemingly separate processes—intersected with and impacted one another. During the interwar years, automobile tourism became a popular leisure activity in France among a French and foreign elite. The rise of automobile tourism coincided with the emergence of the appellation system. It is often assumed that the automobile, even more than the train before it, broke down local boundaries and altered local customs.[7] As mass production standardized goods and as France underwent urbanization, however, the automobile facilitated the creation of a new cultural imaginary around the place of production that catered to tourists as they traveled the countryside in search of authentic experiences.[8] It may be recalled that in the 1930s, a period marked by economic crisis and anxieties about immigration and Americanization, intellectuals and politicians debated the meaning of authentic France. In the wine industry, this authenticity often evoked bucolic, medieval, and European images of the countryside. The automobile helped integrate national and global markets, thereby creating more fluidity in everyday life, but it also helped redefine and fix local boundaries and customs. In this way, automobile and wine tourism helped French people find the "true" France—a European France—in the countryside.

Cars had the capacity to reconnect drinkers to the origins of the wine that they consumed, making both producers and consumers less reliant on the merchants that ruled the industrial wine system. A prestigious association of gourmets known as the Club des Cent (Club of One Hundred), for example, promoted automobile tourism, hotels, mechanics' shops, and local cuisine.[9] According to its founder, the club's mission was "to defend in France the taste of our old national cuisine, threatened by chemical formulas imported from countries where they have never even known how to prepare chicken stew."[10] Legendary eaters such as Maurice Edmond Sailland, better known by his pen-name Curnonsky, published a series of books on French gastronomy to rediscover "the forgotten riches of the *terroirs*."[11] These books aimed to protect local cuisines from foreign influence; however, in doing so, they created a sanitized, middle-class version of them.

Tourist guides encouraged travel to the countryside, where travelers could experience the presumed essence of rural France and its regional cuisines. Guidebooks directed tourists to places where they might find authentic regional dishes, meals that were in fact streamlined to conform to urban tastes. The dishes that became regional specialties were prepared differently, were cooked differently, and consisted of foods rarely eaten by the locals.[12] Tourists came to the countryside in search of traditional dress, folkloric wine festivals, monuments, and an idealized image of tradition. By experiencing the local culture, the tourist could consume a certain idea of French history in an otherwise rapidly changing world. The Michelin guides are perhaps the best-known example of the ways in which the tire and automobile industries encouraged the expansion of regional wine festivals, restaurants, and hotels.[13]

In this context, appellation vine growers, the automobile and tourism industries, folklore scholars, and local politicians marketed regional culture as a way to stimulate the regional economy, enticing automobile tourists with the prospect of an authentic experience. For example, the locals in Gevrey-Chambertin in Burgundy revived the "Feast of King Chambertin" in order to sell wine. American, French, and other European tourists were invited to attend the event, in which King Chambertin would tour the village with two monks and twelve young women whose "charms and feminine graces correspond to the local *terroir* and symbolize the properties of its wines."[14] The Brotherhood of the Knights of the Tastevin held medieval ceremonies as a way to sell wine to tourists, journalists, and American diplomats. In 1937, the first wine route was opened in Burgundy, further linking cars to wine consumption and mobility to the site of production.[15] Brotherhoods and wine routes would open in other regions after World War II.[16] A variety of local actors, many of whom had connections to Parisian elites, thus played a part in the creation and codification of local food and wine.

Automobile tourism was central to the emergence and development of the appellation system and its purpose to link a wine's distinctive qualities to its place of production in mainland France. In a world where food was becoming delocalized and industrialized, thanks in large part to economies of scale and faster transportation, proponents of the appellation system inverted the automobile's use by promoting it as a way to give tourists

access to a supposedly authentic rural experience. The automobile, symbol of mobility and modernity, would help tourists discover the unique
origins of appellation wine, symbol of immobility and tradition.

The Automobile vs. the Industrial Wine System

While the automobile revolution facilitated the appellation revolution,
alcohol-related traffic accidents threatened automobile tourism and the
idyllic images of the countryside that the appellation system promoted.
When, in the interwar years, automobile use had been a preserve of an
elite and not an integral part of everyday life for most French people,
drinking and driving had raised relatively little concern. But after World
War II, the stability between wine and the automobile threatened to
come undone as more French drivers got behind the wheel and accidents
increased. Although only one in every seventeen French inhabitants possessed a car in 1951, car ownership doubled between 1955 and 1970.[17]
The flip side of democratizing the automobile was the social cost of larger
numbers of vehicles on the road. In 1953, state officials recorded 118,881
accidents; by 1970, accidents had nearly doubled.[18] As more tourists traveled the countryside and motor accidents rose, new questions emerged
about the safety implications of the relationship between wine and the
automobile. A new constellation of interest groups emerged to reconcile
car accidents with the imperatives of economic growth and the new consumer society, of which the car and wine industries were a vital part.

   After 1945, just as wine tourism intensified, doctors started raising
alarm over the influence of alcohol on accident victims. Many of these
doctors were also active in combating alcoholism and the industrial
wine system in groups like the HCEIA, the Academy of Medicine, and
the National Committee for the Defense against Alcoholism (CNDCA),
France's largest temperance organization. They claimed that French statistics failed to reflect the real role of alcohol in automobile accidents, especially when compared to statistics produced by other countries. French
studies suggested that as little as 3 percent of accidents were caused by
alcohol.[19] In contrast, American research concluded that 62 percent of
yearly accidents in the United States had occurred under the influence of
alcohol; Swedish studies had recorded 41 percent in Sweden.[20]

Did American and Swedish drivers simply provoke more alcohol-related accidents, or did French officials fail to appreciate alcohol's role in accidents? The evidence leans toward the latter. French law had long held that only observable drunkenness disrupted public order. In 1873, after the unruly Paris Commune, and again during the war mutinies in 1917, the state had enacted legislation against observable drunkenness (*ivresse publique*).[21] The assumption that only overt intoxication disturbed public order informed the first drinking and driving laws of the interwar period. A decree of 1922 against driving "in a state of observable drunkenness" forced the withdrawal of the driver's license of anyone caught in this state. A decree in 1927 gave prefects the option of suspending or canceling licenses in the case of manslaughter or injury.[22] In April 1954, Parliament passed a law against "dangerous drinkers," which authorized the police to screen for "alcoholics" by drawing blood from those guilty of a crime, a misdemeanor, or a road accident. Yet regulations issued in 1955 and 1956 restricted the use of blood tests to cases in which the accident led to injury or death and in which the guilty party appeared to be in an "alcoholic state," a term that was never clarified. If the accident only produced material damage, the culprit had to be found in a state of public drunkenness in order to administer the blood test.[23] Early laws discouraging drinking and driving failed to provide any precision on what constituted the threshold between alcohol use and abuse beyond obvious intoxication.

The way that statistics categorized the causes of driving accidents in France added to the underestimation of alcohol's role in accidents. In 1956, the Ministry of Transportation began publishing statistics about the state of road security.[24] In the causes of accidents, the ministry employed the vague rubric of "under the effect of drink or drugs."[25] As the first responders, police officers had to determine the meaning of "under the effect," which meant that they usually fell back on the idea of overt intoxication. These statistics thus failed to convey the precise role of alcohol in traffic accidents.[26]

The law and its enforcement failed to get at the crux of the problem: the driver who was not observably drunk but whose reflexes were impaired by small quantities of alcohol. In a country that valued wine as an everyday beverage, French drinkers may have had more tolerance toward alcohol than did drinkers in northern Europe, who were known to binge drink.[27] Because the police did not observe overt intoxication in most accidents and because the courts hesitated to convict drivers without absolute proof that their drinking was responsible for the accident, judges rarely implicated alcohol. Moreover, both doctors and gendarmes doubted the efficacy of drawing blood.[28] Finally, if the drinking and driving laws were enforced, convicted drivers could lose their license and be placed in medical care. The 1954 law treated drunken driving as a case of "alcoholism." Given that social security covered alcoholism, enforcing the law would have been a serious burden on the state's coffers. For these reasons, too, alcohol was seldom blamed for accidents.

Unsurprisingly, the alcohol lobbies also threw doubt on the relationship between alcohol and accidents. Given the continued protection of rural interests during the parliamentary Fourth Republic, the lobbies still had a powerful influence over policymaking and the public perception of alcohol. They rightly interpreted any campaign to reduce drinking as a threat to their economic interests. Furthermore, given that newspapers earned money from alcohol advertising, many of them were slow to implicate alcohol in traffic accidents.[29] While French newspapers regularly published statistics explaining the various causes of accidents—the growing number of vehicles on the road, faulty brakes, the increased speed of modern vehicles, or inattention to the rules—they rarely reported on drunkenness.[30] The problem of drinking and driving consequently lacked public visibility.

Parliament hesitated to create a national drinking and driving standard that would threaten their alcohol-producing constituencies and the jurisdiction of the local courts. The Socialist Party was an important political bloc in the Fourth Republic and had a large wine constituency in the Languedoc to look after. In addition, politicians in Parliament interpreted the development of road safety expertise as part of a more general technocratic encroachment on their decision-making power.[31] Establishing a national standard of alcohol use and abuse, which would have helped identify alcohol's responsibility in accidents, would have allowed the state to trample on local networks of power.

Old beliefs about drinking died hard, even when developments in road safety research were beginning to crack the foundations of such beliefs.[32] French drinkers were often confident in their ability to control their drinking and control themselves. "There exists in France," one observer noted, "a tender indulgence for the joyous and glowing drunkard, a genuine admiration for the man who can handle wine well."[33] It was not uncommon in 1950s wine country to find vineyard workers drinking as much as 6 liters of wine and a half liter of wine-based spirits a day.[34] The French pattern of drinking, like the more general Mediterranean style of drinking, tended to be one of small yet repeated doses throughout the day, which meant that drinkers did not usually experience overt intoxication. The public thus balked at the prospects of conforming to the drinking norms of the countries that produced most of the road safety research, countries like Sweden and the United States that had a history of enacting prohibitionist policies. For many French people, the creation of a legal blood alcohol limit recommended by other countries insulted their ability to hold their alcohol. French scientists observed that the "norms . . . have been established in sober countries (Scandinavia, Anglo-Saxon countries), where the consumption of pure alcohol, per individual, is from *five to twenty times inferior to French consumption.*"[35] Who was a Swede or an American to tell a seasoned Frenchman that he had drunk too much? Throughout the 1950s, public opinion was thus slow to embrace the efforts to implement a centralized drinking and driving norm.

Calls for a standardized definition of alcohol use and abuse and a procedure to determine the precise role of alcohol in car accidents spurred the mobilization of economic interests that wished to adjust French drinking habits to a more mobile age. The automobile industry had a twin program of reforming wine production and consumption. Alfred Sauvy wrote stinging criticisms of the alcohol-based "national gasoline" for limiting the inflow of cheaper oil and stunting automobile tourism and economic growth.[36] An automobile magazine excoriated the state for making the driver bear the cost of alcohol surpluses through taxes on the national gasoline.[37] Another automobile magazine asked: "Tourists who are attracted to France in part by the reputation of our wines, will they be chased away by the alcohol in our gasoline?"[38] Indeed, some foreign tourists who traveled the French countryside complained of the national gasoline and threatened to quit visiting France.[39]

The automobile industry joined doctors in combating motor accidents in order to ensure the continuation of automobile tourism. A touring club that opposed the national gasoline could still admit that "it's infinitely less dangerous to ply the motor of a car with alcohol than its driver."[40] Fear of accidents might motivate consumers to take public transportation at a time when the automobile industry was trying to overtake train travel.[41] Driving a car was a riskier behavior than taking a train or an airplane: for every thousand kilometers traveled, the train took the lives of .95 persons; airplanes, 6.8; and automobiles a staggering 42.[42] For the automobile industry, therefore, promoting safety and economic growth were two sides of the same coin.

Given its inability to lend centralized authority to the road safety movement, the Fourth Republic left it largely in the hands of private associations. After the war, the automobile industry and the insurance companies founded a road safety organization called Prévention routière (Road Prevention), which was headed by Georges Gallienne, a former executive at Renault and a vibrant leader of the automobile lobby.[43] Prévention routière worked to encourage automobile use at the same time that it helped prevent accidents (figure 14). Throughout the 1950s and 1960s, the automobile industry vehemently opposed measures to limit speeding and instead preferred to frame the road safety discussion around alcohol. Speed was an important selling point for the automobile industry, and the ability to get places fast was an imperative of a mobile, modern economy.

The insurance companies gave Prévention routière its greatest financial backing.[44] Immediately after the war, the state nationalized most of the insurance companies and implemented the tools of rational economic planning.[45] Insurance experts had alerted the state to the fact that motor accidents were hampering the economy. In 1951, the insurance companies reportedly paid over 39 billion francs in damages, whereas they earned just over 53 billion francs.[46] The insurance companies joined doctors and the automobile industry in trying to establish a solid connection between alcohol and accidents and incite the state to take action on economic grounds.

Some automobile and touring clubs, so crucial to the emergence and development of the appellation system, also supported the campaign against drinking and driving. The Touring Club de France was conscious of the challenges that drinking and driving posed to gastronomic tourism: "It's precisely because we intend to be able, without our conscience being troubled, to continue to vaunt the quality products of the French *terroir* . . . that we refuse to close our eyes. In order to be free to advocate for the use of alcoholic beverages, we must condemn their abuse."[47] A

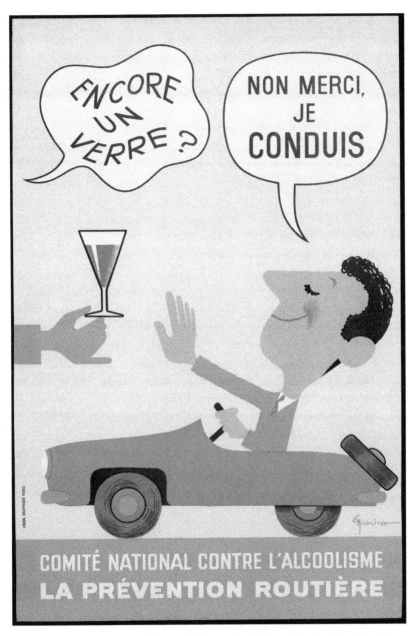

Figure 14. "Another drink? No thank you, I'm driving." Designed by Obrad Nicolitch, propaganda co-sponsored by the CNDCA and Prévention routière, c. 1960. Courtesy of the National Archives of France, Pierrefitte-sur-Seine.

driver's manual pointed out that the road safety movement did not intend "to undermine our national wealth, but we can remind automobilists, motorcyclists, cyclists, and pedestrians also . . . that France is also the country of measure and that a drink too many is perhaps, on the road, one life less."[48] To master the art of driving, one had to master the art of drinking.

In the early 1950s, doctors and technocrats began to raise awareness about the incompatibility between alcohol and automobile use. "The artisanal man of yesterday," one doctor observed, "could be a drinker who did no appreciable harm to others, for he worked on his own, but the technical man of today, through the operation of the machine and the collective service that it imposes, can no longer be a harmless drinker to others."[49] At the same time that road accidents were on the rise, other groups were promoting automobile use and tourism. These potentially conflicting trends became complementary as both road safety activists and the automobile and tourism industries wished to change how the public related to wine in the automobile age. Yet at the end of the 1950s, the road safety movement continued to face the entrenched interests of the courts, the wine lobbies, Parliament, and the drinking public. Each of these groups defended individual rights against the intrusion and extension of state power and the creation of centralized drinking norms. The remainder of this chapter examines how the road safety coalition in particular, and sober revolutionaries more generally, set about creating state-determined norms that would make the roads safer for tourists, root wine in specific metropolitan regions, and sanitize the image of the French drinker and the countryside. The effect would be to separate wine tourism and alcohol-related car accidents in the public consciousness, a necessary effect if the automobile and wine industries were going to thrive in the age of mobility.

International Expertise vs. Parliamentary Power

For the road safety coalition, the inability to pass effective road safety legislation reflected the Fourth Republic's larger parliamentary inefficiency. In the crisis years of 1957 and 1958, as political leaders were trying to find a solution to the Algerian War and harmonize socioeconomic policies within the nascent European Economic Community (EEC), doctors framed drinking and driving, like alcoholism, as a problem of state power. Once again, then, an alcohol-related problem reflected the problems besetting the Fourth Republic and helped justify the need for a more authoritarian republic. Doctor and temperance activist Robert Monod pleaded with Charles de Gaulle, then the Fourth Republic's premier, to act: "The road kills each year more youth than the Algerian war, and more than cancer. It's currently, in the human, social, and economic domains, the number one national scourge."[50] Comparing road accidents to the Algerian War, an increasingly unpopular conflict, provided a moral obligation to do something about the problem. "By laziness, insouciance, or ignorance," the *Courrier de la Nation* asserted about French drinking at the very beginning of the Fifth Republic, "the state has been in the past responsible for a large part of the disastrous situation in which we find ourselves today; it's the state that must now implement the measures of an indispensable recovery."[51]

At the end of the Fourth Republic, Robert Debré, then president of both the HCEIA and the Academy of Medicine, sought to convince state officials to emphasize the human factor in automobile accidents by inviting Édouard Bonnefous, the minister of transportation, to speak to the Academy's medical elite. The Academy's commission on road safety informed Bonnefous that "road accidents aren't especially a problem of the road or the machine, of the engineer or the builder, but above all a problem that concerns the individual's driving, where a whole series of pathological phenomena are at play."[52] The meeting between doctors and transportation interests at the Academy of Medicine marked an important turning point. In the coming months, doctors and automobile tourism stakeholders received support from a new organization established at the Ministry of Transportation called the National Organization of Road Safety (ONSER). Technocrats at Ponts et Chaussées; the automobile, insurance, and tourism lobbies; and representatives of the Ministries of Transportation, Interior, Army, and Public Health participated in this organization. Thus, at the founding of the Fifth Republic, a broad alliance of doctors, technocrats, and automobile-related lobbies began to persuade state officials of the urgency of anti–drinking and driving measures.

Both the HCEIA and the ONSER conducted studies on road safety, mobilized international research, raised public awareness, and took advantage of international networks to undercut French myths about wine. New, more conclusive international research gave their campaign an objective, apolitical air. Since the beginning of the century, international researchers had studied the effects of alcohol on human reflexes and reaction time.[53] In the 1920s, they had expanded this work into the road safety domain. Concerned about the role of alcohol in road accidents and the subjectivity of police examinations, researchers had sought to ascertain alcohol levels by drawing blood with a needle, which proved unpopular. Progress in establishing a precise link between alcohol levels and accidents was made around midcentury when law enforcers in the United States began using the Breathalyzer. The criminologist Robert Borkenstein's major study of 1962 in Grand Rapids, Michigan, forced many of the skeptics of science into retreat.[54] By going beyond laboratory trials into real-life simulation, his work had demonstrated the utility of the breath test and the need to establish a blood alcohol limit of .08.[55] As the international scientific community reached a consensus, it became difficult for national governments to ignore the problem.

The ONSER and the HCEIA not only referred to developments in the United States, which, as they reminded policymakers and the public, was more economically advanced than France, they also took advantage of the emerging EEC. In fact, the impetus for harmonizing European traffic legislation came from France's road safety activists. In 1964, Robert Debré told Prime Minister Georges Pompidou that the drinking and driving problem "has from all evidence an international dimension. Automobile and transport tourism by road is developing rapidly, in particular between the countries of the European community."[56] Soon after, Pompidou called on the European ministries of transportation to study drinking and driving and to recommend a uniform legal blood alcohol limit throughout the EEC.

At the same time, French researchers traveled abroad to study drinking and driving regulations in other European countries. In 1963, for example, they went to West Germany and came away convinced that the breath test was a more effective and humane tool than drawing blood.[57] In Hamburg in 1967, the European Conference of Ministers of Transportation (ECMT) called on member countries to establish a legal blood alcohol level of .08 with the aim of harmonizing the law. England became the first country to follow the ECMT's recommendation when it promulgated its Road Safety Act the same year. The law was said to have reduced road accidents by between 10 and 30 percent, depending on the month and the geographical region.[58]

Road safety advocates thus used the international community to address a thorny political issue at home. Perhaps to a greater degree in France than elsewhere in the EEC, restricting wine consumption was seen as an affront to economic interests and myths about drinking. The combination of more conclusive research and a political regime that lent authority to expertise over political debate slowly isolated the opponents of reform. As the HCEIA wrote in the pages of *Le Nouvel Observateur*, "whereas the majority of economically developed countries (Great Britain, West Germany, Austria, Switzerland, and a large part of the United States, Poland, Yugoslavia, the Scandinavian countries) have set a 'legal blood alcohol limit,' such a measure doesn't exist in French law."[59]

The economic downturn of the late 1960s compelled technocrats in the Ministry of Finance to join the cause of establishing a legal blood alcohol limit. Michel Debré, then the minister of finance, was carrying out his "Rationalization of Budgetary Choices" (RCB), modeled on the management methods of American business and government. As we have seen, as prime minister in 1960, Debré had launched a campaign against alcoholism that had targeted settlers and home distillers. In late 1969, the Debré family found support in the Gaullist prime minister Jacques Chaban-Delmas, who was also serving as mayor of wine-loving Bordeaux, who had close ties with local wine elites, and whose wife would die in an automobile accident one year later. Chaban-Delmas made road security into a national cause as a part of his program for a "New Society."[60] Chaban-Delmas had in his entourage a group of technocrats—Simon Nora, for example, had also helped Pierre Mendès France devise his campaign to promote milk and limit and regulate alcohol production—that viewed automobile accidents as a problem of rational administration and economic growth. Thus a number of economic reformers with a history of combating wine habits came on board in the effort to have the state impose a centralized drinking and driving norm.

The use of the RCB in making the economic waste of road accidents a statistical fact legitimated the movement in favor of a drinking and driving law.[61] In March 1970, the ONSER and the Ministry of Finance estimated that a single road death cost the nation 230,000 francs; a wounded person cost the nation 10,000 francs. They concluded that enacting a legal blood alcohol limit of .08 would save the nation between 300 to 800 million francs.[62] The report noted that of the four principal interests that a drinking and driving law would impact—alcohol, the automobile, the insurance companies, and public health—only the alcohol industry would be adversely affected.[63] The law would also benefit the insurance companies. In the insurance contracts, which were required by a 1959 decree, a clause stipulated the loss of insurance if the insured was found guilty of driving under the influence. But because such a stipulation was harsh and could ruin the livelihoods of certain people who were not covered, judges hesitated to enforce the clause. The creation of a legal blood alcohol limit would mean an automatic conviction. These experts suggested that this clause be suppressed by raising premiums. They estimated that the diminution of the number of accidents would save the insurance companies between 180 and 470 million francs.[64] Implementing a legal blood alcohol limit, the report concluded, would curb alcohol consumption, improve public health and safety, and stimulate economic growth.

Prodded by road safety activists, the international community, and the technocrats' desire for a rational management of the economy, opponents of a legal blood alcohol limit came under pressure to change their position. The Ministry of Justice, longtime defender of individual rights and critic of the state's encroachment on its jurisdiction, fell in line and set about convincing the courts. It sent a circular to public prosecutors in order to gauge their opinion about whether or not to establish a legal limit. Out of the thirty-one district attorney's offices (*parquets*) questioned, twenty-eight came around to the idea of instituting a legal blood alcohol limit. Judicial opinion, however, remained divided on what limit to set.[65] Public opinion was also split. In February 1968, for example, a public opinion poll showed that only 55 percent of drivers believed that a lack of sobriety was one of the principal causes of accidents.[66] Drivers remained somewhat skeptical of alcohol's role in automobile accidents.

Similar to the debate over wine and the home distillers in 1960, the establishment of a legal blood alcohol limit became a site of contention between the supporters of technocracy and the supporters of parliamentary democracy, between the Gaullists and the left-wing opposition. Unlike with so many wine reforms, technocrats chose not to impose a decree establishing a legal blood alcohol level because they wanted to give their campaign a democratic air. They tried to distance the moral critique of drinking by placing the emphasis on separating the acts of drinking and driving rather than prohibiting them. Technocrats knew that political resistance would blacken Parliament's reputation: anyone who questioned an important road safety measure also questioned the value of innocent life and made France look backward in the eyes of the international community. A reform-minded deputy asked the minister of the interior if "official inaction to a blood alcohol level that costs each year more deaths and injuries than the wars in Indochina and Algeria cost France will continue through a lack of courage because of favors granted in the name of a firmly established winegrowing tradition."[67]

Between April and June 1970, just as the European common wine market began to operate, Parliament debated the institution of a blood alcohol limit. The opponents of the bill—those deputies who were Socialist, those from southern vine-growing regions, and those who defended French wine, French law, parliamentary democracy, and older notions of individual rights—tried to knock the wind out of the road safety movement's sails by throwing doubt onto the road safety expertise. A Socialist detractor pointed out that French workers, who were notorious for habitual wine drinking, were rarely the cause of drinking and driving accidents; instead, they blamed the "affluent alcoholism" caused by foreign drinks like whiskey.[68] Other parliamentarians emphasized that the experts were far from unanimous about what limit would impair reflexes and that few countries had in fact implemented the .08 level.[69] They exploited the scientific controversy, underscored national differences in road safety legislation, and emphasized variation in the physiological response to alcohol consumption. "Set the legal blood alcohol level at .08, okay. But in relation to whom?" asked a deputy from Montpellier. "Are you young? Are you old? Are you fat? Are you thin? Are you sick? Are you healthy? Whatever your profession, your alcohol consumption will be legally rationed. Now, for some, that ration will be too much, while for others, it won't be much at all."[70] In general, the opponents of the bill were shocked that, in a democracy, a driver could be pulled over for swerving after driving away from dinner. "For, after all, Mesdames and Messieurs, if after a meal, the police submitted the members of the most serious and most representative of public assemblies to a breath test, I believe . . . that the color green [the color indicating the threshold] would be dominant."[71] The Socialists and the vine-growing deputies saw the breath test device as a manifestation of the government's authoritarianism and its lack of respect for French traditions.[72]

Supporters of the bill bolstered their case with international science and a different conception of liberty. René Pleven, the minister of justice, combated the idea that the anti-drinking and driving measure was a conspiracy against tourism in France: if that were true, "do you think that the prime minister and mayor of Bordeaux would have agreed to propose the bill to Parliament?"[73] Pleven called the blood alcohol level of .08 "the level of science . . . the level of Europe."[74] Treating science as synonymous with Europe made the measure appear apolitical and unclouded by French myths about drinking. Concerned about France's inability to adapt to the new age of mobility, the social reformer Eugène Claudius-Petit asked his fellow parliamentarians: "Have you sometimes noticed that the drivers of school buses stop at the bistro to have a drink? That bus drivers transporting travelers get behind the wheel after consuming a few drinks? Have you observed that our airline companies allow the crew to drink champagne and whiskey when they're flying even though it's forbidden by all the other airline companies in the world?"[75] In his view, France risked being shunned by the international community. Against the argument that the establishment of a legal blood alcohol level would infringe on individual rights, one deputy asked, "under the pretext of defending individual liberty, aren't there numerous examples of basic freedoms being undermined? In this case, the first of freedoms is the liberty to live."[76]

Despite overwhelming evidence that linked alcohol to automobile accidents, French statistics still failed to demonstrate the precise link between them. The Ministry of Transportation showed that a meager 1.7 percent of drivers involved in a bodily accident were in an "alcoholic state." But how would officials know for sure when the alcoholic state had yet to be defined? The statistics of the Gendarmerie and the Ministry of the Interior did little more to flatter the road safety cause. The police continued to screen drivers infrequently.[77] Moreover, the government was still looking for ways to fund the purchase of breath test devices that would minimize the scope for subjectivity. The lack of consensus about the threshold between use and abuse and the lack of funding for breath test devices lay behind the continued inability to know the precise relationship between alcohol and accidents.

Given the doubts thrown on the threshold at which drinking became dangerous, the legal commission of the National Assembly proposed establishing a two-tier system.[78] The ONSER and the HCEIA had reported to the commission that a blood alcohol concentration of .08 or above would impair the driver's ability to drive, but even they agreed that until drivers reached a blood alcohol concentration of .12 they were not always conscious of the effects that the alcohol was having on their driving ability. The ONSER, aware of the obstacles that it faced, admitted that "the choice of the level must nevertheless not only take into account universal physiological facts, but also national characteristics of the concerned population."[79] The legal commission used the scientific uncertainty to plead for a two-tiered law that fit more appropriately with French "national characteristics."

Parliament adopted the law in July 1970 as tourist season hit full swing. The legal commission ultimately won out over those who favored a strict level of .08. The law stipulated that for a blood alcohol concentration between .08 and .12, the driver would be imprisoned for ten days to one month or fined from 400 to 3,000 francs or both; a driver exceeding the .12 blood alcohol level would be imprisoned for one month to one year or fined 500 to 5,000 francs or both.[80] Police could only administer the breath test after an accident or a traffic violation. Now that the state had defined the legal limit, an earlier government decree that canceled the insurance contracts of those convicted of driving in a vague "state of intoxication [*ivresse*]" would become more effective.[81]

The way in which the state established a legal blood alcohol limit demonstrates how it negotiated international road safety imperatives with local power and the development of wine tourism. The legal commission and the wine lobbies managed to water down the government's original drinking and driving bill in order to give some leverage to the courts in penalizing drunk driving. Some of the national press deemed this "French exceptionalism" of "maintaining the prestige of drinking a lot" as downright deplorable.[82] Yet it should be noted that other democratic countries also resisted international norms.[83] What made the French case unique were the particularities of French law, the power of the wine lobbies, and a public that had placed wine at the center of daily life. The wine lobbies doubtless had some impact on the law's outcome, complaining that "there are as many categories of 'drunkenness' as there are experts."[84]

Significantly, Parliament had voted unanimously in favor of the two-tier system, with the exception of one Socialist, Raoul Bayou, ardent defender of the industrial wine system in the Languedoc.[85] It is telling that the political supporters of the industrial wine system, not the appellation system, led the charge against a drinking and driving law. First, the appellation system depended in part on automobile tourism; and second, given their ties to the government, leaders of the National Confederation of Wine and Spirits (CNVS), the National Committee for Wine Promotion (CNPFV), and the National Institute of Appellations of Origin (INAO) could dictate the terms of rational, responsible drinking, which meant a shift away from cheap industrial wines to more expensive appellation wines. The drinking and driving law contributed to the broader technocratic campaign to limit and refine alcohol consumption, eliminate the economic inefficiencies of peasant production, and secure the roads for automobile tourism.

By protesting the connection between drinking and driving, Bayou put his foot down on a slowly changing political landscape. In the 1970s, the Socialist leaders of the Languedoc had begun to abandon their support of vine monoculture in order to develop the region for tourism.[86] This evolution in economic and cultural life was in line with the interests of the appellation system and automobile tourism. Increased mobility and greater exchange across national borders caused greater flux and instability and justified the reformers' attempt to regulate drinking and driving. At the same time, the potentially destabilizing effects of increased automobile use and the freer circulation of goods incited reformers to define a "French" drinking norm around luxury appellation wine that at once lived up to foreign expectations of refined drinking in France, promoted road safety and sobriety, and stimulated economic growth through tourism.

Decolonizing and Refining the French Palate

The campaign against drinking and driving was not only a question of limiting accidents and saving human life; it also contributed to a wider effort to reform consumer behavior in the interests of stimulating economic growth and reinvigorating democracy. In the 1950s and 1960s, the sober revolutionaries—consumer activists, demographers, doctors, economists, engineers, legal experts, statisticians, wine leaders who advocated for the INAO, and the automobile, insurance, and tourism lobbies—negotiated the imperative of becoming a more mobile, industrialized country while acknowledging that France was still quite rural and among the world's largest alcohol producers and consumers. These various groups, in seeking to reform French political institutions and economic arrangements, held the conviction that consumers had an obligation to use self-discipline—as defined by new state expertise rather than by personal or popular belief—when choosing how and what to drink. In their view, greater mobility and international exchange required a new kind of French consumer, one that drank rationally and responsibly, which in a more open economy meant drinking locally. In an era when French consumers had greater access to a wider variety of French and foreign goods and influences, the state set about molding consumers in a way that empowered technocrats over the policymaking process and met the needs of economic growth, public health and safety, and a new national identity as France withdrew from its empire.

Sober revolutionaries wished to adjust everyday life to the demands of international competition. Consumer lobbies like the Federal Union of Consumption (UFC) carried out studies revealing that the key to boosting industrial productivity was to be found in modifying consumer practices. American consumers stood as a model. The UFC noted that "it's thanks to the adoption of small revolutions in daily life that American productivity permits 85 percent of Americans to have a car, telephone, refrigerator, and washing machine, whereas only 15 percent of the French benefit from these things."[87] New consumer goods like automobiles and appellation wine became agents of modernization and challenged older working-class and peasant habits that were seen to stymie economic modernization.

Traditional habits, like industrial wine, were said to stunt economic growth, upward mobility, and the expansion of consumer capitalism. As France underwent urbanization and increased mobility and as work routines shifted from physical labor in fields and factories to sedentary labor in offices, wine habits, it was believed, needed to change. But not everyone agreed that alcohol was hindering French competitiveness. Gustave Deleau, a defender of the small shopkeeper, asked "who could claim that the builders of the fastest trains and commercial planes in the world, and the most modern dams, represent with their technicians, their cadres, their workers, a drunken people?"[88] In his view, France was not a nation of slackers. Wine lobbyist and Senator Georges Portmann even suggested to economists and businessmen that moderate wine consumption boosted productivity![89] When the Americans tried to introduce Coca-Cola to France, a coalition of industrial wine leaders, Communists, and public health activists kept the product at bay on the grounds that it, not wine, endangered public health and national wealth.[90] A wine propagandist in Bordeaux lamented that French youth were spending more on sporting and camping equipment than on wine.[91]

In the emerging society of mass consumption, the state worked to redraw the boundaries between necessities and luxuries. While the automobile was to become a mass consumer good, wine was to become a luxury item. As postwar consumers came to possess the bare necessities to sustain life, they shifted focus to accumulate goods as a means to construct their social status. Reformers used these new consumer aspirations to rally the public against the industrial wine system; they did this by raising wine's price, as we saw in the last chapter, and by disseminating propaganda. The state's slogan "Drink Well, Drink a Little, in order to Drink for a Long Time" could be read as either pro- or anti-wine: those who abstained from alcohol should drink more appellation wine; those who drank to excess should cut down. As one public health reformer put it: "True wine connoisseurs know how to consume in a reasonable way. We're only seeking to habituate the entire French population to do the same."[92]

Sober revolutionaries hoped to gain consent for their cause by demonstrating to citizens that altering their drinking practices would liberate them from the poverty of the past. Against the older view that drinking was a democratic right, technocrats represented drinking as an obstacle to liberty in an age of mobility.[93] The political system, they believed, worked for the industrial wine system and limited consumer access to other goods. Yet this argument also served the interests of the technocrats who wished to seize power from Parliament. Technocrats hoped to deploy state power to set citizens "free" as modern consumers even as they seized control of the policymaking process. Forging a new, "disciplined," yet "free" consumer around automobiles and appellation wine—goods that consumers increasingly wanted—was thus crucial to transforming the structure of power and government.

The perceived liberties of the automobile were placed in opposition to the perceived oppression of industrial wine as a way to alter drinking habits. "It's indeed interesting," one bureaucrat would later recognize, "to combat a well-anchored myth in the collective conscience (alcohol being a symbol of friendship and physical strength), by another popular myth (the automobile)."[94] A decree in February 1958 made automobile insurance mandatory.[95] Then, in January 1959, when Robert Debré's son Michel was prime minister, the government issued a decree that canceled the insurance contracts of those convicted of driving "in a state of intoxication (*ivresse*)," even if "intoxication" had yet to be defined.[96] That the law required each French citizen to have automobile insurance is not without significance. It compelled drivers to behave responsibly or else suffer the consequences of losing their insurance contract and, by extension, their license. As a bureaucrat and road safety activist explained it:

> Given that the present French people feel inferior if they don't have an automobile, I think that one of the preferred domains of our anti-alcohol action must be with automobile drivers, for if we manage to convince them that it's very dangerous to drink and that they thus risk the revocation of their driving license (which can sometimes cause for them the total loss of their livelihood), we will inevitably cause ruptures in habits that could be extremely useful in the struggle against alcoholism.[97]

Road safety advocates built their campaign on the citizen's desire to own and drive an automobile. Through education and threats, drivers would learn to become their "own gendarme."[98]

Through state propaganda, drivers were given the sense that they were exercising their own freedom in separating the acts of drinking and driving. "One Must Choose: Drink or Drive" was one of the main road safety slogans. Robert Debré demonstrated that a half liter of wine with an alcohol content of 11 percent during a meal would not make the individual exceed the legal limit of .08. Drinkers would surpass the threshold, however, if they consumed an aperitif, a quarter liter of wine, and a digestif in a similar time frame.[99] Regardless of how this amount of alcohol might affect different kinds of individuals and their particular physiological conditions, Debré made clear that the new national drinking norm—defined universally from Paris and automatically with a breath test device at between .08 and .12 blood alcohol level—was made antithetical neither to automobile use nor to wine drinking. Turning the automobile revolution and its promise of greater personal mobility and liberty against "excessive" drinking thus became an important strategy in modifying drinking practices.

After World War II, the boundaries of the middle class were arguably more fluid and unstable than at any other period of French history, making the establishment of new consumer norms all the more important.[100] Creating a national drinking norm could help the state regulate this instability and support the development of modern lifestyles around the new middle class. After the war, the number of farmers and small shopkeepers rapidly declined, as these groups moved into a new white-collar class of administrators, engineers, managers, and service employees who worked in offices, relied on mental instead of manual labor, and, compared with peasants, were more integrated into the national and international economy. This new middle class had been shaped by the American productivity missions of the immediate post-1945 era and played a key role in France's economic expansion.[101] French economic growth in the 1950s and 1960s required those who entered this new class to behave in a way that supported a more mobile economy.

With this new class came new expectations for men and women. As men, especially peasant and working-class men, made their way into the new middle class, reformers expected them to abandon their drinking habits, habits that defied the technocrats' entire raison d'être. Daily drinking is usually about pleasures in the moment, occasionally about memories of the past, and seldom about planning for the future. Men needed to become more disciplined, competitive, and interested in upward mobility and status.[102] Technocrats—of which milk-drinking Pierre Mendès France was perhaps the poster child—argued that alcohol both literally and metaphorically emasculated the economy. Statisticians fixated on the excessive mortality of French men. Statistics revealed that the death rate among men between the ages of forty and sixty-five was higher in France than in other countries.[103] Men who spent the productive prime of their lives in a bottle could not contribute to achieving general prosperity.

For reformers, French drinking habits were thus symptomatic of a general crisis of masculinity, a lack of control in an increasingly hostile international environment. As France faced a colonial crisis, new American cultural influences, and the prospects of European integration, reformers feared that men had become too apathetic and powerless to act against these broad historical processes. Interestingly, reformers compared the vigor of colonial man to the vice of metropolitan man. The middle-class magazine *Réalités* represented the Vietnamese man as more sleek, virile, and modern than his more gluttonous and portly French counterpart.[104] Significantly, this depiction was published in July 1954, in the wake of the French defeat at Dien Bien Phu and the signing of the Geneva Accords. As we have seen, when Algeria's war of independence broke out in late 1954, the National Liberation Front (FLN) called on its revolutionaries to abstain from alcohol. From this perspective, colonial men, who were seen to be taking history into their own hands, had become models to follow. Other observers confirmed this comparison between metropolitan and colonial man. In the construction trade, it was reported that employers preferred hiring Algerians to French men because "with the Algerians there are never accidents due to drinking."[105] The message was clear. The working-class man of yesterday, who through rising affluence was becoming the new middle-class man of today, needed to give up his old gluttonous ways and conform to the more disciplined habits that the state was trying to impose. Such quotes also naturalized Algerians as manual laborers, helping demarcate the line between who was French and who was not.

French drinking habits were seen to sap France's international strength. French drinkers were frequently reminded that they consumed ten times more alcohol than an American, Swede, or Dane, five times more than a British citizen, four times more than a Swiss or Belgian; only the Italian compared to the French citizen.[106] A journalist, disappointed in France's recent performance at the Olympics, pointed out that "we could also ask the Olympic committee to plan for 1964 . . . the creation of a drinking competition. France would at last be sure to win a gold medal."[107]

Women, who finally gained the vote by 1945, became potential allies in the campaign to overturn the industrial wine system and open up France to the new world of consumption. Some reformers believed that, as the biggest victims of alcoholism, women would support any measure to curb it. "When parliamentarians travel through their districts they have to listen to the loud voices of the noisy electors who threaten them. But each one of these masculine voices isn't more powerful in the ballot box than the quieter feminine voices."[108] Representing over half the population, women became a powerful political weapon in the sober revolution.

As consumers, women were given a central role in public life just as elites gave them new duties in the home.[109] Responsible for the production and reproduction of social life and for teaching "civilization," they became the managers of everyday life and were expected to teach youth and men about rational consumption. Sober revolutionaries often blamed mothers for France's poor dietary habits. Reports showed that children were accustomed to drinking from an early age. Thus in western France, women allegedly put too much alcohol in the baby bottle.[110] In the Calvados region, eighteen-month-old children reportedly drank hard cider with and without food; in the rural Nord, parents gave beer to six-month-old children; in Lot-et-Garonne, three-year-olds drank pure wine; in the Vendée, children habitually took 50 centiliters of wine with them to school in their lunchbox. The *goutte* (drop) of alcohol was administered as medication. Teachers, those emissaries of the republic, had little luck in replacing wine with milk.[111] From the perspective of reformers, such behavior not only naturalized drinking in everyday life; it also impeded physical and economic growth. In this way, women were burdened with some of the responsibility for France's high rates of alcoholism and economic stagnation.

France's future depended on the civilizing dimension of the household.[112] The emphasis on the nuclear family with its household appliances and cars was to decenter the café from social life.[113] A tidy home could lure men away from the café, a space with a history of radical politics. If women were believed to be responsible for male alcoholism, doctors also saw in women a solution to alcoholism: "The married drinker, whose wife makes sure that he receives nourishment, a capable woman with moral action and also with an appropriate kitchen, has a lot more chance of leading him to an effective cure than the drinker alone does."[114] The anti-alcoholism message reached some women and preoccupied them. Even a leader of the CNVS, no doubt interested in deflecting responsibility away from the alcohol industry for alcohol-related problems, recommended to women to become better role models: "Mesdames, it's definitely you who manages the family budget and like us all you have difficulties in making ends meet. You need a blender, for example, but every month you postpone the purchase of it. Do you know what the price of it is? The equivalent of a few bottles. . . ."[115] This quotation highlights the assumptions that prosperity fell on consumer choices and that consumer choices fell on women.

Women's magazines, which had begun to develop in the 1930s, helped spread the state's modernizing message to diverse regions and establish national consumer norms. For this reason, the HCEIA launched propaganda campaigns in them.[116] In *Femmes d'aujourd'hui*, the HCEIA advised "French women to diminish the abusive consumption of alcoholic drinks and rather to improve the quality of wines that they serve."[117] *Elle* asked women about their greatest fears: having a carousing husband came in second, just after having an unfaithful one.[118] At the beginning of 1964, a large number of women's and youth magazines exposed their readers to the problem of alcoholism. A contest called "Health-Sobriety" encouraged readers to tell their stories. A jury, under the presidency of Robert Debré, granted two prizes to the best submissions to each magazine. The jury, which received eight thousand letters in all, also granted a prize to the best overall letter.[119] The media tried to turn women into state agents that could teach "correct" consumption.

As France modernized, decolonized, Europeanized, and selectively adopted American consumer practices, the modernist wing of the wine industry, groups like the INAO and the CNVS, provided technocrats with a way to induce nostalgia for an ideal French past, one that helped them build legitimacy for their rule and one that conveniently ignored the conflicts of the present. The unpleasant realities of industrial wine were replaced with the sanitized notions of tradition provided by new, appellation wine. The tasting and smelling of these wines provided the sensual pleasure of a particular place and time. Wine was to be "a complex ensemble of sensations and impression, presenting the common feature of being pleasant. . . . It's a pleasure that's exclusive of uniformity and gloomy repetition."[120] The appellation system promoted its time-honored wines as a way to help anchor consumers in a more mobile, unstable world. As French people experienced sweeping change, the wine that they consumed would invoke images of French tradition, a heritage that was rooted in the metropole, not across the sea.

The emphasis on static notions of French wine traditions contradicted France's actual experience of rapid modernization. In this way, the appellation system jibed with the broader intellectual currents of the day. In certain respects, the appellation system had much in common with the Annales school of historiography.[121] Both focused on the premodern and medieval in European history. In this way, they avoided the problems of the present, inconveniences such as rural depopulation and colonial unrest. In 1959, a formative year in state-making, Roger Dion, a geographer connected to the Annales school, published a magisterial history of wine that completely ignored France's acute problems with alcoholism and alcohol-related accidents and largely denaturalized the role of peasants, settlers, and indigenous Algerians to the making of France's modern wine industry.[122] The appellation system, like the Annales school, ignored events and human struggle. These intellectual currents in the social sciences, partially funded by the Americans in an attempt to contain the advance of Marxism, cannot be separated from the ideology of capitalist modernization, an ideology that sought to obscure the social contradictions of economic change through decolonization and European integration.[123] Appellation wine contributed to the ongoing attempts to focus French history around bucolic landscapes and medieval castles, a history that spoke more to the quainter side of medieval localism than to the pitfalls of nationalism, European empires, and global capitalism.

Magazines called on travelers to take to the wine routes in order to receive an education in wine and French history. In this way, consumers could forge a bond with France's diverse regions. In writing about the wine routes of Burgundy and Beaujolais, one magazine affirmed: "Go learn to drink. One is clever when one drinks well. He who doesn't know how to drink knows nothing."[124] The chateaux of Bordeaux were "open to all travelers for whom drinking—reasonably—a good wine remains one of the most normal expressions of living well."[125]

Magazines also taught consumers about the rituals of wine and how to refine their palates. A deputy from the wine-producing Rhône wrote in *Les Échos*, a newspaper that appealed to the new middle class, that "propaganda in favor of the reasonable consumption of quality wine is the best anti-alcohol propaganda."[126] *Réalités* educated its readers about the different wine regions, about pairing wine with food, about how to serve different wines, and about the pomp and circumstance of wine drinking.[127] Magazines sought to refine French wine drinkers through codified wine rituals in order to maintain France's international reputation for "civilized" drinking.

This process of naturalizing the link between luxury wine and metropolitan France was reinforced by the continued importance of automobile tourism after World War II, especially as both the automobile and appellation wines were seen as important to economic renewal.[128] In the first years after the war, France became the world's largest tourist destination.[129] American money, goods, and tourists poured into France. In praising the diversity of French wine and the uniqueness of the French landscape, an American tourist observed that "other countries have land. France has *terroirs* . . . nuances are familiar to the French by privilege of their race. Centuries of tasting have indeed miraculously refined and educated their palates."[130] Americans and other international tourists romanticized French wine and French drinkers, and French wine producers delivered through the creation and promotion of site-specific appellation wines and the education of consumers about how to discern and appreciate them. Numerous wine and gastronomic societies and tourism industry leaders promoted the links between refined taste and the discovery of the French regions.[131]

Appellation leaders continued to ally with the automobile and tourism industries. A cognac producer noted that "these modern things that are the automobile and tourism agree really well with this ancient thing that is wine. The former are eager for progress and change while wine is immobility, tradition. . . . Admirable alliance of the past and the future."[132] The director of the Michelin guide was a member of the esteemed Academy of Wine of France, a group that defended the consumer and promoted appellation wine. Each yearly edition of the Michelin guide showed its readers where to find the best wine regions and wine cellars and how to pair wine with food.[133] Beginning in 1952, the guide presented a chapter entitled "Good Cellars" to help tourists in their search for the best French wines.[134] Michelin and other tourism guides continued to advertise for the wine industry. Automobile rallies also occurred in wine country to familiarize drivers with the local wine industries.[135]

In the 1950s and 1960s, wine routes expanded and the number of folkloric festivals increased. "A trip along the wine route," reported *The Guardian* about the well-known route in Alsace, "will give great pleasure. Peaceful and picturesque scenery, a perfect road, and the remarkable range of fine Alsatian white wines makes this a most rewarding detour" (figure 15).[136] A wine newspaper noted the success of the wine routes, as

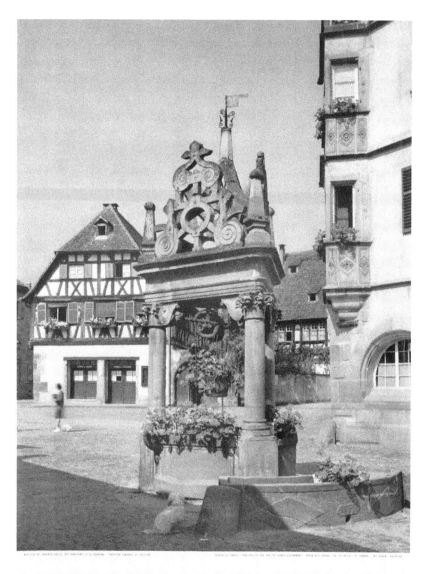

FRANCE *villages Fleuris*

ALSACE : UN VILLAGE SUR LA ROUTE DU VIN

Figure 15. Tourism poster advertising the wine route of Alsace, 1960. Wine producers in Alsace would begin to join the appellation system in 1962. Courtesy of the National Archives of France, Pierrefitte-sur-Seine.

informed tourists could appreciate local food and wine and old monuments and artistic curiosities. "It appears futile, in the century of speed, to advise drivers to stroll about, and yet shouldn't the true tourist search out to know, if not all that is interesting to see, at least the principal historical, archeological, etc. sites of interest of the region, to appreciate the products that make up its originality."[137] The newspaper credited the wine routes for encouraging tourists to appreciate not only the taste of wine but also the beauty of the landscape that produced it, the affability of the wine producers, the variety of the customs, and all the particular aspects of the regions traveled through.

Changes in drinking behavior were a part of France's postwar consumer revolution. The French purchased more automobiles and appellation wine and gradually drank less industrial wine. The consumption of automobiles and appellation wine went hand in hand and symbolized the transformation from neighborly public drinking to a more individualistic, private culture. As *L'Express* noted, "The 1,200,000 vine growers and the 350,000 merchants are drowned by the 15 million individuals with driver's licenses."[138] In this light, citizens' driver's licenses, as well as their insurance contracts, had become powerful tools of government, capable of breaking even the most enjoyably inveterate of habits. The automobile became a key agent in altering French drinking behavior and challenging the political power of the industrial wine system that made France dependent on sun-soaked grapes from first Algeria and then, via the European common market, Italy.

How successful was this campaign to decolonize and refine palates? The period spanning the 1950s and the 1970s should be seen as a threshold between an old and a new wine regime: most people still desired cheap industrial wine for daily consumption, but more and more aspired to the occasional consumption of appellation wines as a sign of bourgeois status. The late 1950s marked the beginning of a long-term decline in industrial wine consumption. In 1957, the annual consumption of industrial wine was an astonishing 140 liters per person; in 1975, however, it decreased to 99 liters and would continue its downward trend.[139] Conversely, the consumption of appellation wine in France increased by 76 percent between 1950 and 1968.[140] "For the moment," one journalist reported in 1963, one year after Algeria's independence, "France is between two wines: the one that it had taken the habit of drinking and that was often mixed with wines coming from Algeria, and the one that we are undertaking to have its people drink tomorrow and that comes from only its own lands."[141] As this observer suggested, the appellation system was as much about the future that elites hoped to build as about a past that they hoped to forget.

France's transition from the old wine regime to the new was far from smooth. Statistics conceal the difficulty of selling appellation wines to the French masses. Invoking taste and tradition appeared natural, but engineering desire for them was deeply political. One journalist confirmed a widely held view that "Algerian wine corresponds to the taste of a certain number of French people."[142] A bureaucrat in the Ministry of Agriculture impatiently asked: "How many times have we heard about this famous and supposed 'taste of *terroir*' that explains all defects; it's as if we're to believe that our good land in France takes pleasure in making monstrosities!"[143] An inhabitant of the industrial wine-producing Languedoc noted that "not only the Aramon but even certain hybrids that face the sun just right and that see good winemaking practices succeed in equaling and even surpassing in quality some of the appellation wines."[144] Not everyone accepted the state as an arbiter of quality and taste.

Although a mass consumer society was firmly established after World War II, class distinctions continued to determine perceptions of wine. One temperance activist reported that her organization "isn't campaigning against good wines because they are too expensive for the average Frenchman to buy."[145] Nor did higher wages necessarily lead to a preference for more expensive appellation wines. Many citizens forged their identities not around the wine itself but around the sociability and solidarity that the act of drinking created. Industrial wine, which was cheap and familiar, was likely a more effective way for people to work through and make sense of fast-paced times than more expensive and esoteric appellation wines. "The disappearance of industrial wine to the benefit of specialized wines isn't without concern for the future of our economy," noted an industrial wine lobbyist. "[I]ndustrial wine . . . is the typical wine of family consumption, which corresponds at once to the tastes, needs, and purchasing power of working-class consumers."[146] That some consumers resisted appellation wines and continued to purchase Algerian wines after independence thwarted the technocrats' efforts to impose a new drinking norm, modernize the economy, and forget the intimate connections that had once fused Algeria to the metropole.

Conclusion

The campaign to reconcile road safety and sobriety with automobile use and tourism in wine country brought together a range of actors who had a stake in strengthening state power over localized practices, liberalizing the economy, and redefining national identity as France retreated from empire and entered the EEC. As we have seen in previous chapters, groups with an interest in freeing up the economy used the Fourth Republic's inability to cope with alcohol surpluses, dietary disorders within the French Union, and alcohol-related accidents as a pretext for centralizing state power and eliminating the perceived inefficiencies and inequities of the industrial wine system. The road safety movement was thus connected to battles over the state's regulatory reach that pitted new expertise against popular beliefs about drinking, beliefs that sustained an outdated structure of production in Algeria and the Languedoc. The desire to promote automobile tourism and road safety widened the scope of the sober revolution.

At the same time that the automobile helped transform France from a country of artisanal production and regional cultures into a country of mass production and national consumer norms, the expanding appellation system promoted a commodified idea of artisanal production and regional cultures as a part of these new norms. The appellation system's idyllic images of French history that it wished to sell to the world conveniently elided many inconveniences in the nation's development, including colonial violence, social conflict in the countryside, alcoholism, and road carnage. The turn toward appellations illustrates how, after Algeria's independence in 1962, producer and consumer norms became more strictly defined and exclusionary even if Algeria lived on through the "alcoholic" consumer's continued commitment to industrial wine.

Whereas the automobile revolution helped technocrats eliminate persisting localisms that prevented economic growth, the appellation revolution helped technocrats root this greater personal mobility in a new cultural imaginary around regional wine production. The automobile and appellation revolutions thus reinforced one another. Mobilizing the appellation system served economic growth and a redefinition of the national heritage that would anchor people in fast-changing times. The automobile revolution did not eliminate a sense of place, nor did it obliterate the past. Instead, supporters of the appellation system harnessed that revolution to help rigidify place, re-create the past, and transport France into the postcolonial age.

5

EUROPEANIZING THE REVOLUTION

In a meeting with his ministers in 1963, President Charles de Gaulle expressed frustration at the government's repeated failure to overcome the industrial wine system, echoing the sober revolutionaries' conviction that the system was an impediment to economic expansion and a drain on state power. "The nature of the discussion has never been framed and controlled," he grumbled. "There have been but stopgap measures. We must produce what we can sell. Quality wine sells very well. Bad quality wine doesn't sell."[1] De Gaulle's sentiment came just as his government was negotiating with the newly independent Algerian state over the future trade relationship between the two countries and the extent to which France would continue to purchase Algerian wine. Concurrently, planners in Brussels were at work devising the European common wine market in which the French wine industry anticipated intense competition from Italy's vineyards of mass production. As France became less imperial and more European, and as cheap Algerian wine was replaced with cheap

Italian wine for use in blending with cheap Languedoc wine, de Gaulle proclaimed that "the reign of plonk is over!"[2]

During de Gaulle's presidency in the 1960s and beyond his term into the 1970s, French debates over the orientation of their wine industry became Europeanized, with two possible effects on the sober revolution.[3] On the one hand, European integration risked outright derailing French efforts to localize wine through the appellation system. The French state's ability to create and safeguard production norms was threatened as the member-states of the European Economic Community (EEC) tried to harmonize their production practices and establish a common wine market. Languedoc vine grower organizations, Italian officials, and the European Commission in Brussels argued that the expansion of the market—from approximately 40 million French to 160 million European consumers—favored higher production levels.[4] Consumers, especially those who had not been trained in or were defiant of the French state's norms, supported the productivist argument. In 1962, the average French person still consumed over 100 liters of Franco-Algerian industrial wine a year, suggesting that the cheapness of the wine retained precedent over its luxury status.[5] Against the state's wishes, the EEC might sustain the industrial wine system.

On the other hand, European integration might advance the sober revolution's goal of economic growth, public health promotion, and cultural renewal. Although the Ministry of Agriculture had been slow to support the appellation system at the expense of the industrial wine system, Edgard Pisani, de Gaulle's dynamic minister of agriculture and one of the masterminds behind the creation of the Common Agricultural Policy (CAP), linked the decline of Algerian wine imports after 1962 and the coming of the more competitive common wine market to the urgent need of localizing wine production within the hexagon and enforcing state-imposed norms.[6] The EEC introduced a new power dynamic that supporters of appellation wine could wield against the industrial wine system. In the 1960s and early 1970s, representatives from the National Institute of Appellations of Origin (INAO), the National Confederation of Wine and Spirits (CNVS), the Ministries of Agriculture and Finance, and the French delegation in Brussels strategically joined forces with the High Commission for Studies and Information on Alcoholism (HCEIA). This coalition for Europe, which sought to maintain and promote the INAO's norms within the EEC, claimed to defend the interests of consumers against the supposedly more money-driven industrial wine system. The Europeanist coalition could also potentially find allies in the Benelux countries and West Germany, which imported more luxury wine than industrial wine and drank less overall. Instead of weakening the French movement to localize and refine wine, then, European integration could further it.

Anxieties about the loss of revenue to the Italian wine industry and about the French state's role in exporting cheap wine—and alcoholism—to neighboring countries incited the Europeanist coalition to become proactive in emphasizing quality over quantity and presenting France as a model for a rational, humanistic, and European way of wine drinking. The reformist journal *Progrès agricole et viticole* suggested that "the Europe of the Six will be either a harmonious construction based on moral values or it will be given over to market forces."[7] Such a discourse could have come from the French handbook on empire-building. The assumption was that France was the land of moral uplift; other European countries, particularly Italy, succumbed to the lure of money. In this way, sober revolutionaries could be seen as part of a long line of French revolutionaries who exported their humanitarian values to the rest of Europe. The fate of the French Revolution, for example, partially hinged on winning over other European countries to the values of liberty, equality, and fraternity and in creating a united front against the Old Regime.

Just as sober revolutionaries exported a "rational" model of French wine production and consumption, they also hoped to turn their European partners against France's own "irrational" producers and consumers. With its claims to an apolitically technocratic vision of governance, the EEC could help sober revolutionaries in their ongoing battle to expose particular aspects of the French worldview as myths and help put to rest a national debate that had begun around 1945: Was wine a dietary staple? Was the peasantry the bedrock of French identity? Was France colonial or continental? In 1962, reformers hoped to settle the first two questions; the third was being answered by the Evian Accords that granted political independence to Algeria. The same year saw the transition from an imperial to a more national France positioned within continental Europe, with major implications for wine. At this juncture, the French state, buttressed by its new European partners, worked to exclude Algerian wine from the new France, on the one hand, and to modernize the Languedoc by local-izing and improving wine production, on the other.

The decolonization of Algeria and European integration marked an important juncture in rebranding wine and rethinking France and its boundaries, myths, and traditions. The INAO's official narrative about the history of French wine—metropolitan with an emphasis on quality—and the experience of tasting wines from so many French districts that just decades before would have been unknown to most consumers out-side of those districts, could help with reimagining France. In 1953, at an exposition on the link between luxury wine and France's national history sponsored by the INAO, the director of the National Archives had argued that "Europe will be unified only when everybody drinks wine . . . French wine."[8] Expressing concern that the EEC would further standardize and mass-produce wine, making wine not regional but European, another INAO member in 1962 cried, "For all of Europe some French wine!"[9] These quotes suggest that European unification and the state-regulated localization of wine and its history could either threaten or strengthen one another. The French state reacted to the EEC's authority by supporting the INAO's narrative of nationhood and regional traditions.[10] Controlling this wine narrative helped the state create a sense of national belonging and occlude the political conflicts that facilitated the INAO's expansion. The INAO's narrative of France's regional diversity and quality products also happened to play on international stereotypes about what France stood for, which made it highly exportable.

From an Imperial to a European Market

From the signing of the Treaty of Rome in 1957 to the beginning of the common wine market in 1970, the member-states of the EEC grappled with how to unite the world's two largest wine producers, France and Italy, and create standardized norms. In 1956, these two countries—including Algeria, then still an administrative unit of France and thus an integral part of the EEC—made up 60 percent of global wine produc-tion.[11] Of the EEC's other four member-states—Belgium, Luxembourg, the Netherlands, and West Germany—only Luxembourg and West Ger-many were major producers. All of these countries held different attitudes about wine. Regulations were stiff in some countries, lax in others. Producers in colder climates like West Germany and northern France could enrich their wine with sugar (through a process known as *chaptalization*), while in warmer climates like Italy and southern France this practice was forbidden. French officials placed strict regulations on vine plantings, whereas the Italians did not. France and Italy followed a Mediterranean drinking pattern that saw wine as a complement to everyday meals, while northern European countries tended to assign luxury status to wine, drinking it more occasionally. New political and cultural dynamics thus emerged that complicated French efforts to establish new norms around the appellation system.

Officials in the INAO and the Ministry of Agriculture worried that Italy's more liberal—French technocrats called it "anarchical"—wine policy would influence the hard-fought French norms that the state was still trying to consolidate. Italian producers could plant vines and sell wines freely, arguing that "wine must be as cheap as possible" and that the EEC should support "the highest yields at the least cost."[12] For this reason, the Italians depended on developing consumption in the EEC. After a French politician called for a limitation of the vineyard area in a debate in the European Parliament in February 1970, his Italian counterpart asserted that "if winegrowing finds itself threatened, it's not the nightmare of overproduction that's behind this threat; rather, because of rising consumption, we'll experience a deficient supply in the near future if we decide today to limit the surface area." Another Italian representative declared that "to accept such a limitation would go against all logic or, if you will, to adopt a crazy logic."[13] A French technocrat showed his apprehension in claiming that "this opinion of Italian viticulture has contaminated . . . the French winegrowing associations and the responsible ministries: Agriculture and Finance."[14] Even more blasphemous for appellation advocates was that some Italian producers had refused to respect the place of production: "what matters is that a given wine has 'the qualities required of chianti . . . without worrying about where it comes from.'"[15] Italy represented an outside influence and new ideas that conflicted with the INAO's norms.

French preparation for the European common market was not totally without precedent. As we have seen, France had created a customs union with Algeria in 1867. In both the imperial market and the new European market, wine flowed freely within the trading bloc while external tariffs hindered goods from coming into it. Yet the EEC presented challenges to the French state that imperial trade had not. In the imperial marketplace, Algeria had been mainland France's main competitor, but Algeria had legally been a part of France; conversely, in the EEC, Italy replaced Algeria as the producer of cheap, colorful, alcoholic wines, but Italy was clearly not under French sovereignty and instead under a shared European sovereignty. The industrial wine system, once reliant on a triangular relationship among Languedoc producers, Algerian producers, and French merchants, was in the future to be dependent on a triangular relationship among Languedoc producers, Italian producers, and French merchants. As a European order supplanted the imperial order, the French state risked losing revenue to foreign blending wines, whether from Algeria or Italy, thus intensifying efforts to consolidate the appellation system within the hexagon. De Gaulle's essentialist ideas of grandeur and national independence would need to come through appellation wine, not industrial wine.

In 1962, the European Council of Ministers issued its first wine regulations when it adopted the French distinction between industrial wine and luxury appellation (AOC) wine. At the European level, industrial wine was categorized as "table wines" (VDT) and luxury wine was classified as "quality wines produced in a determined region" (VQPRD). The two categories of wine would be governed differently. Industrial wines, which constituted 95 percent of European production, fell under European jurisdiction.[16] Significantly, the creation of the VDT made the EEC, not just France, responsible for managing Algerian wine imports and surplus problems within Europe. Therefore, non-wine-producing countries had a hand in determining the fate of industrial wine. The VQPRD, on the other hand, was governed at both the national and European levels. Although local associations and each member-state tended to determine quality norms, these norms had to be approved by the European Commission. The French Ministry of Agriculture complained that the VQPRD was not restrictive enough.[17] Thus during the 1960s, both the Ministry of Agriculture and the INAO sought to ensure that the Commission respected the INAO's norms through the AOC and VDQS classifications, given that "tradition" in the other EEC member-states was not as "old" and as "developed."[18] A vine grower in Burgundy wondered "by what turn of events would France begin selling its wine under the VQPRD label

'Europe' when the word 'France' in wine matters possesses on its own a considerable value."[19] What gradually emerged in the 1960s, then, was a complex series of European regulations that were layered over national wine policies, which constrained each member-state's ability to make decisions about its own wine industry.

The coming of the European common market magnified anxieties about how to protect metropolitan vine growers from merchants who sourced cheap blending wines from abroad. Multinational companies occupied a bigger share of European markets in the 1960s.[20] In 1967, Jean-Jacques Servan-Schreiber published his best-selling book *The American Challenge*, which warned his French readers that the only thing more ominous than cultural influences from the United States was the prospect of American corporations operating in Europe.[21] During this decade, the wine industry experienced an added impulse to de-localize production with the growth in industrial wine companies such as Margnat, Kiravi, Gévéor, Postillon, Préfontaines, and Grap. Combined, these entities held nearly 30 percent of the domestic market for industrial wine.[22] The common market allowed merchants to work across national boundaries to find the cheapest grapes available to concoct their beverages. These merchants, following their consumers' preferences, frequently held little interest in the distinctive qualities of the site of wine production, thereby undercutting the INAO's work. The INAO expressed concern that French wine and spirits companies were installing branch offices in foreign countries in order to make larger profits than they did within France.[23] In the new European context, the INAO repeated its earlier claim that France's quality vineyards "can be compared to sites and historical monuments and equally count in the intellectual or artistic heritage of the country."[24] For the INAO, place mattered as it never had before.

The transnational tendencies of the EEC not only threatened the INAO's efforts to localize wine production within metropolitan France; these tendencies also concerned state officials who saw their jurisdiction over French territory as being severely constrained. Under the German Walter Hallstein, the European Commission's first president, the Commission became active in asserting its power and legitimating its role in the EEC. Debates intensified about whether the EEC should become a supranational or an intergovernmental entity. This debate was most sensationally seen during the Empty Chair crisis of 1965.[25] That summer, de

Gaulle demanded that the French representative in the European Council of Ministers return home in response to what he interpreted as the European Commission's infringements on his authority. The crisis pitted the Commission and its supranationalism against de Gaulle's vision of a Europe of states. Given de Gaulle's resistance, the EEC would remain largely intergovernmental through the 1960s and 1970s. Yet even within an intergovernmental EEC, the French delegation could not fully dictate the terms of its own wine policy.

The French state's power was in some ways reduced as the member-states of the EEC debated a way to harmonize their divergent policies. The Italian delegation had more leverage than the French delegation when it came time to negotiate the terms of the common wine market. Agricultural staples such as grain and milk, markets that France and the Benelux countries dominated, had been integrated into the EEC's CAP before wine.[26] Italy bought three times more agricultural products from its European partners than it sold to them, making wine a key export for Italy.[27] Sicilian vine growers, whose climate and cheap labor gave them a competitive advantage over France, had a vested interest in creating a common market that lifted France's strict regulations and convincing European consumers that wine was an everyday food, not a luxury.

Early on, the Federation of Vine Growing Associations (FAV) and some technocrats in Paris sided with the Italians, suggesting that the common wine market would provide an opportunity to drain France's wine surpluses, a strategy reminiscent of earlier efforts to dump France's surpluses on colonial peoples. The FAV had argued that in the European common market surpluses would no longer present problems.[28] Dr. Étienne May, Robert Debré's colleague, had indicated that the best way to adapt production to consumption would be to "increase reasonable consumption, that's to say to increase the number of consumers."[29] He meant French consumers but also European consumers in the emerging common market.

The European Commission and the European Parliament agreed with this point of view.[30] One study conducted for the Commission, which examined the wine-drinking habits of the member-states in an effort to increase market share in the beer- and spirits-drinking countries of the north, concluded that "pro-wine propaganda mustn't be based only on wine of superior quality but also on industrial wine. It's not a question of inculcating taste in the consumer but rather to incite non-consumers to consume wine by demonstrating that it's a drink like any other and not a luxury item."[31] The report suggested that the wine industry adopt the advertising strategies of the fruit juice and soda industries. Many promoters of the new Europe, then, prioritized quantity over quality and thus blocked France's sober revolution.

The European Commission allied with the advocates of quantity, believing that wine markets should be treated like all other agricultural markets.[32] As a result, it cut down tariff barriers between member-states, offered price supports, purchased surpluses, and refused to regulate vine plantings, all of which conformed to Italian preferences and encouraged high yields. The Commission even suggested an advertising campaign to increase wine consumption.[33] Between 1965 and 1978, vineyard space in Germany grew from 83,000 to 102,000 hectares and in Italy from 943,000 to 1,102,000 hectares. At the same time in France, vineyard space diminished from 1,340,000 to 1,195,000 hectares as a result of the state's policy of uprooting vines and improving quality by incentivizing growers to join the more competitive appellation system.[34] It should be kept in mind, however, that reductions to vineyard area did not necessarily lead to smaller yields. Because of mechanization and other technological advances in viticulture, both French and European production soared. Between the early 1960s and the early 1970s, EEC production rose from 115,772 million hectoliters to 168,422 million hectoliters.[35] In the common wine market, which French officials claimed was "under the influence of Italy and Germany," it was now the case that "an impersonal, 'industrial,' mass-produced wine, one that isn't necessarily natural nor able to be consumed in its natural state, has been favored."[36]

Consolidating French Quality through and for Europe

The creation of a European common wine market and the supranational power dynamics it entailed threatened French efforts to localize and improve wine production. Throughout the 1960s, the French delegation in Brussels pushed to control imports and limit and improve production.[37] Economists in Montpellier, the heartland of industrial wine, forecast that "we'd be making a bad calculation if we hoped that the Germans, the Belgians, the Dutch, and the Luxembourgers would purchase lightly alcoholic wines of mediocre quality."[38] These economists predicted that the consumer trend was toward luxury appellation wines. While the French delegation consequently lobbied officials in Brussels to improve production, local elites in the Languedoc tried to encourage vine growers in the region to become less dependent on Brussels by improving production and joining the appellation system.

As the organization of the common wine market proceeded in the 1960s, creating a locally regulated appellation or joining an existing one could defend vital national interests, just as it had strengthened mainland interests against Algerian interests in the pre-1962 period. Appellations could insulate producers from decisions made in distant Brussels and stem the loss of revenue to the imported Italian blending wines. In addition, high-end producers from esteemed regions could prevent other producers and merchants in their regions from using Italian wine to correct flaws in their own wine; a scandal might erupt if consumers discovered that their expensive burgundy was in fact part Italian! Finally, through appellations, producers and state officials could police the freer-trading EEC and prevent their competitors from using France's famous place-based names. That the EEC now had jurisdiction over industrial wine helps explain why the production of appellation wine and cooperative wineries expanded in the 1960s and 1970s.[39] While cooperatives would not attain the same level of national and international success as the appellation system, both movements gave producers some control over their destiny, whereas the industrial wine system did not.

Yet vine growers in the Languedoc continued to thwart statist efforts to convert them to the appellation system or to other agricultural pursuits. The plan devised in the 1950s under Philippe Lamour to build a canal in the Languedoc, which was supposed to provide irrigation and encourage producers to convert to other crops, merely served the productivist ethos of the 1960s by increasing yields. Officials complained that vine growers used the water from the canal for irrigating vines instead of replacing them with other crops.[40] The Communist press, allied with the Languedoc growers who ignored the state-sponsored uprooting program, reported that the irrigation system was downstream from a nuclear factory; given the radioactivity in the water, the press warned, babies would be born with two heads and six fingers on each hand.[41]

When industry leaders and state officials encouraged Languedoc producers to convert to appellation wine production or to other economic activities, producers saw financial risk, not profit. Because the state continued to subsidize their surpluses, producers sought ever-higher yields. Falling prices led to often violent political protest, which historically meant the state subsidized and protected the producers, which in turn encouraged further surpluses. Oversupply on the one hand and the price system and subsidies on the other fed a vicious cycle. A bureaucrat at the Ministry of Agriculture noted that it is "sometimes more interesting for vine growers to produce wines of an inferior quality, with an elevated productivity, than to care for their vines in order to obtain a better quality."[42] Indeed, growers preferred increasing their yields of wines destined for distillation, which paid at 8.5 francs for each percentage point of alcohol content by volume, than to produce quality wines, of which the yield was limited to 50 or 60 hectoliters per hectare and of which the market price was 10 to 12 francs per percentage point.[43] Given the favorable circumstances to distill surpluses instead of making more competitive wine, the state distilled one-third of total industrial wine production in 1961–1962.[44] Officials could find few outlets for this distilled wine. Wine policy therefore allowed growers "to produce in order to destroy."[45] One frustrated parliamentarian went so far as to say that "wine is better protected than the physically handicapped."[46] State subsidies preserved the winegrowers' way of life and allowed them to avoid the risk-taking venture of joining the appellation movement or converting to other crops.

Faced with the prevailing attitudes within the EEC and in the Languedoc, INAO representatives, the Ministry of Agriculture, and the French delegation in Brussels looked for allies in their bid to localize production. The HCEIA was in a good position to help modify wine norms for the benefit of French interests; in the name of consumer welfare, it could help demonize cheap Italian wine, justify difficult reforms in the Languedoc, and turn consumers toward appellation wines at a time when consumers were being introduced to an array of new goods and influences. From the early 1960s into the 1970s, Robert Debré, president of the HCEIA, called for a partnership between the INAO and public health activists that would simultaneously increase the farmer's standard of living and curb alcoholism. The challenge, as Debré saw it, was how to get European technocrats to listen to the HCEIA's concerns. "We're seeking also to make obvious in the minds of those who represent us in these meetings [whether in Paris or in Brussels] the necessity of adding to their economic effort a public health effort by associating them with the action that we're pursuing."[47] In Debré's view, public health activists and appellation leaders had a common interest: limiting and improving production would increase prices, thereby increasing the producer's standard of living and inhibiting excessive consumption. Economic growth and public health would thus both be served. Europeans, they argued, could not consume surplus wine without potentially falling victim to alcoholism. Thus the wine industry could not follow the course of industrialization that was taking place in other agricultural sectors.

If, in the 1950s, the sober revolutionaries had presented themselves as great liberators of colonial peoples who had fallen victim to the industrial wine system, they now presented themselves as bringing culture and light to all of Europe. Both strategies justified their authority over the policy-making process. The problem for the HCEIA was how to insert public health into the economic discussions on the common wine market and gain the moral high ground over the peasants of the industrial competition, peasants that even some Paris observers saw as virtuous.[48] Furthermore, the priority of the common market was to defend producers, not consumers.[49] Debré complained that "the HCEIA has already searched a million times by what means it could participate in the negotiations of the European community in order to defend the public health point of view."[50] A member of the HCEIA noted that "a certain number of high functionaries . . . are very convinced of the gravity of the problems posed by alcoholism," but because of interest groups, "their preoccupations will above all be of an economic order."[51] To defend quality wine and limit alcoholism, French reformers could refer to Article 36 of the Treaty of Rome, which stipulated that trade liberalization "shall not preclude prohibitions or restrictions on imports, exports, or goods in transit justified on grounds of public morality, public policy, or public security; the protection of health and life of humans, animals or plants; the protection of national treasures possessing artistic historic or archaeological value; or the protection of industrial and commercial property."[52] Reformers also sought to control wine advertising at the European level, noting that "for tactical reasons, this question should be raised by the delegation of a non-wine-producing country (Belgium or the Netherlands)."[53] In this way, the sober revolutionaries invoked the welfare of European consumers and hoped to mobilize France's less biased European partners to localize wine production and combat alcoholism.

To make the sober revolutionaries' voices heard at the European level, the state appointed Philippe Lamour—a leading agricultural expert in the Languedoc and the EEC and the architect of the Delimited Wines of Superior Quality (VDQS) label—to the HCEIA in 1961. Lamour was to become a strategic go-between in the negotiations among appellation leaders, technocrats, and public health activists throughout the 1960s and early 1970s. Lamour had been born in northern France, had been trained as a lawyer, and had become an adamant supporter of state planning in the 1930s. During the German occupation, he had lived in the Languedoc, where he discovered an interest in agriculture and even acquired a vineyard. Significantly, as a northerner in the south, he was an outsider to the Languedoc, who saw the issues facing the region in a different light.

After World War II, Lamour had become a prominent voice in agriculture at the local, national, and later European levels. Locally, Lamour was the president of a chamber of agriculture, the editor of *Le Paysan du Midi*, and president of the Society of the Lower-Rhône Languedoc, which was charged with the region's economic development.[54] Lamour consulted with Jules Milhau, who, as we have seen, was an influential and locally well-respected economist who knew the problems facing southern wine and who used the strategy of participating in the local temperance society in Montpellier as a way to spread the word about the need to modernize the wine industry.[55] Both local economists and local temperance activists wanted to improve the region's wine production, encourage the making of grape juice, and, where necessary, convert mass vineyards to the production of other foodstuffs.[56] As discussed previously, Lamour's principal strategy to modernize southern wine production was to build a canal so that farmers could diversify production.

Nationally, Lamour played a pivotal role in creating the VDQS label and promoting France's economic expansion. In 1947, he became general secretary of the General Confederation of Agriculture (CGA), where he came into contact with the modernizing technocrat and pro-Europeanist Jean Monnet. By the early 1950s, Lamour had become a central figure in the planning commission and the group charged with regional development. Lamour was also a member of the Economic Council's agricultural section, where he collaborated with key alcohol reformers such as Alfred Sauvy and Étienne May and where he advocated for ending France's agricultural protectionism and for competing in a European economic sphere.[57] Through these various contacts, Lamour became aware of the connections that other technocrats were making between wine surpluses and alcoholism.

At the European level, Lamour presided over a commission of industry officials that helped define France's policy in the emerging common wine market and that lobbied the bureaucrats in Brussels. The commission aimed to limit the production of industrial wine and encourage the production of quality wine that held more export potential within the EEC and beyond.[58] Working together, Lamour and the HCEIA were better positioned to push their reform agenda at both the state and EEC levels. To raise awareness about the link between wine production and consumption and to convince others that appellation wine was not only more profitable but also more ethical than industrial wine, the French delegation in Brussels often included a representative of the HCEIA.[59]

Lamour came to the HCEIA at a strategic moment. First, the pro-Europeanist Edgard Pisani was appointed minister of agriculture. He hoped to end the clientelism at the ministry, integrate agriculture into European and global markets, and champion appellation wine.[60] "I'm convinced," Pisani said, "that we won't have enough appellation wine to export in a few years and that we must authorize new plantings in the regions of quality wine."[61] For Pisani, the problem lay in orienting production around exportable appellation wines. Between 1947 and 1965, appellation wine exports increased 349 percent in volume and 917 percent in value.[62] Second, in 1961, European technocrats, many of whom refused to regulate vine plantings and sanctioned high production levels, were about to begin discussions on the organization of the common wine market. Third, the likelihood that Algerian imports would diminish grew, as France struggled to maintain colonial Algeria. In 1961, therefore, forces were pulling both toward and against appellation wine. With Lamour gaining an awareness of the links between wine surpluses and alcoholism from his participation in the HCEIA, he and the French delegation in Brussels could lobby for localizing and refining production in the name of economic efficiency and public health.

The competing interests of appellation leaders, technocrats, and public health activists came together at decisive moments in the construction of the common wine market, particularly during key wine reforms in 1962, 1964, 1970, and 1976. In 1964, for example, the government issued two decrees to organize the wine market and improve production, and it did so in the name of fighting alcoholism.[63] In the lead up to the 1964 decree, the HCEIA was in close communication with Lamour, who also worked at the Ministry of Agriculture.[64] The prime minister also consulted with the HCEIA.[65] Even the Council of State, the government's legal council and supreme court, used the HCEIA's public health discourse.[66] The HCEIA, in generating knowledge about alcoholism and connecting the condition to the industrial wine system, justified the state's intervention in the wine economy to promote authenticity in the common market, which invariably meant locally produced and regulated wines. The evolving EEC regulations of the 1960s served as a fillip for the state to enforce quality production in France in the name of economic growth and consumer welfare.

It is not my intention to suggest any corruption on the part of public health activists but rather to emphasize that they and appellation leaders shared and leveraged the same interests. The promotion of appellation wine served France's political, economic, cultural, and public health interests in the new Europe. Even so, this Europeanist coalition was not foreordained but contingent. Wine and public health interest groups did not always fraternize. For example, in 1966, INAO leaders criticized public health activists for their divide-and-conquer tactics.[67] In 1970, a leader of the CNVS wrote to Prime Minister Jacques Chaban-Delmas to convince him of the "cogency of the protests of all the syndical organizations for viticulture and trade against the manner and tone that has presided for years in the campaign against alcoholism."[68] Yet given that economic imperatives dominated the discussions of the common wine market, public health advocates and the appellation wine trade needed to ally to promote appellation wine over cheaper industrial wine production at home and abroad. This coalition, which had begun to take shape in the late 1950s, became stronger once Algeria achieved independence and once the EEC drew up the plans for a common wine market. As one reformer told his international colleagues, "in France and in several European countries, the viticultural problem is essential in the struggle against alcoholism."[69]

Proponents of appellation wine pitched their cause as serving the "general interests" of both France and Europe. In their mind, French interests and European interests had become one and the same.

Given the strength of the proponents of the industrial wine system, the Europeanist coalition also needed to build international alliances. It is frequently assumed that other countries mimic France's appellation system, but it is less well known that the consolidation of the appellation system in France depended not on the appellation advocacy of a monolithic France but on the advocacy of particular actors and institutions in both France and the international community. In France, we have seen the role played by the INAO, the CNVS, and the HCEIA in refining wine. Internationally, the two most important entities were the nascent EEC and the International Wine Office (IWO), established in 1924.[70] Headquartered in Paris, the French had a predominant influence in the IWO. For much of the pre–World War II period, Édouard Barthe had been its president. From 1949 to 1963, Pierre Le Roy de Boiseaumarié headed the organization. EEC officials regularly consulted with the IWO in developing its wine regulations.[71] Sober revolutionaries needed international support against their domestic and international rivals in solidifying the appellation system.

After 1962, France's European partners began to adopt the appellation system in order to maintain jurisdiction over their reputable wine districts. In this way, they could solidify existing traditions or codify new traditions in winemaking on their own terms without having to abide by the dictates of Brussels. In 1963, Italy created its appellation system, which consisted of the Denominazione di Origine Controllata (DOC) and Denominazione di Origine Controllata e Garantita (DOCG). Germany's unique classification system, which had developed since the late nineteenth century, was based as much on the methods of production—the amount of sugar added to the wine—as on the place of production. To meet the new European distinction between industrial and appellation wine, Germany passed a law in 1969 that based the difference between table and quality wine on whether the wine was artificially sweetened or naturally sweet. Yet like France's appellation system, German producers and state officials delimited zones of production, determined the type of grape varietals that producers could plant, and required producers to abide by recognized viticultural and vinicultural techniques.[72] Despite national variations in rules and classification, all equated quality and authenticity with strict regulations on the place and style of production.

Emulating France's appellation system provided local producers in other countries a space to determine their own distinct traditions and protect their reputation from standardized norms, but this emulation also paid dividends to France's appellation producers. First, it gave the appellation system international legitimacy. Second, France's regional appellations were often better known than those of their neighbors. No amount of money or marketing would allow another bottle of wine to be exactly like a "burgundy" or a "champagne." An appellation producer in Burgundy claimed that "it'd be really stupid of the French to abandon one of their principal commercial advantages in order to go drown in European uniformity."[73] The success of the appellation movement hinged on how the common wine market would operate once it began in 1970.

The Shock of the Local

Although few could have predicted it in 1970, the first years of the common wine market were to be pivotal in excluding Algerian wine from the new Europe, consolidating appellation norms, and reinforcing the image of France as a hexagon. Languedoc vine growers, Italian officials, and the European Commission were slow to acknowledge that wine surpluses were a structural problem. Achieving price stability and sustaining inefficient producers were deemed politically more important than changing the orientation of the industry. Between the implementation of the common wine market in 1970 and the first EEC wine reforms in 1976, a hostile global economic context, a series of abundant harvests, and the continued shift in consumer preferences away from industrial wine compelled European officials to join the sober revolution.

The global economic crisis of the early 1970s put new stress on France and the EEC.[74] The most immediate issue centered on Algeria's status in the new Europe. When French officials had signed the Treaty of Rome in 1957, Algeria was an administrative part of France, which meant that Algeria's vast wine industry would find outlets not just in metropolitan France but in all of the EEC. This situation was altered by Algeria's independence in 1962. The new Algerian government nationalized the vineyards. Although the government was committed to the long-term plan of converting these vineyards to other crops, it still needed to find outlets for its wine abroad in order to generate revenue for the country's industrialization.[75] Wine constituted over half of all Algerian exports to France in the 1960s.[76] French officials promised to continue purchasing Algerian wine to support Algeria's export earnings, about 40 million hectoliters in all between 1964 and 1969.[77] While the French state quickly and conveniently forgot the Algerian impact on French political culture after 1962, it continued to use Algerian wine as a diplomatic tool. French diplomats feared that a failure to purchase Algerian wine would have repercussions on other aspects of Franco-Algerian trade, most notably oil in the Sahara. President Ben Bella reportedly said: "Take my wine, if you want to safeguard your oil interests."[78] For another Algerian official, "wine was as important as oil."[79] French officials promised to purchase some of Algeria's wine surpluses in return for continued access to the Saharan oil fields. France's ties to Algeria complicated the political dynamics of the EEC because they risked undermining Italian efforts to become the cheapest and most competitive wine industry in Europe as well as the Languedoc's efforts to remove one of its largest competitors from the French market.

Wine lobbies in Italy and the Languedoc hoped to block Algerian wine from entering the EEC. Two events in 1971 supported them.[80] First, in February, Algeria nationalized its natural gas and petroleum, which meant that France was less bound to buy Algerian wine. Second, the EEC was confronting a major surplus crisis. Protestors' signs in the Languedoc proclaimed, "The government treats us like slaves. We'll act like bandits [*fellagha*]."[81] *Fellagha* was a reference to the Algerian militants during the war of independence against French rule, which suggested that producers in the Languedoc were about to wage their own war of independence against the French state and the EEC. Significantly, many European settlers of French Algeria had relocated to the Languedoc after 1962, which fanned the flames of both anti-statist and anti-Algerian sentiment in the Languedoc.[82]

In response to the nationalization of the oil fields and to protests from Italian officials and vine growers in the Languedoc, Algeria became a third country to the EEC in October 1971, thus ending its preferential relationship with the EEC at a time when Algeria carried out 80 percent of its trade with the EEC.[83] Interestingly, two months later, an accord reduced

Algerian immigration to France, further hardening the boundaries between France and Algeria.[84] Then, in February 1972, the EEC's Council of Ministers forbade the blending of EEC wines with wines from third countries, officially distancing "Europe" from one of its former colonies.[85] Relations would persist between Algeria, France, and the EEC, but Algeria's wine production continued to diminish, making wine a less important aspect of those relations. The EEC helped France exclude Algeria and its wines; as we will see, the EEC would also support the French state in integrating the Languedoc wine economy more fully into France's appellation norms and into a European idea of France.

Other global economic problems surfaced that would ultimately advance the sober revolution. The end of the Bretton Woods system in 1971 and the global oil shock of 1973 created unfavorable conditions for the common market's first years in operation. After the United States departed from gold, exchange rates fluctuated. France thereafter became particularly susceptible to the impact of Italian wine imports. The general price increases resulting from the oil shock also threatened to put a check on consumption. Given limited markets, producers in the Languedoc demanded protection from what they saw as unfair Italian competition, recalling the historic battles that they had waged against Algeria.

Surpluses and political protest plagued the common wine market throughout the early 1970s.[86] A French diplomat in Germany, having read the local newspapers, asked his superiors in the Ministry of Foreign Affairs: "Will the Community drown in a sea of wine?"[87] Appellation producers, whose markets would be adversely affected by the oversupply, immediately made use of their connections. They called on Jacques Chaban-Delmas, then the prime minister and the mayor of Bordeaux, to push for a dialogue between the wine lobbies and the HCEIA.[88] In a press release, these groups agreed that the fight against alcoholism "consists in combating the abuse of all alcoholic beverages, distilled or fermented, but does not exclude the moderate use in the maximal limits defined by the Academy of Medicine. It must be accompanied by a policy of the improvement of the quality of products leading necessarily to an increase in their price."[89] This statement was an obvious attack on cheaper industrial wines—namely the influx from Italy—and spirits in the new European context. Robert Boulin, the minister of public health and a politician from the winegrowing Libourne, who had formerly been minister of agriculture, also wanted to integrate the wine lobbies into the HCEIA.[90] Collaboration between appellation leaders and the HCEIA would continue to support the expansion of the appellation system and limit the consumption of cheaper Languedoc and Italian wine.

This Europeanist coalition drove home the point that state and European officials could not force consumers to drink more. Unable to force wine surpluses on the population, the political expedient of enacting temporary distillation measures plagued not the French state but European technocrats for the first time in the early 1970s, thereby positioning the EEC against the industrial vine growers of the Languedoc. In 1973, three other non-wine-producing countries—England, Ireland, and Denmark—joined the EEC, making the new Europe potentially even more hostile to using taxpayers' money to subsidize surplus wine. Nevertheless, the EEC paid for and distilled 6.9 million hectoliters of wine in 1971 and 1972, and 19.6 hectoliters of wine from 1973 to 1976. From 1971 to 1975, the bill for subsidies came to 2 billion francs for the French state and the EEC. To be sure, wine represented only a fraction of overall costs for the CAP. Total expenditures on agriculture amounted to about 40 billion, with about 10 billion each going to dairy products and grain.[91] Yet "wine isn't considered a food of first necessity," as a group of young farmers warned, "and the support of the wine market will provoke a growing reaction from the non-producing countries and consumers."[92] As France and Europe experienced a massive rural exodus in the 1960s and 1970s, fewer people were involved in or had ties to the wine trade. Urban people were bitter about subsidizing industrial wine that fewer and fewer people drank. One French journalist asked: "How to convince [the nine EEC member-states] to subsidize the wine surpluses of their neighbors whereas the river of milk already costs them so much? 'Milk is still a basic food,' noted a German minister. 'We can give it to babies. We can send it to underdeveloped countries. But wine?'" (figure 16).[93] As this example suggests, France's neighbors helped sober revolutionaries challenge the French and Italian myth that wine was a food.

Subsidizing surpluses threw the whole European project into question. In 1974 and 1975, producers in the Languedoc blocked Italian wine imports, which mobilized wine merchants, the transportation sector, Italy, and ultimately the EEC against industrial wine. Wine merchants, who

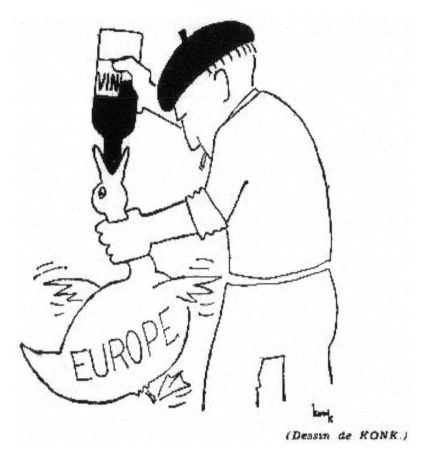

(Dessin de KONK.)

Figure 16. A Frenchman plying a European goose with wine. Cartoon by Laurent Fabre (a.k.a. "KONK"). *Le Monde*, 18 April 1975.

depended on importing both Italy's blending wines, berated producers in the Languedoc for their nationalist tendencies. When these producers disrupted public order and forced the state to put a break on free trade within the EEC, merchants considered themselves to be "victims of terrorist operations and overzealous regulations."[94] Italian customs officers, in an act of retaliation against Languedoc recalcitrance, prevented French vehicles from exporting through Italy, primarily to the Middle East.[95] A bureaucrat in the Ministry of Finance rightly noted that "it was the first time in the history of the common agricultural policy that a member-state had been led to close its borders to its partners."[96] One parliamentarian expressed his disgust "in seeing a very honorable profession block the roads and the ports, tear open the hatch of the wine tanks, forbid Italian wine imports—with the risk of compromising our agricultural exports toward Italy, which have value that is eight or nine times superior to that of the wine that we import. . . . Which will get the upper-hand, the interests of a profession or the interests of the nation?"[97] The European Commission, the Europeanist body par excellence, scolded the French for their nationalistic protection of the Languedoc peasants. In the years following the institution of the common wine market in 1970, the wine glut not only threatened the stability of France but also the movement to unify Western Europe.

While the instability that France had long sought to manage now took a toll on France's non-wine-producing European partners, changes in wine consumption also threw supply and demand out of balance. At the end of a period of prosperity, as a mass consumer society had become firmly entrenched, the Mediterranean drinking pattern underwent a quiet but dramatic revolution. Annual per capita wine consumption in France dropped to 110 liters in the 1970s, after having reached approximately 150 liters in the early 1950s. Similar patterns occurred in Greece, Italy, and Portugal.[98] In the Mediterranean world, wine had long been considered a food. By the 1970s, drinkers in this region began to emulate those in northern Europe and the United States, who tended to view wine as a luxury item to show off one's knowledge and sophistication. Industrial wine was becoming a dirty habit of the past. One vine grower in Provence reported that "they're heaping on wine all the evils, under the name of alcoholism. . . . when certain young people get in accidents, people say they drank. But what did they drink? Certainly it wasn't wine or very little. They drank whiskey, they drank *pastis*, and so on."[99]

As prices collapsed in the early 1970s, Languedoc producers followed custom by blocking the highways and protesting the technocrats in Paris and Brussels and their cold calculations about the future of industrial wine. Even though the Languedoc producers had lost their old allies— the beet growers, the cider producers, the home distillers, the European settlers—they were not isolated. A variety of regional lobbies such as the CGVM and the Regional Committee of Vine Growing Action (CRAV) defended them. Nationally, they continued to find some support from the opposition Socialist Party.[100]

Perhaps most importantly, the producers of the Languedoc had a strong regional identity that they defended from the technocratic "conquest" of Paris and Brussels. In this way, they linked their problems to the entire region, galvanizing the population against centralized authority in the north.[101] In the early 1970s, a regionalist movement to protect Occitan culture mobilized against the centralized state in Paris, hoping "to liberate Occitania from French colonialism."[102] In response to plans to turn the Languedoc economy over to tourism, the radicalized CRAV declared that "we're going to become the 'tanned ass' of industrialized Europe to the sole profit of the powers of money."[103] Vine growers blocked the roads and highways during tourist season in order to show northern European tourists the southern plight. In a novel of the era, a character observed that "financiers, the money grabbers who lead Europe and France, decided that the south was no longer profitable. We have to leave, make place for vacation villages. We won't do it. We're going to show them that this region is still alive."[104] Responding to the state's efforts to modernize the regional wine industry, one mayor in the Languedoc asked despondently: "What kind of inhabitant of Nîmes, what kind of inhabitant of this very Gard department could accept the possibility of substituting modern monuments for our Roman monuments? . . . It's exactly what they propose for our agriculture and viticulture. The only things that escape the general transformation are the vines on the slopes and from the controlled appellations."[105] While structural reform might bring new opportunities like tourism to the region, for the locals it would not necessarily bring a better way of life. Producers in the Languedoc were united in their belief that vine growing was the natural vocation of the region as well as in their sentimental attachment to their Occitan roots.[106]

The patience of France's European partners wore thin. Too much money was being wasted on wine. A major turning point in the EEC's wine policy came in March 1976 when violent demonstrations erupted in the commune of Montredon, recalling the uprisings of 1907. *Volèm viure al païs* (Occitan for "We want to live on our land") was heard throughout the streets.[107] A policeman and a winegrower were shot to death. *Libération* compared the gravity of the crisis in the Languedoc to the Algerian war of the late 1950s, suggesting that the state was losing control over its own territory.[108] Interestingly, José Bové, today a food activist and critic of unfettered globalization, and someone to whom we will return in the conclusion, farmed in Montredon at this time. Under pressure from the demonstrators, the government in Paris tried to block the entry of Italian imports. The EEC forced the state to back down or else Italy would block the importation of French industrial products. France's dynamic sectors that depended on European trade were threatened, and the whole principle of the EEC's existence risked being compromised.[109] The wider belief in the need to support the European project isolated the producers of the Languedoc and ultimately forced them to change their ways.

In the wake of the bloody events of Montredon and faced with the swollen budgetary costs of European wine surpluses, European technocrats recognized the need to reform the wine sector. On 6 March 1976, the ministers of agriculture of each member-state came together and implemented a number of measures to cope with the crisis. Thereafter, the EEC's wine policy more closely resembled France's regulatory practices of subsidizing vine uprooting, distilling surpluses, and promoting quality wine production by placing restrictions on planting rights.[110] During the crisis, Robert Debré lobbied France's Interministerial Committee for Questions of European Economic Cooperation, a disproportionately influential lobby in Brussels, to heed public health warnings.[111] Debré noted that the HCEIA's wine policy informed the program elaborated in Brussels to cope with the surplus crisis.[112] Because of frequent surpluses and the political instability that they caused, European technocrats acknowledged that the wine problem stemmed not from low prices but from the need to reform the industry's structure. In their view, too many small producers participated in vine monoculture and expected subsidies to support their surpluses. The EEC finally accomplished what the French state had struggled to achieve: the EEC bluntly told the cantankerous producers of the Languedoc that the persistence of the old regime was too costly.

The EEC deprived the industrial producers of the Languedoc of their customary means of impacting the political process in Paris, thereby ultimately inciting producers in the Languedoc to change their strategies. Recognizing that the future lay in quality production and that they could achieve more power over the decision-making process in the regionally regulated appellation system, many growers in the Languedoc started to improve their wines. They uprooted their vineyards planted in high-yielding Aramon and unwanted hybrid varieties and reconstituted them with officially recognized ones. AOC labels proliferated: Limoux et Blanquette-de-Limoux in 1975; Côtes-du-Roussillon in 1977; Faugères and Saint-Chinian in 1982; Coteaux-du-Languedoc, Corbières, and Minervois in 1985; and Cabardès in 1998. The majority of French appellations that appeared in the last quarter of the twentieth century belonged to Languedoc-Roussillon.[113] The same trend occurred in the other member-states of the EEC. As more and more producers followed the trend of appellations, European officials noted that overproduction problems were now caused as much by appellation wines as industrial wines. Not all appellation wines were low in yield nor met superior quality standards.[114] As markets Europeanized and globalized in the 1970s, many producers in the Languedoc and other European regions left the industrial wine system to localize production and bottle at the source.

The murderous events at Montredon still left bitter resentment. Distrust remained among southern wine producers toward officials in Paris and Brussels. After the demonstrations of 1976, a bureaucrat in the Ministry of Agriculture, who happened also to be a producer from the south, was asked to name wine's greatest adversaries. He responded, "First the 'technocrats' in Brussels, then the [anti-alcohol] 'lobbies'!"[115] Because of the economic and social challenges that Languedoc producers confronted, the HCEIA promised the government that it would abstain from provoking the producers, going so far as to take down the billboards in the vine-growing regions that cautioned drivers against drinking and driving![116]

By taking to the streets and carrying out acts of violence, the producers of the Languedoc ironically helped shift norms toward the appellation system. The French state mobilized the EEC against them. In the 1970s, the economic, social, and cultural geography of the Languedoc began to change, albeit slowly. The region became increasingly urban. Montpellier became a hub for the tertiary sector.[117] As producers left the land or changed their farming practices and as consumers turned away from industrial wine, the Languedoc lost some of its volatility.[118] Without invoking broader European and consumer interests, the state would have had difficulties asserting its authority over the wine industry.

Producers in the Languedoc were aware of the ironies of the appellation system. They observed that although appellation proponents equated quality with low yields, appellation regions produced more per hectare than the Languedoc. Surpluses beset the producers of bordeaux and champagne; one part of the Champagne region reportedly produced approximately between 1,500 to 1,800 hectoliters per hectare.[119] Languedoc producers also challenged the appellation system's claims to nature and authenticity, pointing out that the EEC allowed appellation producers to add sugar to wines in order to boost production while Languedoc producers could not. Just like appellation producers, the vine growers of the Languedoc presented themselves as the defenders of nature, small landownership, and the local community. Yet the former started to prevail over the latter. The appellation system branded an essentialized idea of the local while being complicit in the modernization and exclusion of local communities.

Conclusion

After 1962, the sober revolution became Europeanized. Algeria's independence and the EEC's first wine decrees in 1962 accelerated the French state's efforts to localize wine production and refine wine consumption through the appellation system. De Gaulle warned that "the fate of our agriculture is from here on out, after the regulation of the Algerian affair, our biggest problem. And if we don't settle it, we might have another Algeria on our own soil."[120] Few farm groups better exemplified defiance to state power than the peasant vine growers of the Languedoc. To diminish Algerian wine imports after Algeria's independence as well as to overcome the continuing resistance of the Languedoc vine growers to reforms, leaders of the Fifth Republic delegated these thorny problems to less democratically accountable European technocrats. These technocrats claimed that the continued coddling of Languedoc producers would undermine the European dream of lasting peace and prosperity. Europeanizing the French struggle over wine laid the groundwork for the establishment of new norms around the appellation system, ones that would lead to a shift to quality production in the Languedoc and to the European Union's adoption of the appellation system for all of agriculture by the century's end. Thus, through decolonization and European integration, the sober revolutionaries ultimately achieved their aim of promoting the more profitable and pacific appellation system. In 1962, France bid adieu to "Greater France" to become "hexagonal France" with its "little homelands" (*petit pays*) and *terroirs*.[121] Hexagonal France was situated in a new Europe that turned its back on empire and an Algerian wine industry that Europeans had created. The rise of the appellation system reflected and facilitated this simultaneous process of localization and Europeanization.

Despite the growing success of the appellation system in the 1970s, its victory was never secure. Algerian and Italian competition had given way to a New World model of "industrial" production based on grape varietals instead of appellations.[122] The strategy that had previously been used by France's luxury wine producers against their European competitors was now being deployed against the New World wine industry. Yet in a blind tasting in Paris in 1976, California wines shockingly triumphed over France's appellation wines.[123] Increasingly after 1976, New World wines would become a force to reckon with.[124] As French wine consumption declined and as anxieties about global capitalism became more acute, one wine writer went so far as to predict the demise of wine. In his view, wine and civilization were inextricably linked. Both were products of the relationship between nature and the human touch: "Wine is at the stage (of development) of its country . . . a people that no longer knows how to drink will soon cease to write, to think, to paint. . . . We've written a lot on wine, to praise it more than to understand it. It passes for a product, whereas it's really an individual. It's a matter more of psychology than of agriculture, of love than of political economy."[125] Such fetishizing reinforced assumptions that wine was a labor of love that could resist the allure of profit and power and that it was incumbent upon France, as the land of quality products, to protect wine from an increasingly money-driven world. This discourse elides the fact that without the diffusion of capitalism through the European common market, the sober revolution might not have succeeded.

Conclusion

Terroir vs. McWorld

In August 1999, just months before the anti-globalization movement erupted on the streets of Seattle during a meeting of the World Trade Organization (WTO), José Bové, a sheep farmer in the Languedoc who produced milk for Roquefort cheese, and the Peasant Confederation (CP), an agricultural union that defends the interests of smallholding farmers, dismantled a McDonald's in Millau, a town in the Languedoc.[1] The act was immediately interpreted as an example of French resistance to the industrial food system and corporate globalization.[2] Activist and journalist Naomi Klein called it an "attack against an agricultural model that sees food purely as an industrial commodity rather than the centerpiece of national culture and family life."[3] Yet interestingly Bové protested in the Languedoc, a region with a history of industrial wine production and whose peasant producers were driven off the land by the very appellation system that Bové was now defending against McDonald's.

Bové's protest came at the end of a decade marked by the deepening and widening of the European Union and by the loosening of regulations

in the international economy. Critics of commodity-driven agriculture responded to end-of-the-century globalization by rallying around
France's appellation system and the notion of *terroir* that it promotes.
A mayor in the Languedoc expressed a common sentiment: "Roquefort
is made from the milk of only one breed of sheep, it's made in only one
place in France, and it's made in only one special way. . . . It's the oppo-
site of globalization. Coca-Cola you can buy anywhere in the world and
it's exactly the same."[4]

Food activists and consumers around the world share the view that
place-based appellation models of production—known in international
law as geographical indications (GIs)—protect the interests of small-scale
farmers and re-connect consumers to the land, to the people who work it,
to time-honored agricultural practices, and to local culture.[5] In the final
decade of the twentieth century, thanks in large part to the influence of
French and European Union policymakers in international trade negotiations, GIs became an international response to unregulated globalization; in this way, they also became a beacon of hope in a world that was
increasingly dominated by industrialized agriculture.

The apparent showdown between industrialized food and the appellation system reinforces common assumptions about how the global—
commonly associated with American-style capitalism, modernization,
standardization, and what might be encapsulated in the term "McWorld"—
conflicts with and even threatens the local—commonly associated with
artisanal products, agricultural traditions, regional diversity, and *terroir*.[6]
Instead of seeing place-based models of production simply as guardians of
the embattled practices of an earlier age, I argue that they can also be seen
as ways for small-scale producers to navigate global change and in fact
profit from it. The rise of the appellation system in the twentieth century
highlights the ways in which the local and the global are not diametrically
opposed but instead interact in dynamic and unexpected ways.

A perspective that places France's wine appellation system on the front
lines of the anti-globalization struggle, then, leads to a misinterpretation of
its rise and how globalization necessarily operates.[7] As this book has suggested, an historical examination of the appellation system suggests that it
has been less a backlash against globalization than a different understanding of how markets should be regulated in a globalized context. "We have
to put the market in its place," Bové asserted, "so that it doesn't control

everything."[8] Today's consumer and scholarly tendencies to sanctify the local and associate France with regional foodways and ethical production leave the impression that small-scale producers are antithetical to global capitalism, which has the effect of eliding their efforts to lobby state and international officials to develop international regulatory institutions that would serve their interests.[9] Wine lobbies like the National Institute of Appellations of Origin (INAO) and farm organizations like the CP have presented their products as an authentic part of the French landscape to be protected from the very economic and political processes that allowed them to gain prominence in the first place. The French movements to localize wine and integrate into global markets were not antagonistic but instead mutually dependent.

The Sober Revolution and the Remaking of France

By now, it should be clear that Bové's critiques of industrialized agriculture and globalization—and his symbolic mobilization of *terroir* against McWorld—were not altogether new or leveled against the United States but instead had their roots in a Franco-French battle between industrialized production and appellation production. The appellation system emerged out of the surplus crises of the Franco-Algerian industrial wine system. It gained prominence in the middle decades of the twentieth century as the result of intense negotiations between French groups that advocated economic modernization and liberalization, on the one hand, and French groups that pleaded with the state to protect the authenticity of agricultural products and promote public health and safety, on the other hand. As the French economy modernized and integrated into the European and world economy after World War II, the state worked to expand its rules and regulations for wine production. The appellation system claimed to promote a more ethical kind of capitalism than the industrial wine system had practiced in the French empire.

A range of groups that supported the appellation system condemned the industrial wine system for causing economic stagnation, political instability, and alcoholism. Yet during the Third and Fourth Republics, industrial vine growers resisted structural reforms that would have driven them off the land. They succeeded because of their large numbers, their organization at the regional level, their ability to influence Parliament, and their claim that they protected the interests of agriculture and French Algeria. Moreover, in the Languedoc and parts of Algeria, wine was the primary agricultural product, making it all the more difficult for technocrats to break up the political power of the system and carry out economic reform. In the late 1950s, only about 15 percent of wine producers participated in the appellation business; the majority, clinging to privileges that they had won in the Third Republic, continued to produce industrial wines and non-market wines and spirits.[10]

To overcome the political power of the industrial wine system and its allies, leaders of the INAO and the National Confederation of Wine and Spirits (CNVS) built alliances with other groups that shared their interest in integrating the French economy into European and global markets and reforming political institutions. The High Commission for Studies and Information on Alcoholism (HCEIA) became a privileged forum for planning reforms because after 1945 a variety of public health activists, technocrats, and lobbies had come around to the idea that changing consumer habits was crucial to modernizing the French wine industry in particular and the economy in general. Although their interests frequently conflicted, they coalesced at strategic moments. Appellation leaders like Pierre Le Roy de Boiseaumarié and Philippe Lamour, given their political connections and their claim to protect consumers from fraudulent products, legitimated changes not only to the wine industry but also and perhaps more importantly to state institutions and economic arrangements.

The transformation of the French wine industry, then, is also a story about building new state institutions that could stimulate economic growth, promote public health and safety, and renew cultural life from the 1930s to the 1970s. It is a story about how the appellation system helped the French rethink the shape and meaning of France as the country decolonized and adjusted to European integration and globalization. My shorthand for these interlocking changes has been the sober revolution. In the wake of World War II, France faced economic ruin and political instability. As politicians, government officials, and industry leaders addressed ways to revive the national economy, leading technocrats like Alfred Sauvy and René Dumont saw the protectionist wine policies of the Third Republic as a main obstacle to renewal. The parliamentary and imperial Third Republic had not only protected wine but also cultivated popular myths about the benefits of habitual wine drinking. Sauvy, Dumont, and other technocrats tried to gain greater legitimacy in public debate, marginalize politicians from the policymaking process, and manage the economy. To technocrats, the wine industry—with reportedly over a million peasant producers influencing Parliament and a settler population unwilling to address the economic and social inequalities in Algeria—exemplified France's backwardness and stymied the development of a stronger state that could prepare the country for the European common market.

At the same time that technocrats sought to rationalize the wine economy, public health activists campaigned against France's high rates of alcoholism. Anti-alcoholism movements had been active in France since the late nineteenth century, but the nature of the debate over alcoholism changed after 1945. Unlike the temperance zealots of earlier eras who had generally claimed that wine was an antidote to alcoholism, public health activists now strategically linked high levels of wine consumption to high levels of production. They saw the industrial wine system, and the institutions that supported it, as the source of a health crisis. These activists thus joined technocrats in stigmatizing the alcohol lobbies and their political allies for causing backwardness, for corrupting democracy, and for allegedly making France the world's most alcoholic nation.

Other sectors that wished to free up the economy—the automobile, insurance, oil, and tourism industries—occasionally joined the fight against alcoholism as a way to overcome the protectionism of the industrial wine system. Subsidized alcohol surpluses had led governments to promote increased wine consumption and turn wine into an ingredient in all sorts of products, including an alcohol-based fuel that proved more expensive than imported oil. The costs of these subsidies fell on consumers, encouraged alcoholism, and threatened the expansion of automobile use. In addition, French wine-drinking habits, combined with the increasing devotion to automobile use and tourism, led to high rates of alcohol-related automobile accidents, threatening tourism at a time when the state depended on generating revenue from international tourists. The automobile, oil, insurance, and tourism industries lobbied the state to promote more responsible drinking habits in order to ensure that tourists would feel safe traveling the roads to experience the various wine regions.

At first, the CNVS and the INAO were either antagonistic or indifferent to technocrats like Sauvy and public health activists like Robert Debré, but as state-directed modernization gained public approval in the 1950s, they championed the causes of political reform, economic restructuring, and public health and safety. Appellation leaders presented themselves, unlike their industrial competitors, as benevolent businessmen who had practical things to offer technocrats and public health activists. They promoted, even if they did not always practice, low yields, thus helping resolve the glut problem. Also, appellation wine production was closely monitored and thus more easily taxed, it commanded a higher price, and it was largely exported, thereby generating much-needed revenue and limiting domestic consumption, especially among peasants and workers. Finally, appellation wine, whose source of production was known, helped protect public health and was free of the violence in the Algerian vineyards. In turn, technocrats and public health activists needed supporters from within the wine industry itself to win over public opinion and legitimize their controversial transformation of production and consumption.

Five structural changes supported the sober revolution. First, the post-1945 years saw the decline of the peasantry and the rise of an ambitious new middle class of office workers. Rising disposable incomes opened the door to new lifestyles based around mass consumption. In the 1950s, however, many French people still centered their social life around the table and preferred Franco-Algerian industrial wines and homemade brandy to consumer goods that would have elevated their social status, thus limiting the appellation system's expansion. In 1954, Pierre Mendès France created the HCEIA to reform drinking habits as part of his broader program to modernize the economy. The HCEIA's declared mission was to raise awareness about alcoholism, yet it quickly became a space where technocrats and wine industry leaders discussed how to reform production. The HCEIA stigmatized producers who arguably symbolized a problem of economic productivity more than a cause of alcoholism; thus it blamed poor and controversial producers—not the appellation system, wine companies like Postillon, or large spirits firms like Ricard—for encouraging the alcoholic condition. Getting consumers to choose appellation drinks and thus to prompt producers to change their ways demanded state intervention and propaganda.

Second, the more favorable regulatory environment of the Fifth Republic after 1958 was an important turning point in the sober revolution. The new constitution gave technocrats in the administration more leverage than politicians in Parliament. Less bound to the electorate, these technocrats found fewer obstacles in restructuring the wine industry. As parliamentary power waned, peasants struggled to influence the policymaking process. A generation of appellation advocates and state reformers, many of whom received formative training in the troubled times of the 1930s, grew in power during the Fifth Republic, men like Sauvy, Debré and his son Michel, Lamour, and Jacques Chaban-Delmas. Technocrats in the Fifth Republic worked to subvert the industrial wine system and cater to the increasingly lucrative appellation system.

Third, the decolonization of Algeria helped clear the path for the sober revolution by eliminating the political power of the European settlers in the wine industry. Into the 1950s, Algeria was the world's largest wine exporter, and nearly all of its production was sold within the French empire and mostly in the metropole. In the early twentieth century, Algeria's contribution to the chronic surplus crisis had compelled wealthy French producers to innovate and distinguish themselves from the industrial wine system.[11] After Algeria's independence in 1962, Algerian wine exports to France and the EEC gradually diminished. Consumer preferences, to a certain degree out of necessity, shifted to appellation wines. The marketing strategy of the appellation system, with its frequent images of folklore, village life, and even a medieval localism that predated nationalism, imperialism, and the inequities of global capitalism, omitted Algeria from the prestigious history of French wine.

Fourth, the political and moral authority of the EEC also played an important role in supporting the sober revolutionaries' cause. As the EEC seized jurisdiction over the industrial wine system in the 1960s and 1970s, those French producers who had the political connections, money, and privileged land created their own locally governed appellation or joined an already existing one. The local and state administrative structure of the appellation system protected producers from supranational governance. In turn, during times of overproduction, French officials could delegate the unpopular task of structural reform to European technocrats, who were less compelled to satisfy the demands of the Languedoc. French officials could even join the industrial vine growers in blaming Brussels for unpopular measures taken against cheap wine. Once they experienced the burdens of subsidies and protest in the Languedoc and recognized the advantages of the appellation system, European technocrats supported efforts underway in France to limit and improve production. The common market also placed barriers around the EEC, thereby restricting the entry of Algerian wines and increasingly competitive New World wines. European officials informed an American diplomat that, in the interests of consumers, imported wine had to carry a GI.[12] The EEC helped French officials draw boundaries, define quality and authenticity, and exclude products that threatened French notions of good taste.

Fifth, Americanization came in many forms after World War II, not least in the influence of mass production and standardization.[13] The middle of the twentieth century witnessed the emergence of the American-led world order and the continued expansion of wine production in the New World, which slowly reduced the demand for French wine abroad. In the 1960s and 1970s, New World wine producers rarely equated quality with the place of production, suggesting instead that technique and the selection of grape varietals determined a wine's taste profile. Because these emerging producers could not yet invoke any longstanding tradition of excellence, they invested less time and money into promoting the place of production. This relative lack of concern for place no doubt reflected a New World marketing strategy. Average consumers rarely showed much interest in the intricacies of a given *terroir*, but they did and still do express their preferences in terms of well-known grape varieties like Cabernet Sauvignon, Chardonnay, and Pinot Noir. The place of production may not be perfectly imitated, but if "quality" wine was determined instead by grape varietals then any producer around the world had a chance to compete. Even more threatening to French vine growers, New World producers often sold their wines under recognizable labels such as bordeaux, burgundy, or champagne.

If the global reach of the United States posed a threat, it also provided an opportunity. Many affluent Americans, looking to escape America's industrial foodscapes, purchased French wines and the worldview they promoted. French wine producers turned toward marketing *terroir* in part to profit from this international sentiment. Starting in the 1970s, popular gastronomic icons like Julia Child, Kermit Lynch, and Alice Waters subscribed to supposedly French values of place and promoted them in the United States.[14] American consumers lapped up these bucolic images of France and even traveled the French countryside to experience them firsthand.[15] Fascinated by France's supposedly traditional local foodways, these American consumers helped expand and consecrate the appellation system.

The appellation system reconciled the postwar imperative of economic liberalization with the protection of small-scale producers and consumers, but it also marginalized those who stood in the way of the state's vision of traditional wine and its vision of France's postcolonial future. Peasant vine growers in the Languedoc, the European settlers of Algeria, the home distillers, and working-class drinkers bore the brunt of state-sponsored economic modernization and anti-alcoholism. The appellation system's imposition of new norms and regulations helped eliminate groups that the state linked to economic backwardness and alcoholism. Writing peasants, workers, and Algeria out of the history of the French wine industry suppressed the violence and other inconveniences that lay at the roots of the appellation system. Yet given the appellation system's exclusionary practices—it participated in the uprooting of the peasantry, it prevented Algerian wines from receiving AOC status and thus from becoming a part of the official national heritage, and it received the support of the overtly racist, authoritarian Vichy regime—today's food activists should be cautious in upholding this French system as simply an exemplar of ethical production. The appellation system may have protected producers and consumers from the uncertainties of global economic forces, but it also essentialized culture and outlawed or marginalized groups that failed to conform to its norms.

The economic crisis of the early 1970s brought the Thirty Glorious Years to a close, but in the last three decades of the twentieth century the consumption of appellation products and related items that marketed *terroir* continued to climb, expanding from wine and spirits into other foods. With the downturn came a general sense of malaise and nostalgia for what was seemingly lost in the postwar transformation: rural landscapes, the peasantry, and an ideal French way of life that was historically hexagonal and European, not imperial.[16] At this time, the appellation system was increasingly associated with *terroir* in a positive way, even though *terroir* was used, and still is used, in contexts independent of the appellation system.[17] Both the system and the idea shared a celebration of the land, the environment, and the culture of a particular place. One reporter observed that from the early 1970s "to be included in the club of gratifying products, we expect alcohol to have certified origins. We demand, in alcohol and wine, 'nature' and '*terroir*.'"[18] Another reporter noted that "for a lot of French people, it [wine] is more than a drink, a lot more than a food, [it is] the means to rediscover one's distant roots . . . to reconnect with nature and the *terroir*."[19] The appellation system had fought since the 1930s to link quality to authenticity and *terroir*; from the 1970s, more and more French consumers were joining them. The appellation system was surpassing the industrial wine system even if it could never totally eliminate industrial wine from the shelves of grocery stores and even though the appellation system helped uproot the world that consumers hoped to re-experience through appellation wine.

Just as the appellation system rode the wave of state-directed modernization, it was also in a strong position to cater to the growing desire for authentic experiences once the public came around to the belief that this statist modernization had gone too far. The very authenticity that the state had promoted through the appellation system since the 1930s was now being used against the state. Tellingly, historian Eugen Weber's classic 1976 book, *Peasants into Frenchmen,* was translated in 1983 as *La fin des terroirs.*[20] The use of *terroir* in the translation was not without significance. Weber argued that in the late nineteenth century the state engaged in an effort to integrate its diverse regions and eliminate local culture. This period supposedly marked, as his French translation suggests, the "end of *terroirs*." In this case, the state and local culture were diametrically opposed. Like any historian, Weber was very much a product of his time. In the 1970s, regional movements, in Languedoc and elsewhere, intensified their criticisms of an overweening state and the impersonal nature of global capitalism.

The state coopted the increased interest in authenticity by declaring 1980 the Year of Heritage, in which officials sought to trace, record, and commemorate significant aspects of French history.[21] The state also started cataloguing the country's regional traditions and *terroirs*.[22] Coincidentally, the appellation system had been in the nostalgia-making business since its inception and thus supported the state's heritage project, what one scholar has called "patrimonialization."[23] In Pierre Nora's massive edited volume *Realms of Memory*, historian Georges Durand argued that the vineyard was an important site of memory, culture, and identity.[24] For Durand, like earlier appellation advocates such as Joseph Capus, appellation wine evoked positive memories of French civilization. Yet significantly, Durand, like earlier advocates, ignored the contribution of Algeria to the history of French wine. Late twentieth-century globalization and multiculturalism did not eliminate place but instead allowed it to become more clearly defined, fixed, and better appreciated, accentuating the positive and silencing the negative. Ironically, French radio at the beginning of the twenty-first century reported on a Muslim Algerian living in Paris who had opened a wine shop because wine had allowed him to discover France, its regions, and its history, and he hoped to impart that knowledge to others.[25]

Globalizing the Revolution

The threat of cheaper wine from Algeria and the EEC—which often bore famous place-based names from Bordeaux, Burgundy, and Champagne—spurred the creation and expansion of the appellation system to defend small-scale vine growers and consumers from the adverse effects of trade liberalization. Thus when globalization accelerated in the 1990s, French wine and agricultural lobbies had a useful strategy at the ready. In recent years, French groups like the CP and the INAO have intensified their efforts to promote GIs in the institutions that govern world trade, namely the European Union and the WTO. Such groups invoke the urgency of protecting farmers and consumers around the world from economies of scale. One of the strengths of this French movement has been to exploit international assumptions about how France is the land of things small and luxurious. In doing so, they have continued with their strategy of simultaneously upholding their model of agriculture as more ethical and undercutting rival visions at home and in international institutions. By treating culture and craftsmanship as beleaguered by unfettered globalization, French farmers and policymakers advance their economic interests at home and around the world.

The 1990s was not the first time that French agricultural interests had tried to promote their model elsewhere. Efforts going back to the late nineteenth century—the Paris Convention of 1883 and the Madrid Agreement for the Repression of False or Deceptive Indications of 1891—addressed but failed to enforce appellations. The spirit of internationalism in the 1920s inspired European and New World wine leaders to create the International Wine Office (IWO), a lobby that promoted and defended each member country's appellation regulations.[26] Perhaps the most significant cooperation came in 1958 with the signing of the Lisbon Agreement for the Protection of Appellation of Origin and their International Registration. The Lisbon Agreement had twenty-two signatories that agreed to the mutual protection of appellations. Despite all these efforts, however, no government matched the French government's enthusiasm in trying to enforce the system. France's strong centralized state gave France a coherent policy orientation that was lacking in other wine-producing countries such as Italy, Portugal, or the United States.

Since the 1990s, France has received increased support from its European neighbors in promoting GIs for agricultural products, particularly from southern European countries that continue to have large rural populations like Greece, Italy, Portugal, and Spain. In 1992, the European Union created its own system to protect GI food products—known in the EU as protected designations of origin (PDOs)—and has promoted this system abroad. The European Commission's "European Authentic Tastes" ("EAT") campaign, which was advertised in magazines and newspapers abroad, praised authentic champagne and condemned usurpers of this place-based labeling system.[27] In a more intense global economic environment, collaboration with other European countries has enhanced France's leverage at the international negotiating table.

The European Union has given French farmers and policymakers more clout in the international arena, helping advance their agenda in organizations like the WTO. In 1994, the year that the WTO came into existence, 111 countries signed the Agreement on Trade-Related Aspects of Intellectual Property Rights, Including Trade in Counterfeit Goods (TRIPS). The TRIPS agreement created a space for multilateral negotiations over defending and promoting GIs, which benefited France and other European countries the most.[28] Significantly, the TRIPS agreement demonstrated that the WTO, at its inception, could acknowledge the legitimacy of GIs, even if it had not yet become fully committed to enforcing them. When this multilateral approach fails, as it still often does, countries that wish to defend their producers' GIs continue to negotiate bilaterally. The European Union, for example, has negotiated bilateral treaties with numerous countries to mutually protect GIs.[29] It has also helped that France's appellation supporters had connections at the WTO. Between 2005 and 2013, the French businessman Pascal Lamy, while director-general of the WTO, argued, as earlier appellation supporters had, that "the future of European agriculture lies not in quantity of exports but quality. . . . That is why we are fighting to stop appropriation of the image of our products and improve protection."[30] As this quote underscores, earlier French discourse had become a European discourse at the global level.

American policymakers have led the opposition to the creation of a global registry for GIs.[31] The United States has a longstanding tradition of promoting corporate brands and trademarks. Whereas corporations can move their production out of a region in order to find cheaper sources of labor, appellations belong to the region itself. American resistance also stems from the fact that many European immigrants settled in the United States and brought with them their culinary techniques and traditions. These immigrants often sold their food and drink with the name of the town from which they came in Europe, the case of Budweiser being perhaps the most well known. Over time, American consumers associated a certain taste with that product. The American cheese lobby has recently fought to maintain names like "feta" and "Parmesan," claiming that the Europeans "are trying to create new barriers to trade by stealing their [cheese] names back."[32]

In pitting "*terroir* against the power of the multinationals," the CP and the INAO claim to protect not only the small-scale farmers and consumers in Europe but those around the world as well.[33] France and the European Union have especially looked to developing countries as potential allies in their bid to change WTO policies. By promoting GIs in the developing world, French farmers and policymakers have tried to deflect criticisms that the defense of GIs is simply another example of French exceptionalism.[34] In recent years, the appellation system has lent support to smaller-scale producers in the developing world who wish to defend local sovereignty and economies against cheaper agricultural imports. Given that nearly 60 percent of the world's population works in agriculture, this strategy could help validate GIs and put France and the European Union at the forefront of defending the developing world, even if at the same time the EU's agricultural trade policies have worked to the detriment of farmers in these regions.[35]

In 2003, through European assistance, producers from around the world created the Organization for an International Geographical Indications Network (oriGIn).[36] Based in Geneva, oriGIn lobbies the WTO. In 2015, oriGIn represented about four hundred producers' associations from forty countries.[37] Its existence demonstrates the ways in which a Europe-led global alliance has emerged to promote and defend GIs around the world. In 2005, the Biotrade Initiative of the United Nations Conference for Trade and Development (UNCTAD) concluded that "more than other major types of intellectual property, GIs have features that respond to norms for use and management of bioresources and traditional knowledge that are characteristic of the culture of many indigenous and local economies."[38] Proponents of the appellation system claim, some say unconvincingly, that appellations defend sovereignty, stimulate rural economies, and protect the environment and public health.[39] France's appellation system and the notion of *terroir* that it promotes has become untethered from its own place of origin to become a global strategy to promote local economies and culture in global markets.

The globalization of wine markets in the twentieth century had the surprising effect of establishing a new kind of localized wine production in France, one that has expanded to other agricultural products and influenced other countries' agricultural practices in recent years. Argan Oil from Morocco, balsamic vinegar from Modena, Basmati rice, Colombian coffee, Darjeeling tea, Kobe beef from Japan, Phu Quoc fish sauce from Vietnam, Stilton cheese, mezcal from Oaxaca, Vermont maple syrup, Willamette Valley wine, and many other agricultural products carry place-based labels.[40] These labels are key to their market value. Clearly, the INAO and the CP have found allies in the international community in globalizing the local. The forces of globalization have unleashed both a homogenizing and differentiating effect on agricultural products.

The media often simplistically presents the debate over wine and agricultural systems as a struggle between "Old World" and "New World" farming practices, consumption habits, and cultural values.[41] In this view, *terroir*, culture, and tradition oppose McWorld, science, and modernity. One area where this clash has occurred is in the debate between *terroir* and grape variety.[42] The proponents of grape varietals, numerous in the

United States, suggest that the advocates of *terroir* exaggerate the importance of the soil and place of production in tasting and experiencing wine. This could be interpreted as a commercial defense of New World wine producers who lack the prestigious place-based names of their European counterparts. But perhaps the attack on *terroir* is based in science as well. Hildegarde Heymann, a sensory scientist at the University of California, Davis, is skeptical of the term.[43] The American wine writer Robert Parker has challenged the subtleties of *terroir* by creating a simple scoring system between 0 and 100. For the average consumer, a score of 90 speaks volumes compared to trying to rate the qualities of a given appellation and its *terroir*.[44] Both grape varieties and "Parkerization" have become synonymous with American-led globalization and challenges to French authority in matters of taste.

What the media sometimes forgets is that American vintners, sommeliers, wine writers, and importers often embrace appellations and *terroir*. In 1980, the first American viticultural area (AVA) was granted in Missouri; since then, American wine appellations have rapidly grown.[45] The wine writer Matt Kramer has argued that "wines express their source with exquisite definition. . . . They allow us to eavesdrop on the murmurings of the earth." Kramer spoke of a specific California vineyard's Chardonnay as "a powerful flavor of the soil: the limestone speaks."[46] Other American wine writers like Eric Asimov and Jon Bonné have helped heighten awareness of American *terroirs*.[47] Since the 1990s, more and more Americans have embraced the idea of *terroir*. In states like California, Oregon, Vermont, and Wisconsin, locavore movements have adopted the idea to promote ethical agriculture.[48]

At the same time that some Americans embrace appellations and *terroir*, some French vintners prefer to market grape varietals and some farmers prefer industrialized agriculture. Interestingly, many of the vine growers who emphasize grape varietals come from the Languedoc. Some of these growers had come from settler families that returned to France after Algeria's independence.[49] France has also had its fair share of debates and conflicts over agribusiness, as we have seen. The National Federation of Farmers' Unions (FNSEA), the country's most powerful agricultural union, has supported the expansion of agribusiness ever since the immediate post-1945 years. Today, France is among the world's largest agricultural producers and exporters. Moreover, one need only shop in a French grocery store to see that corporate products like Danone, Lu, and Ricard line the aisles just as much as place-based products like apples from Normandy or sausage from Toulouse.

Today's global consumer must weigh the pros and cons of the expansion of place-based appellation systems around the world. On the one hand, these systems promise local communities food sovereignty and consumer protection in a largely unregulated world economy that advantages economies of scale to small-scale production.[50] Place-based food strategies resonate culturally in today's fast-changing world as they connect consumers to the land and to the methods of production and tell stories about the product. Place-based products provide consumers with a sense of refinement, as they can learn about the diverse geographies and histories of production. Appellations and the related fascination with *terroir* have sparked new ideas about fair trade in the world economy, creating new solidarities between consumers and producers that transcend the local and the national to become the global and encouraging a new appreciation for the intersections between culture and nature and how we understand, consume, and value food. For all of these reasons, the appellation system can be seen as serving the public good by defending producers and consumers, restoring a respect for the environment and for human relations, and making the act of eating and drinking more meaningful.

On the other hand, the tendency of food activists to glorify the local has the effect of masking the power relations and socioeconomic inequalities that lay behind appellation systems. In Mexico, for example, corporations have coopted time-honored techniques of mezcal and tequila production.[51] Affluent city dwellers have in large part championed local foods in their search for authentic experiences.[52] To earn their living, producers with capital have delivered on these consumer aspirations. Appellations essentialize local culture, keeping what sells and silencing what does not. Producers with fewer political connections and less capital struggle to survive the appellation system's conquest. Appellations have the potential to create new inequalities by driving poorer producers out of business and ratcheting up the price of the end product for consumers.

Moreover, place-based products succumb to the same kind of commodification as industrialized agriculture. In some instances, large corporations invest in appellations as a way to differentiate their products and ensure new markets. LVMH, the multinational luxury goods conglomerate, invested in champagne; similarly, the Lactalis Group invested in some of France's appellation cheeses.[53] Over time, more producers have joined the appellation system in order to meet growing demand. This expansion calls into question the artisanal and small-scale features of the appellation industry.[54] It remains to be seen what the future of the appellation system holds. In recent years, some reputable French wine producers have quit the appellation system because they believe that its state-imposed rules inhibit originality and degrade quality.[55] As local foodways gain greater currency as a critique of or alternative to industrialized agriculture, it is worth recognizing that France's appellation system participated in a broader state-sponsored project of modernization that commodified local wine, spirits, and agricultural production. This modernization eliminated rivals and made small-scale producers more competitive as the country integrated into global markets after World War II.

* * *

The story of the sober revolution offers three counterintuitive lessons about business and market integration. First, European integration and globalization empowered rather than undermined small-scale wine producers through their alliances with the state and other national and international interest groups. Like more conventional actors such as banks and corporations, small-scale farmers also found ways to profit from globalization.[56] Instead of becoming passive recipients or victims of economic modernization, these producers strategized and innovated to remain competitive in global markets by regulating the place and style of production.

Second, European integration and globalization did not eliminate the notion of place but rather created an opportunity for small-scale producers to reposition it. Scholars of globalization speak of a process of deterritorialization that reduces distance, overcomes borders, and diminishes the significance of place.[57] While in some instances transnational processes like European integration and globalization have effaced boundaries, in others these processes have helped make boundaries more important. Both European integration and globalization stimulated anxieties that led to new efforts to define and regulate ownership, identity, and trade. The appellation system has been praised as a protector of local culture at a time when global markets supposedly threaten this culture. In this view, the bordered "local" and the borderless "global" become static, binary opposites. Through appellations, producers and the state successfully imposed regulations in a context of greater mobility and market integration. The solidification of locality thus depended on international actors and processes.

Third, European integration and globalization helped small-scale producers gain ground over industrialized wine and agriculture instead of what might be considered the greater likelihood of industrialization driving them out of business. The appellation system unexpectedly succeeded just when the state became committed to mass production and placed higher value in the idea that bigger is better. As industrialized viticulture and agriculture took off in the early twentieth century, so too did France's appellation system.[58] In the world of wine in twentieth-century France, the new was branded as the old, the small triumphed over the big, and the global gave new meaning to the local.

Between the 1930s and the 1970s, the appellation system grew in response to the economic and social problems associated with an imperial and then a European industrial wine system; it now serves as a critique of a more globalized industrial food system. Like earlier champions of the appellation system, Bové and his followers invoked moral concerns around the unbridled nature of global food chains. In this way, they drew on a rich yet romanticized history of French wine production to demonstrate that agriculture has cultural functions that go beyond economic efficiency even if such rhetoric makes them money. Appellation producers humanized global markets at the same time that they profited from them. In protesting McDonald's and its values, Bové defended the Roquefort appellation: "when a hamburger place springs up, Roquefort cheese dies."[59] In recent years, McDonald's, symbol of the industrial food system and global capitalism, has acted as a foil to the appellation system and to localized food more generally. Was it not the Franco-Algerian industrial wine system that legitimized the appellation system in the first place? Would the appellation system and its promotion of *terroir* have international appeal today without McWorld? Amid today's neoliberal globalization, the sober revolution—in its promotion of a more ethical model of production and consumption that would serve French interests in global markets—continues to resonate in ways that its original protagonists could have barely predicted and of which today's consumers are hardly aware.

NOTES

Introduction

1. Roland Barthes, *Mythologies* (Paris: Seuil, 1957), 83–86. Barthes originally published "Wine and Milk" in *Lettres nouvelles* in April 1955, but this earlier version of his essay did not link French wine-drinking mythologies to the social problems in Algeria, likely because the war had not yet escalated.

2. Gordon Wright makes this claim in *Rural Revolution in France: The Peasantry in the Twentieth Century* (Stanford: Stanford University Press, 1964), 27.

3. For the socioeconomic problems arising from the Algerian wine industry, see, for example, Alistair Horne, *A Savage War of Peace: Algeria, 1954–1962* (New York: New York Review of Books, 2006), 61–64. First published 1977 by Macmillan.

4. Changes in French alcohol consumption since the late 1950s are charted in Catherine Aubey and Daniel Boulet, "La consommation d'alcool en France régresse et se transforme," *Économie et statistique* 176 (April 1985): 47–56. Note that the quantity of wine consumed has declined despite population growth, but such growth was the result of a larger proportion of both children and North African Muslims in the population, two groups that tend to drink less.

5. Leo A. Loubère, *The Wine Revolution in France: The Twentieth Century* (Princeton: Princeton University Press, 1990), 167–168.

6. Notable works on the origins of France's modern wine industry include Kolleen M. Guy, *When Champagne Became French: Wine and the Making of a National Identity* (Baltimore: Johns Hopkins University Press, 2003); Olivier Jacquet, *Un siècle du construction du*

vignoble bourguignon: Les organisations vitivinicoles de 1884 aux AOC (Dijon, France: Éditions Universitaires de Dijon, 2009); Gilles Laferté, *La Bourgogne et ses vins: Image d'origine
contrôlée* (Paris: Belin, 2006); Alessandro Stanziani, "Wine Reputation and Quality Controls:
The Origin of the AOCs in 19th Century France," *European Journal of Law and Economics*
18, no. 2 (2004): 149–167; and Philip Whalen, "'Insofar as the Ruby Wine Seduces Them':
Cultural Strategies for Selling Wine in Inter-war Burgundy," *Contemporary European History*
18, no. 1 (2009): 193–224. To explain the rise of the appellation system through the work of
the INAO alone would be one-dimensional and insufficient, although Florian Humbert has
completed a much-needed work on the history of this agency in "L'INAO, de ses origines à la
fin des années 1960: Genèse et évolutions du système des vins d'AOC," (PhD Diss., Université de Bourgogne, 2011). Giulia Meloni and Johan Swinnen discuss the role of the Algerian
wine industry in spurring the creation of wine regulations in metropolitan France in "The Rise
and Fall of the World's Largest Wine Exporter—and Its Institutional Legacy," *Journal of Wine
Economics* 9, no. 1 (2014), esp. 17–23. For a summary of my perspective on the appellation
system's rise, see "'Drink Better, but Less': The Rise of France's Appellation System in the
European Community, 1946–1976," *French Historical Studies* 37 (Summer 2014): 501–530.

7. Luc Boltanski examines the rise of this new middle class in *The Making of a Class:
Cadres in French Society*, trans. Arthur Goldhammer (New York: Cambridge University Press,
1987). For an understanding of the role of consumption in post-1945 economic modernization, see Rebecca J. Pulju, *Women and Mass Consumer Society in Postwar France* (New York:
Cambridge University Press, 2011). For a cultural analysis of the shift in drinking patterns,
but one where the political dynamics of this transformation are largely absent, see Marion
Demossier, *Wine Drinking Culture in France: A National Myth or a Modern Passion?* (Cardiff: University of Wales Press, 2010); and Pekka Sulkunen, *À la recherche de la modernité:
Consommation et consommateurs d'alcool en France aujourd'hui: le regard d'un étranger*,
Report No. 178 (Helsinki: Social Research Institute of Alcohol Studies, 1988).

8. This phrase is Pierre Bourdieu's. See "Taste of Luxury, Taste of Necessity," in *The
Taste Culture Reader: Experiencing Food and Drink*, ed. Carolyn Korsmeyer (New York:
Berg, 2005), 72–78.

9. I use the words *technocrat* and *expert* interchangeably and acknowledge that these categories, like any category, are fluid. Discussions of the category of technocrat include, among
others, Jackie Clarke, *France in the Age of Organization: Factory, Home, and Nation from
the 1920s to Vichy* (New York: Berghahn, 2011), esp. 8–11; Olivier Dard, "La technocratie,"
in *La France d'un siècle à l'autre, 1914–2000: Dictionnaire critique*, ed. J.-P. Rioux and J.-F.
Sirinelli (Paris: Hachette, 1999), 883–890; Gabrielle Hecht, *The Radiance of France: Nuclear
Power and National Identity after World War II* (Cambridge, Massachusetts: The MIT Press,
2000), 28–38; and Philip Nord, *France's New Deal: From the Thirties to the Postwar Era*
(Princeton: Princeton University Press, 2010), esp. 8–11.

10. It should be noted that the Bordeaux region had created its own classification code
in 1855, but this was based on the name of the chateaux where a given wine was made, not
the larger ecological setting distinctive to each wine. It also remained a model that was specific to Bordeaux, not a nationwide model like the INAO. Bordeaux was unique in that it
could belong to its own classification and to the INAO. For the Bordeaux classification system, see Dewey Markham, *1855: A History of the Bordeaux Classification* (New York: John
Wiley & Sons, 1998).

11. This usage and its ambiguity were inscribed in the appellation laws of the early twentieth century. See Joseph Capus, "Le statut des vins à appellation d'origine: Proposition d'une
nouvelle loi," *Revue de viticulture*, 2 May 1935, 278.

12. The notion of *terroir* predates the INAO and remains partly independent of it. Its
definition has always been contested, but in a general sense, it currently denotes a blend of

soil, weather, and viticultural and vinicultural practices that come from a particular place and that impart unique qualities onto the product. For a scientific understanding of *terroir*, see Charles Frankel, *Terres de vignes* (Paris: Seuil, 2011); Emmanuelle Vaudour, *Les terroirs viticoles: Définitions, caractérisation et protection* (Paris: Dunod, 2003); and James E. Wilson, *Terroir: The Role of Geology, Climate, and Culture in the Making of French Wines* (Berkeley: University of California Press, 1998). Although it would be wrong to see *terroir* as an intrinsic part of French foodways, historical studies of the term in the wine industry and beyond include Jean-Claude Hinnewinkel, *Les terroirs viticoles: Origines et devenirs* (Bordeaux, France: Féret, 2004); Corinne Marache and Philippe Meyzie, eds., *Les produits de terroir: L'empreinte de la ville* (Rennes, France: Presses Universitaires de Rennes, 2015); Mark A. Matthews, *Terroir and Other Myths of Winegrowing* (Oakland: University of California Press, 2015); and Thomas Parker, *Tasting French Terroir: The History of an Idea* (Oakland: University of California Press, 2015).

13. Joseph Capus, *L'évolution de la législation sur les appellations d'origine: Genèse des appellations contrôlées* (Paris: Louis Larmat, 1947), 37.

14. See, for example, the INAO's wine exposition at the National Archives in Paris in 1953, published as *Le vin de France dans l'histoire* by the *Bulletin de l'Institut national des appellations d'origine des vins et eaux-de-vie*, special edition, 1953. This description comes from the agronomist Pierre Fromont, "Splendeurs et misères de la vigne et du vin dans la France moderne," *Le vin de France dans l'histoire*, 45–46.

15. No Algerian district ever received AOC status, but eleven districts obtained the lesser VDQS label in the early 1950s, which suggests the possibility (illusion?) of some Algerian wines attaining AOC status at a future date. Algeria's independence ended that possibility. See Pierre Dussine, *Le statut des vins délimités de qualité supérieure* (Montpellier, France: Causse, Graille, & Castelnau, 1961), no page numbers.

16. For this vulgar expression, which refers to high-yielding vines and which is still in use, see, for example, Jean-François Colomer, "Tempêtes sur le 'gros rouge,'" *Le Figaro*, 14 January 1976.

17. André Leveuf, "Nous vendangerons cette année les 'raisins de la colère,'" *Le Monde*, 10 April 1952.

18. See, for example, Leora Auslander, *Taste and Power: Furnishing Modern France* (Berkeley: University of California Press, 1998); and Whitney Walton, *France at the Crystal Palace: Bourgeois Taste and Artisan Manufacture in the Nineteenth Century* (Berkeley: University of California Press, 1992).

19. Quoted in Jacquet, *Un siècle du construction du vignoble bourguignon*, 105.

20. Roland Barthes, *Mythologies*, trans. Annette Lavers (New York: Hill and Wang, 1972), 61. First published 1957 by Seuil.

21. For another critique of the master narrative, see Céline Pessis, Sezin Topçu, and Christophe Bonneuil, eds., *Une autre histoire des "trente glorieuses": Modernisation, contestations et pollutions dans la France d'après-guerre* (Paris: La Découverte, 2013).

22. The literature on the continuities between the 1930s and the immediate post–World War II era has now become large. A few examples include Herrick Chapman, *State Capitalism and Working-Class Radicalism in the French Aircraft Industry* (Berkeley: University of California Press, 1991); Dard, "La technocratie," 883–890; Stanley Hoffmann, "Paradoxes of the French Political Community," in *In Search of France: The Economy, Society, and Political System in the Twentieth Century*, ed. Stanley Hoffmann et al. (New York: Harper & Row, 1963); Richard F. Kuisel, *Capitalism and the State in Modern France: Renovation and Economic Management in the Twentieth Century* (New York: Cambridge University Press, 1981); Michel Margairaz, *L'État, les finances et l'économie: Histoire d'une conversion, 1932–1952* (Paris: Comité pour l'Histoire Économique et Financière de la France, 1991); Nord,

France's New Deal; Paul-André Rosental, *L'intelligence démographique: Sciences et politiques des populations en France (1930–1960)* (Paris: Jacob, 2003); and Wright, *Rural Revolution in France*.

23. This happy consensus can be found in books as different as Jean Fourastié, *Les trente glorieuses ou la révolution invisible de 1946 à 1975* (Paris: Fayard, 1979); and Thomas Piketty, *Capital in the Twenty-First Century*, trans. Arthur Goldhammer (Cambridge: Harvard University Press, 2014).

24. I agree with Frank Trentmann that values, ideology, and collective representations shape a country's political economic arrangements. See "Political Culture and Political Economy: Interest, Ideology, and Free Trade," *Review of International Political Economy 5* (Summer 1998): 217–251.

25. Kuisel, for example, makes little mention of empire or European integration in *Capitalism and the State in Modern France*.

26. Few scholars have looked at how *both* decolonization and European integration influenced France. For the relationship between these two processes, see Megan Brown, "Drawing Algeria into Europe: Shifting French Policy and the Treaty of Rome (1951–1964)," *Modern and Contemporary France 25*, no. 2 (2017): 191–218; Muriam Haleh Davis, "Restaging Mise en Valeur: 'Postwar Imperialism' and the Plan de Constantine," *Review of Middle East Studies* 44 (January 2011): 176–186; and Peo Hansen and Stefan Jonsson, *Eurafrica: The Untold History of European Integration and Colonialism* (New York: Bloomsbury, 2014). On the relationship between decolonization and the development of modern France, see, among others, Sung-Eun Choi, *Decolonization and the French of Algeria: Bringing the Settler Colony Home* (New York: Palgrave Macmillan, 2016); Amelia H. Lyons, *The Civilizing Mission in the Metropole: Algerian Families and the French Welfare State during Decolonization* (Stanford: Stanford University Press, 2013); Kristin Ross, *Fast Cars, Clean Bodies: Decolonization and the Reordering of French Culture* (Cambridge: The MIT Press, 1995); and Todd Shepard, *The Invention of Decolonization: The Algerian War and the Remaking of France* (Ithaca: Cornell University Press, 2006).

27. Three important histories of the economic relationship between colonial Algeria and the metropole that largely ignore wine are Daniel Lefeuvre, *Chère Algérie: La France et sa colonie, 1930–1962* (Paris: Flammarion, 2005); Jacques Marseille, *Empire colonial et capitalisme français: Histoire d'un divorce* (Paris: Albin Michel, 1984); and Samir Saul, *Intérêts économiques français et décolonisation de l'Afrique du Nord (1945–1962)* (Geneva: Droz, 2016).

28. Ross, *Fast Cars, Clean Bodies*.

29. Steven M. Zdatny examines the fate of French artisans in *The Politics of Survival: Artisans in Twentieth-Century France* (New York: Oxford University Press, 1990).

30. Venus Bivar, "The Ground Beneath Their Feet: Agricultural Industrialization and the Remapping of Rural France, 1945–1976," (PhD Diss., University of Chicago, 2009); José Bové and François Dufour, *The World Is Not for Sale: Farmers Against Junk Food*, trans. Anna de Casparis (New York: Verso, 2002); Steven Laurence Kaplan, *Good Bread Is Back: A Contemporary History of French Bread, the Way It Is Made, and the People Who Make It*, trans. Catherine Porter (Durham: Duke University Press, 2006); and Susan J. Terrio, *Crafting the Culture and History of French Chocolate* (Berkeley: University of California Press, 2000), 32–33.

31. On the shift in the balance of power from merchants to vine growers in the 1930s and 1940s, see Sébastien Durand, "Négociants du Bordelais et de Bourgogne," in *Dictionnaire historique des patrons français*, ed. Jean-Claude Daumas, Alain Chatriot, Danièle Fraboulet, Patrick Fridenson, and Hervé Joly (Paris: Flammarion, 2010), 114–116; and Olivier Jacquet and Gilles Laferté, "Le contrôle républicain du marché: Vignerons et négociants sous

la Troisième République," *Annales: Histoire, science sociales* 5 (September–October 2006): 1147–1170.

32. On such labels, see, for example, "La police de la route aura-t-elle son sérum de vérité?" *France Dimanche*, 28 March 1963.

33. Quoted in Joseph Capus, "Le morcellement de la propriété viticole dans les régions de vins fins," *Bulletin de l'Office international du vin*, September–December 1945, 44. This jurist and politician was Marcel Plaisant.

34. On the trend of calling France "the hexagon" after 1962, see Shepard, *The Invention of Decolonization*, 269–272; and Eugen Weber, "L'Hexagone," in *Les lieux de mémoire*, vol. 2, *La nation*, ed. Pierre Nora (Paris: Gallimard, 1986): 97–116.

35. Here I follow Frederick Cooper, "Provincializing France," in *Imperial Formations*, ed. Ann Laura Stoler, Carole McGranahan, and Peter C. Perdue (Santa Fe: School for Advanced Research Press, 2007), 341–377.

1. Under the Influence

1. For example, J. Couton, "Pour le vente du vin au détail," *Progrès agricole et viticole*, 4 October 1931, 338. Unfortunately, authors who used this figure were not more specific about what role these millions played in the wine industry or how many of them were active in the wine lobbies. For the population of France in 1931, see, for example, A. Cholley, "La population de la France en 1931," *Annales de géographie* 41, no. 234 (1932): 638.

2. "À la Commission interministérielle de la viticulture," *Progrès agricole et viticole*, 29 December 1935, 620. This estimate of the number of Algerian producers in the 1930s comes from Georges Charles, *Le vignoble algérien et sa reconstitution* (Algiers: Jules Carbonel, 1946), 10.

3. Dr. Bourlier, "Les vignerons algériens en face du décret-loi du 30 juillet 1935," *La Voix des colons*, 26 August 1935.

4. Joseph Patouillet, "Le problème viticole et la pénible situation des vins de crus," *L'État moderne*, 3 March 1936, 175.

5. Quoted in Patricia E. Prestwich, *Drink and the Politics of Social Reform: Antialcoholism in France since 1870* (Palo Alto, California: Society for the Promotion of Science and Scholarship, 1988), 17.

6. Michel Augé-Laribé, *La politique agricole de la France de 1880 à 1940* (Paris: Presses Universitaires de France, 1950), 173.

7. Quoted in René Courtin, "La viticulture devant les pouvoirs publics," *Revue politique et parlementaire* 147 (10 June 1931): 454. See note 1.

8. Augé-Laribé, *La politique agricole*, 173; and Charles K. Warner, *The Winegrowers of France and the Government since 1875* (New York: Columbia University Press, 1960), 9.

9. Archives nationales (hereafter AN), F/10/5308. Henri Labroue, "Rapport fait au nom de la Commission des boissons chargé d'examiner le projet de loi sur la viticulture et le commerce des vins," no. 5043, Chamber of Deputies, annex to the minutes of the session of 28 May 1931, 2.

10. Patouillet, "Le problème viticole," 175.

11. On the peasants' republic, see Gordon Wright, "Peasant Politics in the Third French Republic," *Political Science Quarterly* 70 (March 1955): 75–86; on the imperial nation-state, see Gary Wilder, *The French Imperial Nation-State: Negritude and Colonial Humanism between the Two World Wars* (Chicago: University of Chicago Press, 2005); and on the empire-state, see Frederick Cooper, "Provincializing France," in *Imperial Formations*, ed. Ann Laura Stoler, Carole McGranahan, and Peter C. Perdue (Santa Fe: School for Advanced Research Press, 2007), 341–377.

12. Gordon Wright, *Rural Revolution in France: The Peasantry in the Twentieth Century* (Stanford: Stanford University Press, 1964), 13.

13. Quoted in ibid.

14. Ibid.

15. For a discussion of the peasantry in the 1930s, see Shanny Peer, *France on Display: Peasants, Provincials, and Folklore in the 1937 Paris World's Fair* (Albany: State University of New York Press, 1998).

16. For a recent study of the colonization of Algeria, see Jennifer E. Sessions, *By Sword and Plow: France and the Conquest of Algeria* (Ithaca: Cornell University Press, 2011).

17. On the colonial lobby in the early Third Republic, see L. Abrams and D. J. Miller, "Who Were the French Colonialists? A Reassessment of the Parti Colonial, 1890–1914," *Historical Journal* 19 (September 1976): 685–725; C. M. Andrew and A. S. Kanya-Forstner, "The French 'Colonial Party': Its Composition, Aims, and Influence, 1885–1914," *Historical Journal* 14 (March 1971): 99–128; and Stuart Michael Persell, *The French Colonial Lobby, 1889–1938* (Stanford: Hoover Institution Press, 1983).

18. Rudolph A. Winnacker, "Elections in Algeria and the French Colonies under the Third Republic," *American Political Science Review* 32 (April 1938): 266.

19. Hildebert Isnard, "Vineyards and Social Structure in Algeria," trans. James H. Labadie, *Diogenes* 7 (1959): 76–77. See also Fiona Barclay, Charlotte Ann Chopin, and Martin Evans, "Introduction: Settler Colonialism and French Algeria," *Settler Colonial Studies* (2017): 1–16; and David Prochaska, "The Political Culture of Settler Colonialism in Algeria: Politics in Bone (1870–1920)," *Revue de l'Occident musulman et de la Méditerranée* 48–49 (1988): 293–311.

20. Léon Archimbaud promoted the idea of "Greater France" in *La Grande France* (Paris: Hachette, 1928).

21. Rod Phillips, *French Wine: A History* (Oakland: University of California Press, 2016), 142.

22. Michel Augé-Laribé was among the first to chart the development of France's industrialized viticulture in *Le problème agraire du socialisme: La viticulture industrielle du Midi de la France* (Paris: V. Giard & E. Brière, 1907). James Simpson has more recently described it in *Creating Wine: The Emergence of a World Industry, 1840–1914* (Princeton: Princeton University Press, 2011), esp. 53–57.

23. On these factors in the growth of the Algerian wine industry, see Giulia Meloni and Johan Swinnen, "The Rise and Fall of the World's Largest Wine Exporter—and Its Institutional Legacy," *Journal of Wine Economics* 9, no. 1 (2014): 5–12.

24. Leo A. Loubère, *The Wine Revolution in France: The Twentieth Century* (Princeton: Princeton University Press), 177.

25. On the phylloxera crisis, see George D. Gale, *Dying on the Vine: How Phylloxera Transformed Wine* (Berkeley: University of California Press, 2011); and Gilbert Garrier, *Le phylloxéra: Une guerre de trente ans (1870–1900)* (Paris: Albin Michel, 1989).

26. Meloni and Swinnen, "The Rise and Fall of the World's Largest Wine Exporter," 8.

27. On the Algerian wine industry, see Susanna Barrows, "Alcohol, France, and Algeria: A Case Study in the International Liquor Trade," *Contemporary Drug Problems* (Winter 1982); Omar Bessaoud, "La viticulture oranaise, au coeur de l'économie coloniale," in *Histoire de l'Algérie à la période coloniale*, ed. Abderrahmane Bouchène, Jean-Pierre Peyroulou, Ouanassa Siari Tengour, and Sylvie Thénault (Paris: La Découverte, 2012), 425–428; Kolleen M. Guy, "Culinary Connections and Colonial Memories in France and Algeria," *Food and History* 8 (Spring 2011): 219–236; Elizabeth Heath, "The Color of French Wine: Southern Wine Producers Respond to Competition from the Algerian Wine Industry in the Early

Third Republic," *French Politics, Culture, and Society* 35 (Summer 2017): 89–110; John Strachan, "The Colonial Identity of Wine: The Leakey Affair and the Franco-Algerian Order of Things," *Social History of Alcohol and Drugs* 21 (Spring 2007): 118–137; Owen White, "The Bottle of Algiers: A Vineyard in French Algeria, 1869–1963," paper presented at Stanford University, 26 April 2012; and also White, "Roll Out the Barrel: French and Algerian Ports and the Birth of the Wine Tanker," *French Politics, Culture, and Society* 35 (Summer 2017): 111–132. For an informative analysis of the Algerian wine industry that is nevertheless closer to the events, see Hildebert Isnard, *La vigne en Algérie: Étude géographique*, 2 vols. (Gap, France: Ophrys, 1951 and 1954); for another useful study that expresses some nostalgia for French Algeria, see Paul Birebent, *Hommes, vignes et vins de l'Algérie française, 1830–1962* (Nice, France: Jacques Gandini, 2007).

28. Hildebert Isnard, "Vigne et colonisation en Algérie," *Annales de géographie* 58, no. 311 (1949): 216–217.

29. Ibid., 217. Italics in the original.

30. See, for example, V. des C., "A propos du nouveau Statut de la viticulture," *La Voix des colons*, 27 July 1931. Originally published in the Bordeaux newspaper *La Petite Gironde*.

31. Isnard, "Vigne et colonisation en Algérie," 217.

32. Isnard, "La viticulture algérienne: Erreur économique?" *La revue africaine* 50 (1956): 466–467.

33. For the barrel-makers, dockworkers, and shippers, see White, ""Roll Out the Barrel."

34. Hildebert Isnard, "Vigne et colonisation en Algérie (1880–1947)," *Annales: Économies, sociétés, civilisations* 2, no. 3 (1947): 299–300.

35. Quoted in P. Gallet, "L'approvisionnement de Paris en vin," *Annales de géographie* 48, no. 274 (1939): 359.

36. For an example of the violence of colonization, see Benjamin C. Brower, *A Desert Named Peace: The Violence of France's Empire in the Algerian Sahara, 1844–1902* (New York: Columbia University Press, 2009).

37. Isnard, "Vigne et colonisation en Algérie (1880–1947)," 299.

38. For one of those intellectuals, see Isnard, "Vigne et colonisation en Algérie (1880–1947)," 295–296. The doctor and agronomist Jules Guyot had described the relationship this way. Quoted in Isnard, *La vigne en Algérie: Étude géographique*, vol. 1, 5.

39. For an extensive study of the social ramifications of this vineyard transformation, see Gaston Galtier, *Le vignoble du Languedoc méditerranéen et du Roussillon. Études comparatives d'un vignoble de mass*, 3 vols. (Montpellier, France: Causse, Graille & Castelnau, 1960); Geneviève Gavignaud-Fontaine, *Le Languedoc viticole, la Méditerranée et l'Europe au siècle dernier (XXe)* (Montpellier, France: Publications de l'Université Paul-Valéry, 2000); and Rémy Pech, *Entreprise viticole et capitalisme en Languedoc Roussillon: Du phylloxera aux crises de mévente* (Toulouse, France: Publications de l'Université de Toulouse-Le Mirail, 1975). Other local studies of this vineyard transformation include Laura Levine Frader, *Peasants and Protest: Agricultural Workers, Politics, and Unions in the Aude, 1850–1914* (Berkeley: University of California Press, 1991); and J. Harvey Smith, "Work Routine and Social Structure in a French Village: Cruzy in the Nineteenth Century," *Journal of Interdisciplinary History* 5, no. 3 (1975): 357–382.

40. "Aramon," in *The Oxford Companion of Wine*, 3rd ed., ed. Jancis Robinson (Oxford: Oxford University Press, 2006), 28.

41. Marcel Lachiver, *Vins, vignes et vignerons: Histoire du vignoble français* (Paris: Fayard, 1988), 582–583.

42. Warner, *The Winegrowers of France*, 9.

43. Ibid., 10.

44. For a study of property in the Languedoc at the time of the French Revolution, see Noelle Plack, *Common Land, Wine, and the French Revolution: Rural Society and Economy in Southern France, c. 1789–1820* (Surrey, UK: Ashgate, 2009).

45. Pech, *Entreprise viticole et capitalisme en Languedoc-Roussillon*, 64.

46. Frader, *Peasants and Protest*, 67.

47. Ibid., 67.

48. This big estate was the Compagnie des Salins du Midi. See Simpson, *Creating Wine*, 53–57.

49. Lachiver, *Vins, vignes et vignerons*, 465.

50. The large merchants and wine companies have been studied much less than the vine growers, in part because their archives are harder to track down. For the role of merchants in the Languedoc wine industry, see Stéphane Le Bras, "La domination du marché viticole par le négoce des vins languedociens en temps de crise (1925–1939)," *Siècles* 35–36 (2012): 1–12.

51. Loubère, *The Wine Revolution in France*, 118.

52. Philippe Roudié, *Vignobles et vignerons du Bordelais (1850–1980)* (Paris: Centre National de la Recherche Scientifique, 1988), 208.

53. Lachiver, *Vins, vignes et vignerons*, 491.

54. Didier Nourrisson, *Le buveur du XIXe siècle* (Paris: Albin Michel, 1990), 36.

55. Adrien Berget, *Les vins de France: Histoire, géographie et statistique du vignoble français* (Paris: Germer Baillière, 1900), 177–182; and Antoinette Volck, *Le problème viticole franco-algérien* (Paris: Domat-Montchrestien, 1934), 85–86.

56. Leo A. Loubère, *The Red and the White: A History of Wine in France and Italy in the Nineteenth Century* (Albany: State University of New York Press, 1978), 296.

57. Ibid., 294–295.

58. Warner, *The Winegrowers of France*, 14.

59. Roudié, *Vignobles et vignerons du Bordelais*, 208.

60. On the liberal order during the Third Republic, see Richard F. Kuisel, *Capitalism and the State in Modern France: Renovation and Economic Management in the Twentieth Century* (New York: Cambridge University Press, 1981), 1–30.

61. Isnard, "La viticulture algérienne: erreur économique?," 462.

62. For the tariff structure of the French wine trade, see Giulia Meloni and Johan Swinnen, "Bugs, Tariffs, and Colonies: The Political Economy of the Wine Trade, 1860–1970," American Association of Wine Economists Working Paper 206 (October 2016): 1–43. On the political dynamics of tariff protection in the early Third Republic, see, for example, Herman Lebovics, *The Alliance of Iron and Wheat in the Third French Republic, 1860–1914* (Baton Rouge: Louisiana State University Press, 1988).

63. Quoted in Warner, *The Winegrowers of France*, 196.

64. Ibid., 34.

65. Ph. Gringberg, "Le régime des alcools et les branches organisées de l'économie agricole française," *Revue d'économique politique* 52 (March–April 1938): 407–408.

66. Thierry Fillaut, *Les Bretons et l'alcool (XIXe–XXe siècle)* (Rennes, France: École Nationale de la Santé Publique, 1991), 194.

67. Ibid., 196.

68. For more information on the home distillers, see Olivier Verdier, "Action politique et défense des intérêts catégoriels: André Liautey et le monde des groupes de pression (1919/1960)," (PhD Diss., Université Paris X, 2009).

69. Robert O. Paxton, *French Peasant Fascism: Henry Dorgères's Greenshirts and the Crises of French Agriculture, 1929–1939* (New York: Oxford University Press, 1997), 25.

70. Nourrisson, *Le buveur du XIXe siècle*, 81.

71. Like the merchants, the commercial distillers are somewhat murky in the historical record.

72. "Où vont les milliards de l'alcool," *L'Express*, 5 September 1953, 6–7.

73. On the global wine industry in the late nineteenth and early twentieth centuries, see Simpson, *Creating Wine*; on the impact of globalization on the southern wine producers, see Elizabeth Heath, *Wine, Sugar, and the Making of Modern France: Global Economic Crisis and the Racialization of French Citizenship, 1870–1910* (New York: Cambridge University Press, 2014).

74. The revolt of 1907 has inspired many studies. See, for example, Georges Ferré, *1907, la guerre du vin: Chronique d'une désobéissance civique dans le Midi* (Portet-sur-Garonne, France: Loubatières, 1997); Félix Napo, *1907, la révolte des vignerons* (Toulouse, France: Privat, 1982); and Jean Sagnes, Monique Pech, and Rémy Pech, *1907 en Languedoc-Roussillon* (Montpellier, France: Espace Sud, 1997).

75. Joseph Capus, "Le statut des vins à appellation d'origine: proposition d'une nouvelle loi," *Revue de viticulture*, 2 May 1935, 278–279.

76. Harry Paul, *Science, Vine, and Wine in Modern France* (New York: Cambridge University Press, 1996), 105; and Giulia Meloni and Johan Swinnen, "The Political Economy of Wine Regulations," *Journal of Wine Economics* 8, no. 3 (2013): 262.

77. Paul Lukacs, *Inventing Wine* (New York: Norton, 2012), 212; and Loubère, *The Wine Revolution in France*, 119–121.

78. Capus, "Le statut des vins à appellation d'origine," 280.

79. Ibid., 278.

80. Loubère makes this claim in *The Wine Revolution in France*, 130. On the statist experiment in agriculture in the 1930s, see Alain Chatriot, Edgar Leblanc, and Édouard Lynch, eds., *Organiser les marchés agricoles: Le temps des fondateurs des années 1930 aux années 1950* (Paris: Armand Colin, 2012).

81. *Bulletin d'information de l'Union fédérale de la consommation*, September–October 1952, 16.

82. Quoted in Warner, *The Winegrowers of France*, 129.

83. Quoted in ibid.

84. Quoted in ibid.

85. As remembered in "La Fédération des Associations viticoles contre la solidarité des ruraux," *Le Bouilleur de France*, December 1951.

86. Quoted in Warner, *The Winegrowers of France*, 128.

87. Quoted in ibid., 129.

88. Gaston Defossé, *La place du consommateur dans l'économie dirigée* (Paris: Presses Universitaires de France, 1941), 103–104.

89. Prestwich, *Drink and the Politics of Social Reform*, 208.

90. Gringberg, "Le régime des alcools," 429.

91. Tom Kemp, *The French Economy, 1913–39: The History of a Decline* (New York: St. Martin's Press, 1972), 140.

92. Quoted in Sarah Howard, "Selling Wine to the French: Official Attempts to Increase French Wine Consumption, 1931–1936," *Food and Foodways* 12, no. 4 (2004): 204.

93. Capus, "Le statut des vins à appellation d'origine," 281.

94. Ibid., 283.

95. For French responses to hybrids, see Paul, *Science, Vine, and Wine in Modern France*, 65–120.

96. "La loi viticole," *La Voix des colons*, 20 July 1931.

97. Prestwich, *Drink and the Politics of Social Reform*, 200.

98. See, for example, René Pinon, "Les nouvelles conceptions de l'État," *Revue économique internationale* 4 (October 1929): 9; or the series of articles in *L'État moderne* on 12 December 1929 and 3 March 1936.

99. Quoted in Howard, "Selling Wine to the French," 204.

100. Jean Sagnes, "Viticulture et politique dans la 1re moitié du XX siècle: Aux origines du statut de la viticulture," in *La viticulture française aux XIXe et XXe siècles*, ed. Jean Sagnes (Béziers, France: Presses du Languedoc, 1993), 56; and Capus, "Le statut des vins à appellation d'origine."

101. Florian Humbert, "L'INAO, de ses origines à la fin des années 1960: Genèse et évolutions du système des vins d'AOC," (PhD Diss., Université de Bourgogne, 2011), 100.

102. For the debate about the true France, see Herman Lebovics, *True France: The Wars over Cultural Identity, 1900–1945* (Ithaca: Cornell University Press, 1992).

103. Gilles Laferté, *La Bourgogne et ses vins: Image d'origine contrôlée* (Paris: Belin, 2006).

104. Gilles Laferté, "The Folklorization of French Farming: Marketing Luxury Wine in the Interwar Years," *French Historical Studies* 34 (Fall 2011): 679–712; and Philip Whalen, "'Insofar as the Ruby Wine Seduces Them': Cultural Strategies for Selling Wine in Inter-war Burgundy," *Contemporary European History* 18, no. 1 (2009): 67–98.

105. Quoted in J.-L. Gaston Pastre, "Le problème du vin," *Revue des deux mondes*, 15 November 1935, 365–366.

106. Gabriel Taïx, *La faillite de la viticulture est-elle pour demain?* (Bordeaux, France: Delmas, 1934), 48. Italics in the original.

107. For a discussion of how agronomists, demographers, economists, and state officials started to doubt the viability of French Algeria in the 1930s, see Daniel Lefeuvre, *Chère Algérie: La France et sa colonies, 1930–1962* (Paris: Flammarion, 2005).

108. See, for example, Volck, *Le problème viticole Franco-Algérien*, 53–55.

109. Quoted in Augé-Laribé, *Politique agricole*, 428.

110. Quoted in Lefeuvre, *Chère Algérie*, 74.

111. Édouard Kruger, *Les bienfaits de l'Union douanière métropole-Algérie et la question vinicole* (Oran, Algeria: Syndicat du Commerce des Vins en Gros de Département d'Oran, 1933). See also AN, F/10/5360. Letter from Doctor Bourlier, president of the General Confederation of Algerian Vine Growers to the prime minister, 16 August 1935, 3. On the construction of French identity in Algeria, see Jonathan K. Gosnell, *The Politics of Frenchness in Colonial Algeria, 1930–1954* (Rochester: University of Rochester Press, 2002), especially pp. 13–40.

112. Alfred Sauvy, *Histoire économique de la France entre les deux guerres*, vol. 2 (Paris: Economica, 1984), 160.

113. Nathan Pedigo, "The Struggle for *Terroir* in French Algeria: Land, Wine, and Contested Identity in the French Empire," (PhD Diss., Southern Illinois University, 2015), 165.

114. Sully Ledermann, *Alcool, alcoolisme, alcoolisation: Données scientifiques de caractère physiologique, économique et social* (Paris: Presses Universitaires de France, 1956), 34.

115. Ibid., 74.

116. For a discussion of this wine propaganda committee in the 1930s, see Bertrand Dargelos, *La lutte antialcoolique en France depuis le XIXe siècle* (Paris: Dalloz, 2008), 186–201; and Howard, "Selling Wine to the French," 197–224.

117. Phillips, *French Wine*, 197.

118. Quoted in ibid., 195.

119. Quoted in ibid., 199.

120. Quoted in Howard, "Selling Wine to the French," 212.

121. Quoted in ibid., 213.

122. AN, F/10/5383. Jean Prats, "La consommation et la protection des vins français dans nos colonies et pays de protectorat," no date but likely 1932 or 1933.

123. Quoted in Howard, "Selling Wine to the French," 213.

124. Kim Munholland, "*Mon docteur le vin*: Wine and Health in France, 1900–1950," in *Alcohol: A Social and Cultural History*, ed. Mack P. Holt (New York: Berg, 2006), 77–90.

125. Quoted in Howard, "Selling Wine to the French," 212.

126. On the British school meal service, see James Vernon, *Hunger: A Modern History* (Cambridge, Massachusetts: The Belknap Press of Harvard University Press, 2007), 161–180.

127. Prestwich, *Drink and the Politics of Social Reform*, 216–224.

128. See, for example, Susanna Barrows, "'Parliaments of the People': The Political Culture of Cafés in the Early Third Republic," in *Drinking: Behavior and Belief in Modern History*, ed. Susanna Barrows and Robin Room (Berkeley: University of California Press, 1991), 87–97; and W. Scott Haine, *The World of the Paris Café: Sociability among the French Working Class, 1789–1914* (Baltimore: Johns Hopkins University Press, 1996).

129. Nourrisson, *Le buveur du XIXe siècle*, 7–10.

130. Prestwich, *Drink and the Politics of Social Reform*, 23.

131. W. Scott Haine discusses café life in the 1930s in "Drink, Sociability, and Social Class in France, 1789–1945: The Emergence of a Proletarian Public Sphere," in *Alcohol: A Social and Cultural History*, 121–144.

132. On the Vichy regime and its prehistory, see, for example, Robert O. Paxton, *Vichy France: Old Guard and New Order* (New York: Alfred A. Knopf, 1972); and Julian Jackson, *France: The Dark Years, 1940–1944* (New York: Oxford University Press, 2001).

133. Quoted in M. C. Cleary, *Peasants, Politicians, and Producers: The Organization of Agriculture in France since 1918* (New York: Cambridge University Press, 1989), 92.

134. Quoted in Barthe, *Le combat d'un parlementaire sous Vichy: Journal des années de guerre, 1940–1943*, introduction, notes, and postface by Jean Sagnes (Gap, France: Singulières, 2007), 157.

135. Munholland, "'Mon docteur le vin,'" 85.

136. Léon Douarche, *Le vin et la vigne dans l'économie nationale française* (Paris: Cahiers de la Réorganisation Économique, 1943), 96–97.

137. Léon Douarche, *La vigne française et l'Europe* (Paris: Rassemblement National Populaire, 1941).

138. Warner, *The Winegrowers of France*, 162.

139. Gavignaud-Fontaine, *Le Languedoc viticole*, 121.

140. Ibid., 121–122.

141. AN, 80AJ/71. Jean Branas, "La production viticole française en 1954: rapport au Conseil supérieur de l'agriculture (Section Union française)," 5 September 1954, 106.

142. Pedigo, "The Struggle for *Terroir* in French Algeria," 218.

143. Stéphane Le Bras, "Négoce et négociants en vins dans l'Hérault: Pratiques, influences, trajectoires (1900–1970)," vol. 1 (PhD Diss., Université de Montpellier III—Paul Valéry, 2013), 294.

144. On Vichy's corporatism in agriculture, see Isabel Boussard, *Vichy et la Corporation paysanne* (Paris: Presses de la Foundation Nationale des Sciences Politiques, 1980).

145. Douarche, *Le vin et la vigne dans l'économie nationale française*, 67.

146. For an understanding of the Interprofessional Committee of the Wine of Champagne (CIVC), see Florian Humbert, "La Champagne viticole au prisme du national, de la mise en place des AOC à la création du CIVC," in *La construction des territoires du*

Champagne (1811–1911–2011), ed. Serge Wolikow (Dijon, France: Éditions Universitaires de Dijon, 2013), 197–205.

147. Phillips, *French Wine*, 244.

148. In 1938 and 1939, doctors at several medical schools drew a link between habitual wine drinking and alcoholism. See Prestwich, *Drink and the Politics of Social Reform*, 238–242.

149. M. Lapicque, "L'abus du vin (cri d'alarme)," session of 27 February 1940, *Bulletin de l'Académie de Médecine* (1940): 156.

150. M. Lapicque, "Au nom de la Commission du vin," session of 28 May 1940, *Bulletin de l'Académie de Médecine* (1940): 427.

151. On Vichy's anti-alcoholism, see Marc Boninchi, *Vichy et l'ordre moral* (Paris: Presses Universitaires de France, 2005).

152. Munholland, "'Mon docteur le vin,'" 84.

153. Ibid., 85.

154. Warner, *The Winegrowers of France and the Government*, 158.

155. Ibid.

156. Michele Cépède, *Agriculture et alimentation en France durant la IIe Guerre mondiale* (Paris: Éditions Génin, 1961), 360.

157. Don Kladstrup and Petie Kladstrup, *Wine and War: The French, the Nazis, and the Battle for France's Greatest Treasure* (New York: Broadway Books, 2001), 58–60.

158. Ibid., 89.

159. On black markets during the occupation, see Fabrice Grenard, *La France du marché noir (1940–1949)* (Paris: Payot, 2008); Kenneth Mouré, "Food Rationing and the Black Market in France, 1940–1944," *French History* 24, no. 2 (2010): 262–282; and Paul Sanders, *Histoire du marché noir* (Paris: Perrin, 2001).

160. Jules Milhau, "L'avenir de la viticulture française," *Revue économique* 4, no. 5 (1953): 720.

161. Humbert, "L'INAO, de ses origines à la fin des années 1960," 341.

162. Prestwich, *Drink and the Politics of Social Reform*, 251.

163. Warner, *The Winegrowers of France*, 161.

164. AN, F/10/5362. "Procès-verbal de la réunion du Comité national du 4 juin 1942 à Paris," 4.

165. For Sauvy's recollections of the wartime experience, see "Problème de l'alcoolisme," *Bulletin du Conseil économique*, 22 January 1959, 28.

166. AN, 72AJ/247. "Programme constructif de lutte contre l'alcoolisme," 1945, 8–9.

167. AN, 72AJ/247. "Note sur la création et l'organisation d'un Ministère de la Population et de l'Hygiène," 1945, 13.

168. Gavignaud-Fontaine, *Le Languedoc viticole*, 122.

169. Jules Milhau, *Le problème français du vin* (Montpellier, France: Causse, Graille, & Castelnau, 1945), 15. Quoted in Gavignaud-Fontaine, *Le Languedoc viticole*.

170. Quoted in Prestwich, *Drink and the Politics of Social Reform*, 17.

2. The Imperative of Intervention

1. "Le nombre des alcooliques a triplé en France en 6 ans," *Combat*, 5 December 1951.

2. "Proportionnellement à son revenu, le Français boit dix fois plus d'alcool que l'Américain et cinq fois plus que le Britannique," *Le Monde*, 20 February 1954. It is worth noting that the WHO did not include statistics on Russian drinking habits.

3. Jean Claude, "Le coût de l'alcoolisme," *Le Figaro*, 12 January 1951.

4. For a list of the lobbies allied against alcohol at this time, see Alfred Sauvy, *De Paul Reynaud à Charles de Gaulle: Un économiste face aux hommes politiques, 1934–1967* (Paris: Casterman, 1972), 185.

5. On the continued domination of Parliament by rural interests in the 1950s, see Mattei Dogan, "La Représentation parlementaire du monde rural," in *Les paysans et la politique dans la France contemporaine*, ed. Jacques Fauvet and Henri Mendras (Paris: Armand Colin, 1958), 207–227.

6. For the French position on alcoholism at the WHO, see the Archives of the World Health Organization (hereafter AWHO), 461/1/3. Dr. A. Cavaillon, "Report on Alcoholism," 30 August 1947. For an understanding of how the WHO influenced French notions of alcoholism, see Centre des Archives contemporaines (hereafter CAC), 19920020, art. 28. Jean Crozier, "L'activité du Comité national français de défense contre l'alcoolisme," *5ème cours d'été d'études scientifiques pour la prévention de l'alcoolisme* (22 June–3 July 1959). French researchers challenged some of the observations of the Yale Center of Alcohol Studies, where E. M. Jellinek, one of the leading alcohol researchers at the WHO at this time, worked. See, for example, Paul Perrin, "Les travaux du Centre américain de Yale," *Études anti-alcooliques*, April–June 1950, 30.

7. Alfred Sauvy, "Le vin et l'économie française," *La Journée vinicole*, 4 August 1953.

8. Pierre Le Roy de Boiseaumarié, "Il faut en finir . . . ," *La Journée vinicole*, 6 July 1954. These articles originally appeared in *Midi libre*, the most widely circulated newspaper of the Languedoc. Significantly, they would be reproduced in INED statistician Sully Ledermann's influential *Alcool, alcoolisme, alcoolisation: Données scientifiques de caractère physiologique, économique et social* (Paris: Presses Universitaires de France, 1956).

9. "Le combat contre les paysans," *Alcool et dérivés*, October 1954, 11. Originally published in *L'Union agricole du Loir-et-Cher*.

10. G. de Magnin, "Tout va très bien, M. le Baron!" *L'Algérie agricole et viticole*, 6 September 1952.

11. Giulia Meloni and Johan Swinnen, "The Rise and Fall of the World's Largest Wine Exporter—and Its Institutional Legacy," *Journal of Wine Economics* 9, no. 1 (2014): 23.

12. René Cercler, "Le marché du vin: une défaite du dirigisme," *L'Information*, 23 April 1953.

13. Centre des Archives économiques et financières (hereafter CAEF), 4A/2251/1. Jacques Bonnet de la Tour, Gabriel Pallez, and Jean Saint-Geours, "Note générale sur le problème de l'alcool," 1953, 31, 46.

14. Ibid., 1.

15. Gilbert Noël, *Du pool vert à la politique agricole commune: Les tentatives de la Communauté agricole européenne entre 1945 et 1955* (Paris: Economica, 1988).

16. Alan S. Milward, *The Reconstruction of Western Europe, 1945–1951* (Berkeley: University of California Press, 1984), 443; and Noël, *Du pool vert à la politique agricole commune*, 424–426.

17. Alan S. Milward, *The European Rescue of the Nation-State* (Berkeley: University of California Press, 1992), 291–292.

18. On the relationship between technocrats and peasants, see Pierre Muller, *Le technocrate et le paysan. Essai sur la politique française de modernisation de l'agriculture, de 1945 à nos jours* (Paris: Les Éditions Ouvrières, 1984).

19. "La bataille de l'alcool," *Alcool et dérivés*, June 1953, 5. The article was written by Jean Closier and originally published in *L'Union agricole*.

20. Sauvy, "Le vin et l'économie française."

21. Archives nationales (hereafter AN), 80AJ/55. René Dumont, "Le vignoble languedocien et le canal du bas-Rhône," 25 November 1952. See also Dumont's articles "Alcool, ou

lait et viande? Étude technique et économique d'orientation agricole et alimentaire," *Population* 8, no. 1 (1953): 57–72; and "Remontons la vigne sur les coteaux," *Bulletin des transports*, February 1953.

22. See, for example, René Dumont, *Le problème agricole français: Esquisse d'un plan d'orientation et d'equipement* (Paris: Les Éditions Nouvelles, 1946).

23. Alfred Sauvy, *Histoire économique de la France entre les deux guerres (1931–1939): De Pierre Laval à Paul Reynaud*, vol. 2 (Paris: Fayard, 1967), 378.

24. Dumont, "Alcool, ou lait et viande?" 70. Italics in the original.

25. For French responses to Americanization after 1945, see Richard F. Kuisel, *Seducing the French: The Dilemma of Americanization* (Berkeley: University of California Press, 1993).

26. Dumont, "Alcool, ou lait et viande?," 67. See note 1.

27. Robert Debré and Alfred Sauvy, *Des Français pour la France* (Paris: Gallimard, 1946), 20.

28. See, for example, Dumont, *Le problème agricole français*, 101.

29. André Chaudières, "Le vin: richesse nationale," *Syndicalisme*, October 1952.

30. On these feudal interests, see, for example, Georges Malignac and Robert Colin, *L'alcoolisme* (Paris: Presses Universitaires de France, 1954), 88.

31. Dumont, *Le problème agricole français*, 99–100.

32. Jules Milhau, "L'avenir de la viticulture française," *La Revue économique* 4, no. 5 (1953): 700.

33. Ibid., 724.

34. Nessim Znaien, "Le vin et la viticulture en Tunisie coloniale (1881–1956): Entre synapse et apartheid," *French Cultural Studies* 26, no. 2 (2015): 149. See note 2.

35. See Dumont's "Alcool, ou lait et viande?"

36. AN, 80AJ/55. Philippe Lamour, "Note introductive relative à l'économie viticole dans le deuxième plan de modernisation," 4 March 1953.

37. For Lamour's story, see Jean-Robert Pitte, *Philippe Lamour, 1903–1992: Père de l'aménagement du territoire en France* (Paris: Fayard, 2002); see also his autobiography, *Le cadran solaire* (Paris: Robert Laffont, 1980).

38. On the Economic Council proposition, see Charles K. Warner, *The Winegrowers and the Government since 1875* (New York: Columbia University Press, 1960), 189.

39. AN, 80AJ/55. René Dumont, "Le vignoble languedocien et le canal du bas-Rhône," 25 November 1952, 13. Italics in the original.

40. Daniel Lefeuvre, *Chère Algérie: La France et sa colonie, 1932–1962* (Paris: Flammarion, 2005), 327–365.

41. See, for example, Georges Charles, *Le vignoble algérien et sa reconstitution* (Algiers: Jules Carbonel, 1946), 13–14.

42. Gaston Galtier, *Le vignoble du Languedoc méditerranéen et du Roussillon: Étude comparative d'un vignoble de masse,* vol. 3 (Montpellier, France: Causse, Graille & Castelnau, 1960), 170.

43. CAEF, 4A/2261/1. Jacques Mayoux, "Note sur les conclusions d'une enquête menée parmi les négociants en vin de Paris," September 1953.

44. For the settler position, see, for example, Édouard Kruger, "L'Algérie et la vigne: Simple réponse à un paragraphe de l'article de M. Alfred Sauvy," *La Journée vinicole*, 27 August 1953. To gain a sense of the grinding poverty, hunger, and everyday struggle that many indigenous people experienced under French rule, see Mohammed Dib's novel *L'incendie* (Paris: Seuil, 1954).

45. Louis Leroy, "Statut de l'alcool: Problème de l'orientation à donner à la production agricole et des mesures propres à organiser un nouveau statut de l'alcool," sessions of 11 and 12 July 1950, *Journal officiel de la République française: Avis et rapports du Conseil économique*, 13 July 1950; and Gabriel Taïx, "Étude des problèmes posés par les excédents d'alcool," session of 8 July 1953, *Journal officiel de la République française: Avis et rapports du Conseil économique*, 21 July 1953.

46. Sauvy, *De Paul Reynaud à Charles de Gaulle*, 185.

47. AN, CE/429. Commission of Industrial Production, Working Group for the Study of the Problem of Petroleum Products, "Procès-verbal de la séance du jeudi 7 mai 1953 à 10 heures 30."

48. *Bulletin d'information de l'Union fédérale de la consommation*, September–October 1952, 16.

49. On the importance of being small in the luxury wine industry, see Joseph Capus, "Le morcellement de la propriété viticole dans les régions de vins fins," *Bulletin de l'Office international du vin*, September–December 1945, 42–44.

50. Ledermann, *Alcool, alcoolisme, alcoolisation*, 27.

51. AN, 80AJ/71. Viticultural Group, Agricultural Sub-Commission, Committee on the Section of Metropolitan-Overseas Economic Integration, General Commissariat of the Plan, "Compte rendu de la réunion du vendredi 18 février 1955," 8.

52. René Cercler, "La vérité sur nos exportations de boissons," *L'Information*, 14 February 1952.

53. Mis de Lur-Saluces, "Les grands vins de France," *Revue des deux mondes*, 15 March 1953, 286.

54. See, for example, Jean-François Gravier, *Paris et le désert français: Décentralisation, équipement, population* (Paris: Le Portulan, 1947).

55. CAEF, 4A/2261/1. Jacques Mayoux, "Note sur le projet de loi #5827, relatif à l'orientation de la production viticole," November 1953, 2.

56. On the French temperance movement, see Bertrand Dargelos, *La lutte antialcoolique en France depuis le XIXe siècle* (Paris: Dalloz, 2008); and Patricia E. Prestwich, *Drink and the Politics of Social Reform: Antialcoholism in France since 1870* (Palo Alto, California: Society for the Promotion of Science and Scholarship, 1988).

57. On how the wine lobbies benefited from the return of Parliament, see Léon Dérobert, "Alcoolisme et législation," *Alcool ou santé* 3 (1952): 7–8; and M. Laignel-Lavastie, "Note abrégée sur l'alcoolisme en France, de 1912 à 1944," session of 4 December 1945, *Bulletin de l'Académie de Médecine* (1945): 679.

58. André Monnier, "Un meurtrier en liberté," *Alcool ou santé* 3 (1951): 9.

59. Dumont, *Le problème agricole français*, 101.

60. Ibid., 99–100.

61. AN, F/10/5383. "Tract de l'Association de propagande pour le vin financé par le Comité national."

62. Malignac and Colin mention this in *L'alcoolisme*, 80.

63. *Alcool ou santé* 4 (1952): 33.

64. Albert Michot, "Le problème du lait en France," *Population* 2, no. 1 (1947): 69.

65. Mlle Serin, "L'alcoolisme des enfants," session of 22 June 1954, *Bulletin de l'Académie de Médecine* (1954): 325–326.

66. Michot, "Le problème du lait en France," 78.

67. This issue came before the Economic Council in 1952. See Serpos Tidjani, "Fabrication, importation, vente et consommation des boissons alcooliques en AOF, AEF, Cameroun et Togo," session of 20 May 1952, *Journal officiel de la République française: Avis et rapports du Conseil économique*, 21 May 1952.

68. Gabriel Taïx, "Étude des problèmes posés par les excédents d'alcool," session of 8 July 1953, *Journal officiel de la République française: Avis et rapports du Conseil économique,* 21 July 1953, 522.

69. Warner, *The Winegrowers and the Government,* 195.

70. See, for example, Emmanuel La Gravière, "L'alcoolisation des populations d'outre-mer," in *Problèmes sociaux: La prostitution, l'alcoolisme, le logement* (Paris: Fayard, 1954).

71. Étienne May, "Le problème de l'alcoolisme en France," sessions of 12 and 14 January 1954, *Journal officiel de la République française: Avis et rapports du Conseil économique,* 30 January 1954, 187.

72. Taïx, "Étude des problèmes posés par les excédents d'alcool," 522.

73. Dumont, "Remontons la vigne sur les coteaux," 108.

74. Sauvy, "Le vin et l'économie française."

75. Henri Géralin, "Le problème de l'alcoolisme dans les territoires d'outre-mer," *Population* 8, no. 2 (1953): 310.

76. Prestwich, *Drink and the Politics of Social Reform,* 263.

77. Georges Létinier, "Éléments d'un bilan national de l'alcoolisme," *Population* 1, no. 2 (1946): 319.

78. Quoted in May, "Le problème de l'alcoolisme en France," 180.

79. May, "Le problème de l'alcoolisme en France," 180–181.

80. For the INED's role in the campaign against alcoholism, see Luc Berlivet, "Les démographes et l'alcoolisme: Du 'fléau social' au 'risque de santé,'" *Vingtième Siècle* 95 (July–September 2007): 93–113. On the INED, see Paul-André Rosental, *L'intelligence démographique: Sciences et politiques des populations en France (1930–1960)* (Paris: Odile Jacob, 2003). For an understanding of the technocrats at the Ministry of Finance, albeit one that excludes any discussion of alcoholism, see Aude Terray, *Des francs-tireurs aux experts: L'organisation de la prévision économique au ministère des Finances, 1948–1968* (Paris: Comité pour l'Histoire Économique et Financière de la France, 2002).

81. Dr. De Leobardy, "Le vin et le foie," *Le progrès agricole et viticole,* 29 March 1953, 182.

82. For the relationship between public health and the economy in postwar France, see Daniel Benamouzig, *La santé au miroir de l'économie: Une histoire de l'économie de la santé en France* (Paris: Presses Universitaires de France, 2005).

83. See, for example, Léon Dérobert, *L'économie de l'alcoolisme* (Paris: Institut National d'Hygiène, 1953).

84. May, "Le problème de l'alcoolisme en France," 185.

85. See, for example, Jacques Sylvain Brunaud, *Rapport sur le coût annuel et la prévention de l'alcoolisme* updated and revised (Paris: Comité Central d'Enquête sur le Coût et le Rendement des Services Publics, 1955); Malignac and Colin, *L'alcoolisme*; and Ledermann, *Alcool, alcoolisme, alcoolisation.*

86. Malignac and Colin, *L'alcoolisme,* 87.

87. This claim is based on my assessment of the newspaper clippings in the private archives of the Association nationale de prévention en alcoologie et addictologie (hereafter ANPAA), S512.

88. See, for example, G. Pilliet, "L'alcoolisme grève de 20% le coût de notre production," *La Vie française,* 24 September 1954; and Georges Kletch, "Douze décrets contre l'alcoolisme," *La Vie française,* 26 November 1954.

89. Alfred Sauvy, "Faits et problèmes du jour," *Population* 5, no. 1 (1950): 8.

90. *Journal officiel de la République française: Débats parlementaires, Assemblée nationale,* 22 October 1952, 4296.

91. *Le Monde*, 22 October 1952.

92. For peasant attitudes toward consumerism, see, for example, Laurence Wylie, *Village in the Vaucluse* (Cambridge, Massachusetts: Harvard University Press, 1957, 1974), esp. 153–184. For working-class consumer aspirations in the interwar years, see Tyler Stovall, *The Rise of the Paris Red Belt* (Berkeley: University of California Press, 1990). For post-1945 housing, see Kenny Cupers, *The Social Project: Housing Postwar France* (Minneapolis: University of Minnesota Press, 2014); and Nicole C. Rudolph, *At Home in Postwar France: Modern Mass Housing and the Right to Comfort* (New York: Berghahn Books, 2015).

93. Three of these experts were René Dumont, Alfred Fabre-Luce, and Jean Morard. See Henri Fontanille, "Le vin, principal agent de la suralcoolisation?" *Algérie agricole et viticole*, 30 May–6 June 1953. Originally published in *Le Monde*.

94. Henri Fontanille, "Perspectives algériennes," *Algérie agricole et viticole*, 23 May 1953. Originally published in *Le Monde*, 8 May 1953.

95. Marcel Niedergang, "Avant le Congrès international contre l'alcoolisme," *Réforme*, 30 August 1952.

96. Jacques Delbo, "Les vrais responsables de l'alcoolisme: ce sont les parlementaires," *L'Aurore*, 27 December 1953.

97. For female consumers in the early Third Republic, see Lisa Tiersten, *Marianne in the Market: Envisioning Consumer Society in Fin-de-Siècle France* (Berkeley: University of California Press, 2001). For the role of women in post-1945 consumerism, see, for example, Rebecca J. Pulju, *Women and Mass Consumer Society* (New York: Cambridge University Press, 2011).

98. Cited in *Alcool ou santé* 2 (1952): 11.

99. Marcel Bresard, "L'opinion publique et l'alcoolisme," *Population* 3, no. 3 (1948): 548.

100. Henri Bastide, "Une enquête sur l'opinion publique à l'égard de l'alcoolisme," *Population* 9, no. 1 (1954): 42.

101. Bastide, "Une enquête sur l'opinion publique à l'égard de l'alcoolisme," 15.

102. Jean-Raymond Guyon, *Le régime économique de l'alcool* (Bordeaux, France: Delmas, 1950), 22.

103. See, for example, 2nd session of Friday, 31 March 1950, *Journal officiel de la République française: Débats parlementaires, Assemblée nationale*, 1 April 1950, 2727–2728.

104. Jean-Raymond Guyon, *Le problème de l'alcool: Les travaux de la Commission extraparlementaire* (Bordeaux, France: Delmas, 1952), 8.

105. Henri Cayre, "L'agriculture présente du nouveau," *Alcool et dérivés*, October 1952, 1.

106. E.-J. Dauphin, "Réflexions sur la réponse du Statut viticole et . . . la démocratie," *La Journée vinicole*, 28 August 1953. See also Lucien Daumas, "Halte à la dictature viticole," *Midi vinicole*, 28 February 1953.

107. For the full story, see Bernard E. Brown, "Alcohol and Politics in France," *American Political Science Review* 51 (December 1957), 988–989; see also Malignac and Colin, *L'alcoolisme*, 90–91. Jean Meynaud also noted that rural interests contributed to Mayer's fall in *Les groupes de pression en France* (Paris: Armand Colin, 1958), 312.

108. Jean Closier, "La bataille de l'alcool," *Alcool et dérivés*, June 1953, 5. Originally published in *L'Union agricole*.

109. "Décret #53-703 du 9 août 1953 relatif au régime économique de l'alcool et portant organisation d'un plan sucrier," *Journal officiel de la République française: Lois et décrets*, 10 August 1953, 7042–7045.

110. Georges Malignac, "Le nouveau statut de l'alcool," *Alcool ou santé* 10 (1953): 11.

111. Malignac and Colin, *L'alcoolisme*, 49.

112. May, "Le problème de l'alcoolisme en France," 185.

113. AN, C/15606. Family, Population, and Public Health Commission, "Séance du mercredi 21 juillet 1954."

114. Session of 10 August 1954, *Journal officiel de la République française: Documents parlementaires, Assemblée nationale,* annex no. 9126, 1661–1662.

115. For these different groups, see *Alcool ou santé* 9 (1953): 23–27; "Adoption d'un voeu au nom de la Commission de l'alcoolisme," session of 30 June 1953, *Bulletin de l'Académie de Médecine* (1953): 383; and Brown, "Alcohol and Politics in France," 993.

116. Session of 10 August 1954, *Journal officiel de la République française: Documents parlementaires, Assemblée nationale,* annex no. 9126.

117. 2nd session of Tuesday, 10 August 1954, *Journal officiel de la République française: Débats parlementaires, Assemblée nationale,* 11 August 1954, 4067–4068.

118. See, for example, Archives de l'Institut Pierre Mendès France (hereafter IPMF), Carton 1 (Économie). "Rapport du Groupe du Travail Gruson, juillet 1954: Annexes: Premières mesures d'application," B5-B6; and AN, F/10/7148. General Commissariat of the Plan, "Préparation d'un programme d'action économique: Questions agricoles," 2 July 1954.

119. AN, F/10/5386. "Décret #54-955 du 14 septembre 1954 relatif à l'assainissement de la production viticole," from *Journal officiel,* 24 September 1954. Jean-Robert Pitte discusses this canal project in *Philippe Lamour, 1903–1992,* 180–182.

120. Pierre Mendès France, "La reconversion de l'économie française et le problème de l'alcool: Discours prononcé à l'inauguration de la foire-exposition d'Annecy, 26 septembre 1954," in *Oeuvres complètes: Gouverner c'est choisir, 1954–1955,* vol. 3 (Paris: Gallimard, 1986), 352.

121. Ibid. For a political analysis of Mendès France's sweetened milk campaign, see Joseph Bohling, "The Mendès France Milk Regime: Alcoholism as a Problem of Agricultural Subsidies, 1954–1955," *French Politics, Culture, and Society* 32 (Winter 2014): 97–120; and Annie Collovald, "Le verre de lait de Pierre Mendès France ou l'oubli des origines politiques," in *La Santé dans tous ses états,* ed. Alain Garrigou (Biarritz, France: Atlantica, 2000), 35–54. For a cultural history of Mendès France's milk program, see Didier Nourrisson, "Le lait à l'école. Pédagogie de la voie lactée," in *A Votre Santé! Éducation et santé sous la IVe République,* ed. Didier Nourrisson (Saint-Étienne, France: Publications de l'Université de Saint-Étienne, 2002), 85–96.

122. IPMF, Carton 4 (Économie). "Conférence de presse—Lepicard & Génin—La FNSEA (Fédération nationale des syndicates d'exploitants agricoles) estime que le marché rural est le facteur décisive du relèvement de l'économie nationale, 22 août 1954."

123. On the politics of the French dairy industry, see Denis Pesche, *Le syndicalisme agricole spécialisé: Entre la spécificité des intérêts et le besoin d'alliances* (Paris: L'Harmattan, 2000), esp. 152–156.

124. IPMF, Carton 4 (Économie). "Conférence de presse—Lepicard et Génin."

125. IPMF, Carton 4 (Économie). "Déclaration du Président Lepicard à l'émission 'Paysans de France,' les 25 août et 1er septembre 1954," 2.

126. IPMF, Carton 4 (Économie). Letter from the Prefect of the Eure to Pierre Mendès France, 17 January 1955.

127. For a discussion of Mendès France's local politics, see Dominique Franche and Yves Léonard, eds., *Pierre Mendès France et la démocratie locale: Actes du colloque du conseil général de l'Eure* (Rennes, France: Presses Universitaires de Rennes, 2004), esp. 157–174. See also Françoise Chapron, "Pierre Mendès France à l'écoute des agriculteurs," in *Pierre Mendès France et l'économie: Pensée et action,* ed. Michel Margairaz (Paris: Odile Jacob, 1989), 443–447.

128. Pierre Mendès France, "Développer la distribution de lait dans les écoles, le 16 novembre 1937," *Oeuvres complètes: S'engager,* vol. 1 (Paris: Gallimard, 1984), 272–273.

129. AN, 80AJ/71. Jean Branas, "La production viticole française en 1954: rapport au Conseil supérieur de l'agriculture (Section Union française)," 5 September 1954, 40.

130. IPMF, Carton 4 (Économie). Letter from J. Nester to Pierre Mendès France, 9 December 1954.

131. IPMF, Carton 4 (Économie). Letter from the Eure Prefect to Pierre Mendès France, 20 January 1955.

132. Jean Bène, "Le lait et le vin," *La Journée vinicole,* 4 January 1955. Originally published in *Le Midi libre.*

133. "Un communiqué du Comité national de défense contre l'alcoolisme," *Alcool et dérivés,* November 1954. The CNDCA sent its press release to *Alcool et dérivés.*

134. On the politics of home distillation in the twentieth century, see Olivier Verdier, "Action politique et défense des intérêts catégoriels: André Liautey et le monde des groups de pression (1919/1960)," (PhD Diss., Université Paris X, 2009).

135. *Bouilleur de France,* August–September 1954.

136. André Liautey, "Les décrets-lois au service des trusts: Le gouvernement va-t-il supprimer les bouilleurs de cru?" *Bouilleur de France,* October 1954.

137. "La lutte anti-alcoolique," *La Défense des distillateurs & bouilleurs ambulants,* January 1955.

138. "Lettre de M. Liautey à M. Mendès-France," *Bouilleur de France,* January 1955.

139. On Poujade and Dorgères and their respective movements, see, for example, Robert O. Paxton, *French Peasant Fascism: Henry Dorgères's Greenshirts and the Crises of French Agriculture, 1929–1939* (New York: Oxford University Press, 1997); and Romain Souillac, *Le mouvement Poujade: De la défense professionnelle au populisme nationaliste (1953–1962)* (Paris: Les Presses de Sciences Po, 2007).

140. Pierre Poujade, *J'ai choisi le combat* (Saint-Céré, France: Société Générale des Éditions et des Publications, 1955), 114.

141. IPMF, Carton 4 (Économie). *La Gazette agricole,* 8 January 1955.

142. IPMF, Carton 4 (Économie). Letter from the Eure Prefect to Mendès France, 20 January 1955.

143. Maurice Nicolas, *Avec Pierre Poujade sur les routes de France* (Les Sables-d'Olonne, France: Les Éditions de l'Équinoxe, 1955), 170.

144. Janet Flanner, *Paris Journal, 1944–1965* (New York: Atheneum, 1965), 254.

145. Malignac and Colin, *L'alcoolisme,* 125.

146. Pierre Mendès France, "Divergence avec les socialistes sur la méthode de gouvernement, non sur les buts," radio speech on 13 November 1954, in *Gouverner c'est choisir, 1954–1955,* vol. 3 (Paris: Gallimard, 1986), 461.

147. On Mendès France's relationship to the public, see Pierre Laborie, "Le gouvernement Mendès France et l'opinion: La logique de l'exceptionnel," in *Pierre Mendès France et le mendésisme: L'expérience gouvernementale (1954–1955) et sa postérité,* ed. François Bédarida and Jean-Pierre Rioux (Paris: Fayard, 1985), 165–174. On Mendès France's use of the radio, see André Jean Tudesq, "Pierre Mendès France et la radiodiffusion," in *Pierre Mendès France et le mendésisme,* 205–211.

148. *Sondages* 1 (1955): 19.

149. Ibid., 20.

150. Ibid., 19–20.

151. Ibid., 60–61.

152. Archives départementales de Seine-Saint-Denis (hereafter ADSSD), "Archives du Parti communiste," 2 NUM 4/2. "Réunion du Bureau politique du 4/12/1954," 1.

153. ADSSD, "Archives du Parti communiste," 2 NUM 4/2. "Réunion du Bureau politique du 31/12/1954," 4.

154. ADSSD, "Archives du Parti communiste," 2 NUM 4/3. Waldeck Rochet, "Note sur les ravages de l'alcoolisme, les moyens de les combattre et les dernières mesures gouvernementales à ce sujet," 5 January 1955, 6. To learn about Waldeck Rochet's life, see Jean Vigreux, *Waldeck Rochet: Une biographie politique* (Paris: La Dispute, 2000).

155. *Le Betteravier français*, special edition, February 1955. Pierre Leclercq was president of the CGB.

156. For their commonalities in the Fourth Republic, see Philip M. Williams, *Crisis and Compromise: Politics in the Fourth Republic* (London: Longmans, 1964), 353–359.

157. 2nd session of Friday, 4 February 1955, *Journal officiel de la République française: Débats parlementaires, Assemblée nationale,* 5 February 1955, 782–783.

158. Colette Coutaz, *Bistros, bouilleurs & cie* (Paris: Les Éditions du Centurion, 1956), 39. Other authors have also claimed that the alcohol lobbies supported the Algeria lobby in bringing down the Mendès France government. See Michel Louis Lévy, *Alfred Sauvy: Compagnon du siècle* (Paris: La Manufacture, 1990), 144; and Jean-Pierre Rioux, "1954: la croisade antialcoolique," *Enjeux*, September 2004, 117.

159. ANPAA, S7. "Les indépendants paysans ne voteront les pouvoirs spéciaux que si le décret "betteravier" de M. Mendès France est abrogé," *France-Soir*, 5 March 1955.

160. For this analysis, see Brown, "Alcohol and Politics in France," 990.

161. This observation is based on my reading of *Le Betteravier français*.

162. Sauvy, *De Paul Reynaud à Charles de Gaulle*, 184.

163. Bastide, "Une enquête sur l'opinion publique," 15–17, 31–32.

164. On the rebellious role of drink in the early Third Republic, see Susanna Barrows, "'Parliaments of the People': The Political Culture of Cafés in the Early Third Republic," in *Drinking: Behavior and Belief in Modern History,* ed. Susanna Barrows and Robin Room (Berkeley: University of California Press, 1991), 87–97. On the concern about postwar passivism, see *Alcool ou santé* 3 (1951): 12.

3. Quantity or Quality?

1. Archives de l'Institut Pierre Mendès France (hereafter IPMF), "Questions sociales." Pierre Mendès France, "Appel à toutes les femmes de ce pays," no date but sometime after the fall of his government in 1955.

2. For the official number of vine growers, see "Importance du vin dans l'économie française," *Bulletin de l'Institut national des appellations d'origine des vins et eaux-de-vie,* July 1959, 27; for the number of home distillers, see Étienne May, "Problème de l'alcoolisme," *Journal officiel de la République française: Avis et rapports du Conseil économique,* 19 February 1959, 192.

3. "Les appellations d'origine contrôlée et la qualité," *Bulletin de l'Institut national des appellations d'origine des vins et eaux-de-vie,* January 1957, 88. Originally published in the *Bulletin d'information du Ministère de l'Agriculture,* 29 September 1956.

4. *Journal officiel de la République française: Lois et décrets,* 20 November 1954, 10,898.

5. For Robert Debré's connections, see Paul-André Rosental, *L'intelligence démographique: Sciences et politiques des populations en France (1930–1960)* (Paris: Odile Jacob, 2003), 84.

6. Barjot and Hirsch would become members of the HCEIA in the late 1950s.

7. Archives nationales (hereafter AN), 80AJ/55. René Dumont, "Le vignoble languedocien et le canal du bas-Rhône," 25 November 1952, 3.

8. Jacques Sylvain Brunaud, *Rapport sur le coût annuel et la prévention de l'alcoolisme* reviewed and updated (Paris: Comité Central d'Enquête sur le Coût et le Rendement des Services Publics, May 1955), 91.

9. For this language, see, for example, Centre des Archives contemporaines (hereafter CAC), 19940020, art. 18. Letter from Jean Durand to Robert Debré, 14 April 1959.

10. And for this language, see, for example, CAC, 19940020, art. 18. Letter from the director of the INAO to Robert Debré, 24 December 1958.

11. For many of Portmann's speeches, see his *Son activité, parlementaire, scientifique, économique et sociale* (Bordeaux, France: Delmas, 1959).

12. Philippe Lamour noted Robert Debré's love of wine in *Le cadran solaire* (Paris: Robert Laffont, 1980), 418.

13. AN, F/10/5385. "Le Comité national de propaganda en faveur du vin: création, composition, financement, activité," no date but likely 1954 or 1955, 2.

14. G. de Magnin, "Drôle de propagande . . . ," *L'Algérie agricole et viticole*, 4 October 1952.

15. AN, F/10/5385. "Le Comité national de propaganda en faveur du vin: Création, composition, financement, activité," 7.

16. Archives du Sénat (hereafter AS), 33/S7. Drinks Commission, "Séance du jeudi 14 mars 1957," 4.

17. Quoted in Bertrand Dargelos, *La lutte antialcoolique en France depuis le XIXe siècle* (Paris: Dalloz, 2008), 204.

18. Alexandre Baurens, "La campagne anti-alcoolique vue par . . . ," *Bulletin de Presse de la Santé de la France*, March 1958, 27.

19. Archives départementales de Gironde (hereafter ADG), 69J. Private Papers of Jean-Max-Eylaud. Georges Portmann, "Les qualités alimentaires et hygièniques du vin," *La feuille vinicole*, 1 December 1957.

20. For a discussion of the role of wine in popular medicine and for these quotations, see Harry W. Paul, *Bacchic Medicine: Wine and Alcohol Therapies from Napoleon to the French Paradox* (Amsterdam: Rodopi, 2001), 11–13.

21. Jean-Max Eylaud, *Vin et santé: Vertus hygièniques et thérapeutiques du vin* (Soissons, France: La Diffusion Nouvelle du Livre, 1960).

22. CAC, 19940020, art. 18. Georges Portmann, "Les vins de Bordeaux sont vins de santé," *Études médicales et scientifiques sur le vin et le raisin* (May 1956), 5.

23. Sully Ledermann, *Alcool, alcoolisme, alcoolisation: Données scientifiques de caractère physiologique, économique et social* (Paris: Presses Universitaires de France, 1956), 159.

24. Roger Andrieu, "1958 marque une nouvelle chute spectaculaire de l'alcoolisme," *L'Industrie hôtelière de France et d'Outre-Mer*, April 1959.

25. Jacques Borel, *Le vrai problème de l'alcoolisme: Étude médico-sociale, ses conditions, ses limites, mensonges des statistiques, réfutation d'un mythe* (Villejuif, France: Chez l'Auteur, 1957), 159.

26. ADG, 69J. E.-J. Dauphin, "Où est la vérité sur l'alcool et l'alcoolisme," newspaper not noted but likely *La Journée vinicole*.

27. CAC, 19940020, art. 26. IFOP, *Alcool: opinion du corps médical sur l'alcoolisme* (December 1959): 5.

28. CAC, 19940020, art. 18. Georges Portmann, "Les vins de Bordeaux sont vins de santé," *Études médicales et scientifiques sur le vin et le raisin* (May 1956): 4.

29. Portmann, *Son activité*, 77.

30. Michel Cépède, "La question viticole et l'alcoolisme," *Les Cahiers économiques* (February 1955).

31. AN, F/10/5385. J. Deramond, "Propagande et publicité en faveur du vin et du raisin et étude des marchés," 7th International Congress on the Vine and Wine, Rome, 12–20 September 1953, 1.

32. Archives de l'Association nationale de prévention en alcoologie et addictologie (hereafter ANPAA), N145. Paul Pagès, "Vin et alcoolisme," report presented at the International Congress for the Scientific Study of Wine and Grapes, Bordeaux, 11–13 October 1957, in "Le Centre interdépartemental d'éducation sanitaire démographique et sociale de Montpellier vous invite à prendre connaissance d'une série d'articles et rapports traitant de l'alcoolisme."

33. CAC, 19940020, art. 32. "Allocution prononcée à Montpellier le 20 juin 1957 par M. Gilbert Nicaud, Secrétaire général de Santé de la France," 2.

34. Roland Sadoun, Giorgio Lolli, and Milton Silverman, *Drinking in French Culture* (New Brunswick, New Jersey: Rutgers Center of Alcohol Studies, 1965), 51.

35. CAC, 19940020, art. 26. IFOP, *L'opinion publique française devant l'alcoolisme* September–December 1955, 9.

36. ANPAA, A1/I. Alain Barjot, *Aspects sociologiques du phénomène de l'alcoolisme et leurs conséquences dans l'élaboration d'une politique antialcoolique* (Geneva: 3e Cours d'Études Scientifiques pour la Prévention de l'Alcoolisme, 1957), 8.

37. Quoted in Colette Coutaz, *Bistros, bouilleurs & cie* (Paris: Les Editions du Centurion, 1956). The quote is on the back cover.

38. AN, C/15598. Drinks Commission, National Assembly, "Séance du mercredi 16 mars 1955."

39. *Journal officiel de la République française: Débats parlementaires, Assemblée nationale*, 1st session of 16 March 1955, 1514.

40. CAC, 19940020, art. 1. "Note sur les crédits du Haut Comité d'étude et d'information sur l'alcoolisme," 5 August 1958, 1.

41. CAC, 19940020, art. 9. Letter from Robert Debré to Paul Reynaud, 25 June 1957.

42. CAC, 19940020, art. 1. "Note du Secrétaire général sur l'activité du Haut Comité d'étude et d'information sur l'alcoolisme en 1956 et les perspectives de 1957," 31 December 1956, 8.

43. CAC, 19940020, art. 1. Letter from Eugène Forget to Alain Barjot, 3 January 1957.

44. Portmann, *Son activité*, 66, 68.

45. CAC, 19940020, art. 18. Letter from Alain Barjot to Jean Riou of *La Journée vinicole*, 9 November 1956.

46. CAC, 19940020, art. 18. Letters from Robert Debré to M. le Baron Le Roy, president of the INAO, and to Jean Bourcier, honorary president of the CNVS, 5 August 1958.

47. "Importance du vin dans l'économie française," 27.

48. Marcel Lachiver, *Vins, vignes et vignerons: Histoire du vignoble français* (Paris: Fayard, 1988), 538.

49. "Les appellations d'origine contrôlée et la qualité," 86.

50. CAC, 19940020, art. 8. Letter from the undersecretary of state in the office of the prime minister who was responsible for the HCEIA, to the secretary of state in the Ministry of Agriculture who was charged with the general direction of agricultural production, 19 September 1957.

51. ADG, 69J. Jean Riou, "Bordeaux, congrès international de médecine pour l'étude scientifique du vin et du raisin: Compte rendu des communications (suite)," *La Feuille vinicole*, 17–18 October 1957.

52. Quoted in "Hommage au Dr Étienne May," *Alcool ou santé* 4/5 (1962): 3.

53. Ann-Christina L. Knudsen, *Farmers on Welfare: The Making of Europe's Common Agricultural Policy* (Ithaca: Cornell University Press, 2009), 59.

54. CAC, 19940020, art. 18. "La Confédération nationale des vins & spiritueux, réunie en congrès les 10, 11 et 12 juin 1958."

55. CAC, 19940020, art. 11. Letter from Jean Fraisse, president of the CNVS, to Robert Debré, 16 September 1958.

56. CAC, 19940020, art. 18. Letter from the premier to Félix Martin, president of the APV, 19 April 1957.

57. Pierre Le Roy de Boiseaumarié, "La viticulture française devant son avenir," *La Journée vinicole*, 8 March 1952. Reproduced in *Alcool ou santé* 3 (1952): 18. CAC, 19940020, art. 18. Letter from Robert Debré to Marcel Lugan, 13 November 1956.

58. Quoted in P. Bridonneau, "La liberté de tuer," *Le Monde*, 7 May 1970. From what I can gather, Mauriac made this statement in 1959.

59. Archives d'histoire contemporaine (hereafter ADC), Papers of Michel Debré, 2DE52. Robert Escarpit, "Qui a bu boira," *Le Monde*, 5 May 1960.

60. ANPAA, S512. François Muselier, "S'ils avaient vu ces visages . . . ," *L'Express*, 9 November 1955.

61. *Le Bouilleur de France*, May 1955.

62. Coutaz, *Bistros, bouilleurs & cie*; and Marise Querlin, *Les chaudières de l'enfer: Le problème de l'alcoolisme en France* (Paris: Gallimard, 1955).

63. Pierre Fromont, "L'agriculture algérienne et ses problèmes," *Le Figaro*, 21 June 1955. Reprinted in *Algérie agricole et viticole*, 22 June 1955. On Fromont's support of the INAO, see Pierre Fromont, "Splendeurs et misères de la vigne et du vin dans la France moderne," in *Le vin de France dans l'histoire*, published by the *Bulletin de l'Institut national des appellations d'origine des vins & eaux-de-vie*, special edition, 1953.

64. Hildebert Isnard, "La viticulture algérienne: Erreur économique?" *La revue africaine* 50 (1956): 465.

65. Ibid., 463.

66. Ibid., 462.

67. Hildebert Isnard, "Vineyards and Social Structure in Algeria," *Diogenes* 7 (1959): 70.

68. Quoted in Paul Sicard, "Nouveau front d'attaque contre l'Algérie," *L'Algérie agricole et viticole*, 3 March 1956. Originally published in *Le Monde*, 15 February 1956.

69. For the "insane extension" quote, see "Conférence du Baron Le Roy à la Société des Agriculteurs de France," *Revue du vin de France*, April–June 1955, 32. The other quote comes from "Le problème viticole algérien," *L'Algérie agricole et viticole*, 5 March 1955.

70. For references to alcohol prohibition during the war, see Mouloud Feraoun, *Journal, 1955–1962: Reflections on the French-Algerian War*, trans. Mary Ellen Wolf and Claude Fouillade (Lincoln: University of Nebraska Press, 2000).

71. Mahfoud Bennoune, *The Making of Contemporary Algeria, 1830–1987: Colonial Upheavals and Post-Independence Development* (New York: Cambridge University Press, 1988), 79.

72. See the frequent commentary in *L'Algérie agricole et viticole* during the war.

73. Quoted in Kolleen M. Guy, "Culinary Connections and Colonial Memories in France and Algeria," *Food and History* 8, no. 1 (2010): 227; and Alistair Horne, *A Savage War of Peace: Algeria, 1954–1962* (New York: New York Review of Books, 2006), 57. First published 1977 by Macmillan.

74. Albert Camus, "Réflexions sur la guillotine," in Albert Camus and Arthur Koestler, *Réflexions sur la peine capitale* (Paris: Calmann-Lévy, 1957), 155–156.

75. AN, F12/11802. *Groupe d'étude des relations financières entre le Métropole et l'Algérie* (Algiers: Imprimerie Officielle, June 1955), 10. For a sketch of Maspétiol's career trajectory, see Isabel Boussard, "Roland Maspétiol, une figure marquante de l'économie rurale," *Économie rurale* 223 (1994): 3–5.

76. AN/F12/11802. Charles Frappart, André Valls, and Claude Cheysson, "Quelques données du problème algérien," June 1957. For the Frappart report in relation to other reports, see Phillip C. Naylor, *France and Algeria: A History of Decolonization and Transformation* (Gainesville: University Press of Florida, 2000), 19.

77. For an analysis of French public opinion on the Algerian war, see John Talbott, "French Public Opinion and the Algerian War: A Research Note," *French Historical Studies* 9 (Autumn 1975): 354–361.

78. CAC, 19940020, art. 11. Letter from Alain Barjot to Bernard Lafay, minister of public health, 20 July 1955.

79. AHC, 2DE52. IFOP, *L'opinion française et les bouilleurs de cru*, May 1960.

80. "Les Jeunes et les bouilleurs de cru," *Bulletin de liaison des Comités départementaux et locaux*, March–April 1960, 1–2.

81. ANPAA, P39/b. Letter from M. Martraire to André Mignot, general director of the CNDCA, 25 November 1958.

82. CAC, 19940020, art. 11. Letter from Robert Monod to Prime Minister Michel Debré, 2 May 1960.

83. *Alcool ou santé*, 6 (1959): 2.

84. Archives du Comité départemental de défense contre l'alcoolisme du Finistère (hereafter CDDCA du Finistère). See also Thierry Fillaut, *Les Bretons et l'alcool (XIXe–XXe siècle)* (Rennes, France: École nationale de la santé publique, 1991), 247–250.

85. Pierre Fontaine, "Les cultivateurs algériens ne sont pas tous des 'féodaux,'" *La Tribune agricole*, 22 June 1956.

86. As reported in "Vin et 'Réalités,'" *Bulletin de l'Institut national des appellations d'origine des vins et eaux-de-vie*, October 1957, 53. Written by L. Bourgeois and originally published in *La Journée vinicole*.

87. See, for example, J.F., "À propos des vins de coupages," *L'Algérie agricole et viticole*, 19 March 1955.

88. AN, 80AJ/71. Viticultural Group, Committee of the Section on the Economic Integration of the Metropole and the Overseas Territories, "Compte rendu de la réunion du vendredi 18 février 1955," 5.

89. "Une richesse et un fléau: le point de vue agricole," *Le Figaro*, 6–7 November 1954.

90. CAC, 19940020, art. 11. "Appel du Bureau national des bouilleurs de cru," 10 February 1957.

91. J. Roulleaux-Dugage, "Le canal de Suez et les bouilleurs de cru," *Le Bouilleur de France*, September 1956.

92. "Faites-vous une opinion sur la campagne antialcoolique," *Paris-Presse L'Intransigeant*, 28–29 July 1957.

93. Guy Beaufrère, "La presse anti-bouilleur contre l'alcool français," *Le Bouilleur de France*, September 1956.

94. Jean Meynaud, *Les groupes de pression en France* (Paris: Armand Colin, 1958), 260. See the quote in note 3 as well.

95. André Mignot, *Le privilège des bouilleurs de cru . . . ou un scandale qui nous coûte plus de 50 milliards par an* (Paris: Allain SICAR Elbeuf, 1958), 4.

96. AHC, 2DE52. Michel Bosquet, "Les rois de l'alambic," *L'Express*, 10 December 1959.

97. On the tightening of fiscal policy at the beginning of the Fifth Republic, see Frédéric Tristram, *Une fiscalité pour la croissance: La Direction générale des impôts et la politique fiscal en France de 1948 à la fin des années 1960* (Paris: Comité pour l'Histoire Économique et Financière de la France, 2005), 491–559.

98. On the early Fifth Republic's important contribution to agricultural modernization, see John T. S. Keeler, *The Politics of Neocorporatism in France: Farmers, the State, and Agricultural Policy-Making in the Fifth Republic* (New York: Oxford University Press, 1987).

99. Quoted in John T. S. Keeler, "The Corporatist Dynamic of Agricultural Modernization in the Fifth Republic," in *The Fifth Republic at Twenty,* ed. William G. Andrews and Stanley Hoffmann (Albany: State University of New York Press, 1981), 273.

100. See Debré's autobiography, *Gouverner: Mémoires, 1958–1962* (Paris: Albin Michel, 1988); see also Serge Berstein, Pierre Milza, and Jean-François Sirinelli, eds., *Michel Debré: Premier Ministre, 1959–1962* (Paris: Presses Universitaires de France, 2005).

101. For the precursors to the Constantine Plan, see Phillip C. Naylor, "A Reconsideration of the Fourth Republic's Legacy and Algerian Decolonization," *French Colonial History* 2 (2002): 159–180.

102. "Le plan de Constantine et la viticulture," *L'Algérie agricole et viticole,* 26 March–2 April 1960.

103. For the importance of wine to the Algerian economy in the late 1950s, see Keith Sutton, "Algeria's Vineyards: A Problem of Decolonization," *Méditerranée* 65, no. 3 (1988): 57; or Michel Launay, *Paysans algériens: La terre, la vigne et les hommes* (Paris: Seuil, 1963), 42.

104. Lachiver, *Vins, vignes et vignerons,* 587.

105. CAC, 19940020, art. 18. "Exposé de M. Roland Maspétiol, Institut des vins de consommation courante," 8 March 1957, 2.

106. *Rapport sur les obstacles à l'expansion économique* (Paris: Imprimerie Nationale, 1960), 62.

107. Jaume Bardissa made this claim in *Cent ans de guerre du vin* (Paris: Tema-Éditions, 1976), 74.

108. CAC, 19940020, art. 18. Letter from Jean Durand, president of the Departmental Federation of Mass-Consumed Wines, to Robert Debré, 14 April 1959.

109. CAC, 19940020, art. 2. Meeting between the HCEIA and the CNVS, 3 November 1958.

110. "Rapport d'ensemble," *Rapport au Premier Ministre sur l'activité du Haut Comité d'étude et d'information sur l'alcoolisme* (Paris: La Documentation Française, 1962), 137.

111. ANPAA, N192. *Le Bien public,* 25 May 1959.

112. ANPAA, N192. *L'Alsace,* 27 May 1959.

113. *Alcool ou santé,* 2 (1959): 30.

114. CAC, 19940020, art. 18. C. M. Bertrand, "Propositions soumises aux administrateurs du CNDCA," July 1959, 2.

115. CAC, 19940020, art. 18. "Déclarations de quelques administrateurs à la réunion du 28/9/1959," 1 bis. Italics in the original.

116. "Une lettre du ministre des finances," *Bulletin de l'Institut national des appellations d'origine des vins et eaux-de-vie,* April 1959, 186.

117. "Le vin trop cher?" *L'Algérie agricole et viticole,* 20 December 1958.

118. Waldeck Rochet, "Un décret qui sacrifie consommateur et le petit vigneron," *L'Humanité,* 22 May 1959.

119. "Protestation du Syndicat national des producteurs de VDN et VDL à appellation contrôlée," *Bulletin de l'Institut national des appellations d'origine des vins et eaux-de-vie,* January 1959, 66.

120. Andrew W. M. Smith, *Terror and Terroir: The Winegrowers of the Languedoc and Modern France* (Manchester, UK: Manchester University Press, 2016), 77–79.

121. "Il ne sera bientôt possible de garantir l'ordre public affirment les vignerons du Midi," *Le Monde*, 14 May 1959.

122. Annie Moulin, *Peasantry and Society in France since 1789*, trans. M. C. Cleary and M. F. Cleary (New York: Cambridge University Press, 1991), 173.

123. Quoted in Benjamin Stora, *Algeria, 1830–2000: A Short History*, trans. Jane Marie Todd (Ithaca: Cornell University Press, 2001), 76.

124. AHC, 2DE/52. *Le Monde*, 25 November 1959.

125. AHC, 2DE/52. Michel Bosquet, "Les rois de l'alambic," *L'Express*, 10 December 1959.

126. AHC, 2DE52. *Libération*, 19 July 1960.

127. "Lutte contre certains fléaux sociaux," 1st session of Monday 18 July 1960, *Journal officiel de la République française: Débats parlementaires, Assemblée nationale*, 19 July 1960, 1958.

128. These senators were Pauzet, Grégory, Brun, Sinsout, Grand, Monichon, Portmann, and Pams. See "Lutte contre certains fléaux sociaux," session of Thursday 21 July 1960, *Journal officiel de la République française: Débats parlementaires, Sénat*, 22 July 1960, 1043. For the need to protect the wine statute of 1953, see AHC, 2DE52. "L'alcoolisme," 23 November 1960, 2.

129. "La viticulture et les fléaux sociaux," *Le Progrès agricole et viticole*, 31 July 1960, 37.

130. Fillaut, *Les Bretons et l'alcool*, 247.

131. May, "Problème de l'alcoolisme," 189.

132. Ibid., 192.

133. "Le groupe d'études fiscales institué par l'arrêté du 9 février 1959 se prononce pour le maintien, en 1959, de la fiscalité actuelle des vins et alcools et demande avec insistance la suppression du privilege des bouilleurs de cru dès 1960," *Bulletin d'informations du HCEIA*, May–June 1959, 29.

134. ANPAA, P39/a. Guy Beaufrère, "Proxénètes, homosexuels et bouilleurs de cru," *Le Bouilleur de France*, September–October 1960.

135. ANPAA, P39/a. See, for example, the article "Dernière heure: L'ordonnance sur les bouilleurs va être promulgué à bref delai," *Le Bouilleur de France*, July–August 1960.

136. ANPAA, P39/a. "Le Senateur Henri Prêtre demande au Gouvernement de tenir ses promesses," *Le Bouilleur de France*, September–October 1960.

137. "Ordonnance #60-907 du 30 août 1960 relative au régime des bouilleurs de cru," *Journal officiel de la République française: Lois et décrets*, 31 August 1960, 8039–8040.

138. *Alcool ou santé*, 6 (1959); and *Le Monde*, 5 December 1959.

139. Stéphane Banessy, "Seul record français qui ne soit pas près d'être battu: L'alcoolisme," *Carrefour*, 7 September 1960.

140. "Décret #60-1257 du 29 novembre 1960 modifiant le code des débits de boissons et des mesures de lutte contre l'alcoolisme (deuxième partie, règlements d'administration publique et décrets en conseil d'Etat)," *Journal officiel de la République française: Lois et décrets*, 30 November 1960, 10,712–10,713.

141. See, for example, ANPAA, P39/b. Letter from Pierre Bories, general administrative assistant of the Regional Interprofessional Committee for the Brandies of the Languedoc, to Jules Milhau, member of the Economic Council, 17 January 1959.

142. Alfred Sauvy, *Ce que serait la France sans l'alcoolisme* (December 1956): 14.

4. Drinking and Driving

1. "Le Ministre du Tourisme parle," *Touring Club de France*, May 1953, 171.

2. François Toché, "Stop à l'accident routier," *Touring Club de France*, May 1953, 173.

3. For a history of the French automobile, see Mathieu Flonneau, *L'automobile au temps des trente glorieuses: Un rêve d'automobilisme* (Carbonne, France: Loubatières, 2016); and Jean-Louis Loubet, *Histoire de l'automobile française* (Paris: Seuil, 2001). On tourism in France, see, for example, Ellen Furlough, "Making Mass Vacations: Tourism and Consumer Culture in France, 1930s–1970s," *Comparative Studies in Society and History* 40 (1998): 247–286; Stephen L. Harp, *Marketing Michelin: Advertising and Cultural Identity in Twentieth-Century France* (Baltimore: Johns Hopkins University Press, 2001); Harp, *Au Naturel: Naturism, Nudism, and Tourism in Twentieth-Century France* (Baton Rouge: Louisiana State University Press, 2014); and Eric Reed, *Selling the Yellow Jersey: The Tour de France in the Global Era* (Chicago: University of Chicago Press, 2015).

4. The Ecole Nationale des Ponts et Chaussées is the world's oldest civil engineering school and has been responsible for building France's infrastructure. See Jean-Claude Thoenig, *L'ère des technocrates: Le cas des Ponts et Chaussées* (Paris: Les Éditions d'Organisation, 1973).

5. Archives de l'Association nationale de prévention en alcoologie et addictologie (hereafter ANPAA), S2. "20 ans d'antialcoolisme officiel estime le 'Comité interprofessionnel de défense des boissons nationales,'" *Le Moniteur vinicole*, 20 January 1968.

6. On the battle against drinking and driving in France, see Anne Kletzlen, *De l'alcool à l'alcool au volant: La transformation d'un problème public* (Paris: L'Harmattan, 2007); and Marie-Claire Jayet, *Prévention du risque "alcool au volant" dans un pays producteur de vin, 1960–1990* (Arcueil, France: Institut National de Recherche sur les Transports et leur Sécurité, 1994). On the equivalent process in the United States, see Barron H. Lerner, *One for the Road: Drunk Driving since 1900* (Baltimore: Johns Hopkins University Press, 2011); and for Britain, see Bill Luckin, "A Kind of Consensus on the Roads? Drink Driving Policy in Britain, 1945–1970," *Twentieth Century British History* 21, no. 3 (2010): 350–374.

7. On how trains transformed perceptions of time and space, see Wolfgang Schivelbusch, *The Railway Journey: The Industrialization of Time and Space in the Nineteenth Century* (Oakland: University of California Press, 2014). First published 1979 by Urizen Books.

8. Kolleen M. Guy discusses the relationship between Fordism and *terroir* in "Silence and Savoir-Faire in the Marketing of Products of the Terroir," *Modern and Contemporary France* 19 (November 2011): 459–475.

9. Gilles Laferté, *La Bourgogne et ses vins: Image d'origine contrôlée* (Paris: Belin, 2006), 90.

10. Quoted in Harp, *Marketing Michelin*, 253.

11. Quoted in Catherine Bertho Lavenir, *La roue et le stylo: Comment nous sommes devenus tourists* (Paris: Odile Jacob, 1999), 237. On food in regional tourism, see Julia Csergo, "The Emergence of Regional Cuisines," in *Food: A Cultural History*, trans. A. Sonnenfeld, ed. Jean-Louis Flandrin and Massimo Montanari (New York: Columbia University Press, 1999), 497–511.

12. To learn more about how authenticity was staged in the French regions, see Philip Whalen, "'Insofar as the Ruby Wine Seduces Them': Cultural Strategies for Selling Wine in Inter-war Burgundy," *Contemporary European History* 18, no. 1 (2009): 67–98; and Patrick Young, *Enacting Brittany: Tourism and Culture in Provincial France* (Burlington, Vermont: Ashgate, 2012)

13. On the role of the Michelin guide in French wine and automobile tourism in the inter-war years, see Harp, *Marketing Michelin*, 225–268.

14. Quoted in Whalen, "'Insofar as the Ruby Wine Seduces Them,'" 85.

15. Olivier Jacquet and Gilles Laferté examine the emergence of the wine route in interwar Burgundy in "La route des vins et l'émergence d'un tourisme viticole en Bourgogne dans l'entre-deux-guerres," *Cahiers de géographie du Québec* 57, no. 162 (2013): 425–444.

16. This observation is based on my reading of *La Revue du vin de France*.

17. Jacob Meunier, *On the Fast Track: French Railway Modernization and the Origins of the TGV, 1944–1983* (Westport, Connecticut: Praeger, 2002), 50.

18. Jacques Vallin and Jean-Claude Chesnais, "Les accidents de la route en France. Mortalité et morbidité depuis 1953," *Population* 3 (1975): 445.

19. "La circulation routière en 1955: les accidents corporels, leurs causes connues et méconnues," *Alcool ou santé* (March–April 1957): 12. See also Sully Ledermann, *Alcool, alcoolisme, alcoolisation: Données scientifiques de caractère physiologique, économique et social* (Paris: Presses Universitaires de France, 1956), 196.

20. Henri Rouvillois and Léon Dérobert, "Alcool et accidents de la circulation," session of 27 November 1951, *Bulletin de l'Académie de Médecine* 1 (1951): 597.

21. "Loi tendant à réprimer l'ivresse publique et à combattre les progrès de l'alcoolisme," *Journal officiel de la République française: Lois et décrets*, 4 February 1873, 801–802.

22. For these different decrees, see Jean Orselli, "Usages et usagers de la route, mobilité et accidents, 1860–2008," (PhD Diss., Université de Paris I, 2009).

23. "Le dosage d'alcool dans le sang," *Le Figaro*, 17 May 1955.

24. This publication was *Les accidents corporels de la circulation routière*.

25. Direction of Roads and Traffic, Ministry of Public Works, Transportation, and Tourism, *Les accidents corporels de la circulation routière en 1954*.

26. This would continue to be the case into the 1970s. See, for example, "Sécurité routière," *Alcool ou santé* 2 (1976).

27. "L'alcool et la sécurité routière," *Nouvelles de la Prévention routière*, January 1953, 3.

28. On doctors, see E.M., "Les automobilistes ayant causé un accident et soupçonnés d'avoir absorbé trop d'alcool seront soumis à un prélèvement de sang," *Le Monde*, 15 February 1956; on gendarmes, see Robert Monod, "La fatigue et l'alcoolisme: causes essentielles des accidents de la route," *Prévention routière*, May–June 1960, 4.

29. Georges Malignac and Robert Colin, *L'alcoolisme* (Paris: Presses Universitaires de France, 1954), 84.

30. Henri Rouvillois and Léon Dérobert, "Alcool et accidents de la circulation," session of 27 November 1951, *Bulletin de l'Académie de Médecine* 1 (1951): 596.

31. Delphine Dulong analyzes the conflicts between politicians and experts in *Moderniser la politique: Aux origines de la Ve République* (Paris: L'Harmattan, 1997).

32. For some of these beliefs, see, for example, "Qui vit, qui meurt de l'alcool," *L'Express*, 23 January 1954.

33. Quoted in Roland Sadoun, Giorgio Lolli, and Milton Silverman, *Drinking in French Culture* (New Brunswick, New Jersey: Rutgers Center of Alcohol Studies, 1965), 48.

34. "L'alcoolisme en France: faut-il sévir ou éduquer," *Carrefour*, 27 May 1959.

35. H. Hinglais and M. Hinglais (Presentation by M. Justin-Besançon), "Alcoolémie et définition légale de l'alcoolisme. Bases de l'intérpretation médico-légale. Conséquences particulières en France," session of 10 July 1956, *Bulletin de l'Académie de Médecine* 1 (1956): 431. Italics in the original.

36. See, for example, Alfred Sauvy, "Excédents agricoles et alcool carburant," *Bulletin des transports*, August–September 1950; or his articles in *Revue française de l'énergie* in 1949, 1950, and 1953.

37. "Encore l'alcool carburant!" *L'Action automobile et touristique*, February 1953.

38. "Tourisme anti-alcoolique," *L "Auto-Journal*, 15 March 1953. Reprinted in *Alcool et dérivés: Livre blanc de la campagne de presse contre l'alcool* 1(1953): 23.

39. See, for example, R. Debonder, "Tourisme anti-alcoolique," *L'Auto-Journal*, 15 March 1953. Reprinted in *Alcool et dérivés: Livre blanc de la campagne de presse contre l'alcool* 1(1953), 23.

40. André Defert, "Le flot qui monte," *Touring Club de France*, March 1955, 108.

41. On the competition between road and rail, see Joseph Jones, *The Politics of Transport in Twentieth-Century France* (Montreal: McGill-Queen's University Press, 1984); Meunier, *On the Fast Track*, 43–73; and Nicolas Neiertz, *La coordination des transports en France: De 1918 à nos jours* (Paris: Comité pour l'Histoire Économique et Financière de la France, 1999).

42. "Problèmes de sécurité routière: Étude présentée par la section des travaux publics, des transports et du tourisme sur le rapport de M. Claude de Peyron le 3 juillet 1968," *Journal officiel de la République française: Avis et rapports du Conseil économique et social*, 26 November 1968, 866.

43. "La Prévention routière," *Nouvelles de la Prévention routière*, July 1952, 1. For a discussion of Prévention routière and the early postwar road safety movement, see Séverine Decreton, "Les trois temps de la communication de sécurité routière," *Quaderni* 33, no. 1 (1997): 85–98.

44. Marcel Henry, "Les sociétés d'assurances et la *Prévention routière*," *L'Argus des assurances*, 13 July 1958.

45. On the nationalization of the insurance companies, see Claire Andrieu, "Les assurances, pour quoi faire?" in *Les nationalisations de la Libération: De l'utopie au compromis*, ed. Claire Andrieu, Lucette Le Van, and Antoine Prost (Paris: Presses de la Fondation Nationale des Sciences Politiques, 1987), 339–351.

46. "Augmentation alarmante des accidents de la circulation," *Alcool ou santé* 9 (1953): 13.

47. André Defert, "Le flot qui monte," *Touring Club de France*, March 1955, 108.

48. François Toché, *L'art de bien conduire* (Paris: Flammarion, 1954), 139.

49. Centre des Archives contemporaines (hereafter CAC), 19940020, art. 28. Dr. A. Requet, "Problème de la tolérance dans les pays développés," *26ème congrès international sur l'alcool et l'alcoolisme*, 1–5 August 1960, 404–405.

50. CAC, 19780409, art. 1. Letter from Robert Monod to General de Gaulle, 12 July 1958.

51. "L'alcoolisme, problème de gouvernement," *Courrier de la Nation*, 11 September 1958.

52. "Allocution de M. R. Debré, Président de l'Académie," session of 14 January 1958, *Bulletin de l'Académie de Médecine* (1958): 33.

53. On this topic, see Anson Rabinbach, *The Human Motor: Energy, Fatigue, and the Origins of Modernity* (Berkeley: University of California Press, 1990).

54. For the history of drinking and driving research, see Lerner, *One for the Road*, 14–63.

55. Robert F. Borkenstein, *A Practical Experiment on the Effects of Alcohol on Driving Skill: A Report on the Driving Tests Conducted by the Participants of the Seminar on Alcohol and Road Traffic at the Southern Police Institute, February 23, 1956* (Louisville: Southern Police Institute, University of Louisville, 1956).

56. CAC, 19940020, art. 14. Letter from Robert Debré to Georges Pompidou, 23 May 1964.

57. Georges Pequignot, "Études relatives aux relations entre l'alcool et la sécurité routière," *Rapport au Premier Ministre sur l'activité du Haut Comité d'étude et d'information sur l'alcoolisme* (Paris: La Documentation Française, 1972).

58. CAC, 19880442, art. 1. Léon Fleck, general secretary of the HCEIA, "Voeu adressé à M. le Premier Ministre à la suite de la séance du Haut Comité d'étude et d'information sur l'alcoolisme du 15 janvier 1969," 1.

59. HCEIA, "Alcool et conduite," *Le Nouvel Observateur*, 23 June 1969.

60. For an understanding of Chaban-Delmas's "New Society," see Pierre Guillaume, "Un projet: la 'Nouvelle société,'" in *Jacques Chaban-Delmas en politique*, ed. Bernard Lachaise, Gilles Le Béguec, and Jean-François Sirinelli (Paris: Presses Universitaires de France, 2007), 185–199.

61. CAC, 19880510, art. 15. Michel Ternier, engineer at Ponts et Chaussées, "Présentation de la RCB," 27 January 1970. This document explains Ternier's use of the RCB.

62. Michel Ternier, Jean L'Hoste, and Jérôme Lion, "Les aspects économiques de la mise en place d'un taux légal d'alcoolémie," *L'alcoolisme en France*, notes and documentary studies (Paris: La Documentation Française, 1970), 53–54.

63. Ibid., 55.

64. Ibid.

65. CAC, 19950317, art. 84. Direction of Criminal Affairs and Pardons (*grâces*), Ministry of Justice "Conduite d'un véhicule sous l'empire d'un état alcoolique: Résultats de la consultation organisée par la Chancellerie auprès des Parquets généraux au sujet de l'application actuelle et de la modification éventuelle de l'article L1 du Code de la route," January 1969, 10. See also Kletzlen, *De l'alcool à l'alcool au volant*, 115.

66. "La réglementation des 'restoroutes,'" *Bulletin d'informations du HCEIA*, March–May 1968, 42.

67. CAC, 19880442, art. 2. "Question écrite #7.551, posée le 6 mars 1968, par M. Frys, député, a/s de l'application plus stricte de l'alcootest aux automobiliste."

68. "Taux légal d'alcoolémie," session of Thursday, 16 April 1970, *Journal officiel de la République française: Débats parlementaires, Assemblée nationale*, 17 April 1970, 1105.

69. Ibid., 1110.

70. Ibid., 1112.

71. Ibid.

72. Ibid., 1106.

73. "Taux légal de l'alcoolémie," session of Friday, 12 June 1970, *Journal officiel de la République française: Débats parlementaires, Sénat*, 13 June 1970, 796.

74. "Le Garde des Sceaux explique sa position: Lors du 2ème débat à l'Assemblée nationale (21 avril 1970), M. René Pleven, Garde des Sceaux, expose les raisons pour lesquelles le gouvernement s'opposera à l'amendement de la Commission des lois instituant un double taux d'alcoolémie," *Alcool ou santé* 4 (1970): 17.

75. "Taux légal d'alcoolémie," session of Tuesday, 21 April 1970, *Journal officiel de la République française: Débats parlementaires, Assemblée nationale*, 22 April 1970, 1194.

76. "Taux légal d'alcoolémie," session of Thursday 16 April 1970, *Journal officiel de la République française: Débats parlementaires, Assemblée nationale*, 17 April 1970, 1110.

77. CAC, 19880442, art. 1. Commission of Constitutional Law, Legislation, and General Administration of the Republic, National Assembly, "Communiqué à la presse," 25 February 1970, 4.

78. "Rapport Mazeaud au nom de la Commission des lois," *Journal officiel de la République française: Documents parlementaires, Assemblée nationale*, no. 1038, 2 April 1970.

79. CAC, 19950317, art. 83. ONSER, *L'alcool et la conduite*, ONSER Document no. 1 (January 1969).

80. "Loi du 10 juillet 1970 sur le taux légal d'alcoolémie," *Bulletin d'informations du HCEIA*, July–September 1970, 3. See also "Loi #70-597 du 9 juillet 1970 instituant un taux légal d'alcoolémie et généralisant le dépistage par l'air expiré," *Journal officiel de la République française: Lois et décrets*, 10 July 1970, 6463–6464.

81. "Décret #59-135 du 7 janvier 1959 portant règlement d'administration publique pour l'application de la loi #58-203 du 27 février 1958 instituant une obligation d'assurance

en matière de circulation de véhicules terrestres à moteur," *Journal officiel de la République française: Lois et décrets*, 9 January 1959, 655.

82. P. Bridonneau, "La liberté de tuer," *Le Monde*, 7 May 1970.

83. See, for example, André Mignot's comments in the Senate, "Taux légal d'alcoolémie," session of Friday, 12 June 1970, *Journal officiel de la République française: Débats parlementaires, Sénat*, 13 June 1970, 787. Mignot was a temperance activist and reporter for the legal commission of the Senate.

84. On the influence of the wine lobbies, see Michel Debord, "Le 83ème congrès de la CNVS," *Le Moniteur vinicole*, 4 July 1970. For the quote, see "Le projet de fixation du taux légal d'alcoolémie," *La Journée vinicole*, 24 March 1970.

85. "Mise au point au sujet d'un vote," session of Wednesday, 23 April 1970, *Journal officiel de la République française: Débats parlementaires, Assemblée nationale*, 24 April 1970, 1242.

86. Jaume Bardissa, *Cent ans de guerre du vin* (Paris: Tema-Éditions, 1976), 91.

87. *Bulletin d'information de l'Union fédérale de la consommation*, February–March 1952, 32.

88. The Health of France, *Bulletin de Presse*, 15 May 1960, 656. The *cadres* refers to the new middle class that arose in the middle of the twentieth century.

89. Georges Portmann, *Son activité, parlementaire, scientifique, économique et sociale* (Bordeaux, France: Delmas, 1959), 99. Portmann made this assertion in *Production française* in 1957.

90. For this story, see Richard F. Kuisel, "Coca-Cola and the Cold War: The French Face Americanization, 1948–1953," *French Historical Studies* 17, no. 1 (1991): 96–116.

91. *Alcool ou santé* 3 (1951): 5–6.

92. CAC, 19940020, art. 6. Letter from J. Jacquemin to M. Delaquier (in the Gard), 10 July 1961.

93. See, for example, Archives de l'Institut Pierre Mendès France (hereafter IPMF), carton 4 (speeches). "Discours prononcé par M. Mendès France, Président du Conseil, à la radio, le 13 novembre 1954," 2.

94. Archives nationales (hereafter AN), 5AG3/2177. Pierre Richard, "Note à l'attention de Monsieur le Président de la République," 15 November 1977, 2.

95. "Loi #58-208 du 27 février 1958 instituant une obligation d'assurance en matière de circulation de véhicules terrestres à moteur," *Journal officiel de la République française: Lois et décrets*, 28 February 1958, 2148.

96. "Décret #59-135 du 7 janvier 1959 portant règlement d'administration publique pour l'application de la loi #58-203 du 27 février 1958 instituant une obligation d'assurance en matière de circulation de véhicules terrestres à moteur," *Journal officiel de la République française: Lois et décrets*, 9 January 1959, 655.

97. "M. Alain Barjot, président de séance," following Paul Robillard, "Le coût de l'alcoolisme pour les compagnies d'assurances," "Les actes du congrès de Versailles contre l'alcoolisme, octobre 1969, II," *Alcool ou santé* 1/2 (1970): 35.

98. CAC, 19880442, art. 3. "Conférence de presse donnée par le Professeur Robert Monod de l'Académie de Médecine, Président du Comité national de défense contre l'alcoolisme, le 29 janvier 1964: Pour la sécurité de la route: Opération Seine-et-Oise," 2.

99. CAC, 19880442, art. 1. Commission of Constitutional Law, National Assembly, "Communiqué à la presse," 25 February 1970, 1.

100. Rebecca J. Pulju, *Women and Mass Consumer Society in Postwar France* (New York: Cambridge University Press, 2011), 151.

101. On the development of the new middle class, see Luc Boltanski, *The Making of a Class: Cadres in French Society*, trans. Arthur Goldhammer (New York: Cambridge University Press, 1987); see also Pulju, *Women and Mass Consumer Society*, 149–161.

102. Marcel Bresard, "L'abus du vin et les chances de promotion sociale," *Bulletin d'informations du HCEIA*, February–March 1958, 9.

103. See especially Sully Ledermann, *Alcool, alcoolisme, alcoolisation: Mortalité, morbidité, accidents du travail* (Paris: Presses Universitaires de France, 1964), 19–159.

104. *Réalités*, July 1954, 32.

105. Raymond Girard, "Les Français malades de l'alcool," *Réalités*, September 1957, 71.

106. Georges Malignac, "La consommation d'alcool en France et à l'étranger," *Population* 8, no. 4 (1953): 770. Newspapers also published these comparisons.

107. Stéphane Banessy, "Seul record français qui ne soit pas près d'être battu: L'alcoolisme," *Carrefour*, 7 September 1960.

108. Malignac and Colin, *L'Alcoolisme*, 93.

109. On the role of French women in consumerism after 1945, see Pulju, *Women and Mass Consumer Society*; Kristin Ross, *Fast Cars, Clean Bodies: Decolonization and the Reordering of French Culture* (Cambridge, Massachusetts: The MIT Press, 1995); and Susan Weiner, *Enfants Terribles: Youth and Femininity in the Mass Media in France, 1945–1968* (Baltimore: Johns Hopkins University Press, 2001).

110. See reports in *Alcool ou santé* throughout the 1950s.

111. For an account of drinking among children, see Mlle Serin, "L'alcoolisme des enfants," session of 22 June 1954, *Bulletin de l'Académie de Médecine* (1954).

112. For examples of the "civilizing" role of consumption in the late nineteenth and early twentieth centuries, see Leora Auslander, *Taste and Power: Furnishing Modern France* (Berkeley: University of California Press, 1996); and Lisa Tiersten, *Marianne in the Market: Envisioning Consumer Society in Fin-de-Siècle France* (Berkeley: University of California Press, 2001).

113. Ross, *Fast Cars, Clean Bodies*, 51–54.

114. *La Presse médicale*, 11 April 1953.

115. CAC, 19940020, art. 18. Letter from Maurice Seguin to Michel Taupignon, general secretary of the HCEIA, 23 November 1972.

116. For magazines that were included in the 1961 campaign, see "Campagnes du Haut Comité dans les journaux féminins," *Bulletin de liaison des Comités départementaux et locaux*, May 1961, 20–21.

117. CAC, 19940020, art. 6. Letter from Léon Fleck, general secretary of the HCEIA, to M. Plauzolles, Salles d'Aude (Aude), 5 December 1961.

118. ANPAA, S1. "Les joies et les soucis de la femme," *Elle*, 28 January 1957.

119. "Livre blanc sur l'alcoolisme," *Bulletin d'informations du HCEIA*, November–December 1964.

120. Quoted in "Splendeurs et misères de la vigne et du vin dans la France moderne," *L'Algérie agricole et vinicole*, 20 June 1953.

121. On the relationship between the social sciences and modernization in France, see Ross, *Fast Cars, Clean Bodies*, 176–196.

122. Roger Dion, *Histoire de la vigne et du vin en France des origines au XIX siècle* (Paris: Clavreuil, 1959). Kolleen M. Guy observes the lack of a discussion of Algeria in Dion's work in "Culinary Connections and Colonial Memories in France and Algeria," *Food and History* 8, no. 1 (2010): 236.

123. Ross, *Fast Cars, Clean Bodies*, 186.

124. "Routes des grands vins: Bourgogne-Beaujolais," *L'Action automobile et touristique*, September 1963, 15.

125. Jean Linnemann, "La route des vins de France: Le Bordelais," *L'Action automobile et touristique*, November 1963, 19.

126. Cited in *Bulletin d'Informations du HCEIA*, October 1956, 14.

127. J.N.-N., "Les vins de France: Tout ce qu'il faut savoir sur la façon de les choisir, de les conserver, de les server et de les boire," *Réalités*, March 1953.

128. See, for example, J. Pouget, "Le tourisme et notre redressement," *Cuisine de France*, July 1947, 9.

129. Pierre Andrieu, "M. André Morice Ministre des Travaux Publics nous parle du tourisme," *La Journée vinicole*, 1–2 February 1953.

130. Claude Bonvin, *Un Art de France: Le Savoir-Boire* (Marseille, France: La Tartane, 1948), 10, 18.

131. These groups included, for example, the Academy of Wine and the Michelin Guides.

132. "Discours de reception de M. Bourdon-Michelin par Gaston Briand," *Revue du vin de France*, January–March 1950, 30.

133. *Guide Michelin*, 1947, 1950, 1954, 1962, 1964, 1965, 1970.

134. As reported in "Le Guide Michelin et les bonnes caves," *La Journée vinicole*, 31 May and 1 June 1953.

135. See, for example, "IIe rallye automobile des vins d'Anjou et de Samur," *Revue du vin de France*, April–June 1956.

136. O. W. Loeb, "La Route du vin," *The Guardian*, 22 November 1960.

137. "Routes et 'autoroutes des vins,'" *Le Moniteur vinicole*, 3 January 1970.

138. Monique Mounier, "La route du vin est coupée," *L'Express*, 20 April 1970.

139. Jean-Philippe Martin, "Les syndicates de viticulteurs en Languedoc (Aude et Hérault) de 1945 à la fin des années 1980," (PhD Diss., Université Paul-Valéry-Montpellier III, 1994), 131.

140. "Revue de presse," *Bulletin de l'Office international du vin*, February 1970, 194.

141. Y. Le Vaillant, "La France entre deux vins," *Témoignage chrétien*, 29 August 1963.

142. Ibid.

143. Charles Quittanson, "Le vin dans la restauration," *La Revue du vin de France*, October–December 1958, 26.

144. "A propos des 'vins de café': Lettre d'un lecteur du Gard," *La Journée vinicole*, 16 June 1953.

145. Art Buchwald, "Drinking Is Not a Vice," *New York Herald Tribune*, 6 June 1959.

146. CAC, 19940020, art. 18. Letter from Jean Durand, president of the Departmental Federation of Mass-Consumed Wines in Bordeaux, to Robert Debré, 14 April 1959.

5. Europeanizing the Revolution

1. French Council of Ministers, "Comme toujours, dans les systèmes compliquées, il y a des gens qui trouvent leur compte, ce sont les initiés," 21 August 1963, in Alain Peyrefitte, *C'était de Gaulle: "La France reprend sa place dans le monde,"* vol. 2 (Paris: Fayard, 1997), 364.

2. Ibid.

3. More research needs to be done on the impact of European integration on the French wine industry. For a seminal start, see Maria X. Chen, "Wine in Their Veins: France and the European Community's Common Wine Policy, 1967–1980," (PhD Diss., London School of Economics and Political Science, 2013); for a more general understanding of the evolution of wine policy in the common market, see Antonio Niederbacher, *Wine in the European Community* (Luxembourg: Office for Official Publications of the European Communities, 1988).

4. For the number of European consumers, see "Un exposé de M. de Longueau, directeur de la Fédération internationale des industries et du commerce en gros des vins et

spiritueux à l'Assemblée générale des négociants en vins fins des Côtes du Rhône," *Bulletin de l'Institut national des appellations d'origine des vins et eaux-de-vie*, April 1958, 97.

5. Jean-Pierre Deroudille, *Le vin face à la mondialisation: L'exception viticole contre la globalisation des marchés?* (Paris: Hachette, 2003), 85.

6. Edgard Pisani's response to "Question #2565, du 7 mai 1963, de M. Raoul Bayou, député," *Bulletin d'informations du HCEIA*, September–October 1964, 32.

7. "Les voies de l'harmonisation," *Le Progrès agricole et viticole*, 30 April 1962, 186.

8. Charles Braibant, "Le vin de France dans l'histoire," *La Journée vinicole*, 15 January 1953.

9. Henri Delagrange, "Le vin de qualité Europe?" *Bulletin de l'Institut national des appellations d'origine des vins et d'eaux-de-vie*, April 1962, 18.

10. The regions have long been important to French nation-state building. For just two examples, see Caroline Ford, *Creating the Nation in Provincial France: Religion and Political Identity in Brittany* (Princeton: Princeton University Press, 1993); and Kolleen M. Guy, *When Champagne Became French: Wine and the Making of a National Identity* (Baltimore: Johns Hopkins University Press, 2003).

11. For this figure, see "Un exposé de M. de Longueau," 98.

12. J.K., "Le vin français et le marché commun," *Perspectives*, 17 January 1970, 6. Originally published in *Cahiers de la CE*, May 1962.

13. Centre des Archives contemporaines (hereafter CAC), 19940020, art. 18. Quoted in Georges Malignac, "Le marché commun et la lutte contre l'alcoolisme," 1971, 2.

14. CAC, 19940020, art. 18. Malignac, "Le marché commun et la lutte contre l'alcoolisme," 2.

15. *Bulletin de l'Office international du vin*, June 1947, 163. Originally published in Rome's *La Gazeta vinicola*, 26 May 1947.

16. For a summary of these policies, see Andy Smith, Jacques de Maillard, and Olivier Costa, *Vin et politique: Bordeaux, la France, la mondialisation* (Paris: Presses de la Fondation Nationale des Sciences Politiques, 2007), esp. 78–87.

17. Michel Cointat, "Le vin et le marché commun," *Bulletin de l'Institut national des appellations d'origine des vins et d'eaux-de-vie*, July 1965, 62.

18. The quote comes from Edgar Faure in F.-M. d'Athis, "Le président Edgar Faure répond à nos questions," *Revue du vin de France*, June 1966, 10. On the INAO's efforts to protect its norms within the EEC, see, for example, Michel Cointat, "Le vin et le marché commun," *Revue du vin de France*, June 1965.

19. Delagrange, "Le vin de qualité Europe?," 17.

20. Charles de Gaulle, for example, notoriously challenged American corporate influence in France in the 1960s. On this topic, see Richard F. Kuisel, *Seducing the French: The Dilemma of Americanization* (Berkeley: University of California Press, 1993), 154–184. For a discussion of multinationals in the alcohol industry, see Teresa da Silva Lopes, *Global Brands: The Evolution of Multinationals in Alcoholic Beverages* (New York: Cambridge University Press, 2007).

21. Jean-Jacques Servan-Schreiber, *Le défi américain* (Paris: Denoël, 1967).

22. "France's Grapes of Wrath," *The Economist*, 22 July 1967, 339.

23. "Mémoire en réponse aux critiques formulées à l'égard du régime des appellations d'origine contrôlée," *Bulletin de l'Institut national des appellations d'origine des vins et d'eaux-de-vie*, July 1963, 36.

24. Henri Pestel, "La protection des produits originaux dans la CEE," *Bulletin de l'Institut national des appellations d'origine des vins et d'eaux-de-vie*, January 1963, 19.

25. On the Empty Chair Crisis, see N. Piers Ludlow, "Challenging French Leadership: Germany, Italy, the Netherlands and the Outbreak of the Empty Chair Crisis of 1965–1966," *Contemporary European History* 8 (July 1999): 231–248.

26. On agricultural politics in the common market, see Ann-Christina L. Knudsen, *Farmers on Welfare: The Making of Europe's Common Agricultural Policy* (Ithaca: Cornell University Press, 2009).

27. Historical Archives of the European Commission (hereafter BAC), 48/1984/1132. European Commission, "Le marché européen du vin," February 1978, 6.

28. Archives nationales (hereafter AN), 80AJ/103. "Observations de la Fédération des associations viticoles sur le rapport présenté par M. J. Long, directeur de l'IVCC," April 1957, 7–8.

29. Étienne May, "Problème de l'alcoolisme," sessions of 20 and 21 January 1959, *Journal officiel de la République française: Avis et rapports du Conseil économique,* 19 February 1959, 205.

30. CAC, 19940020, art. 18. Malignac, "Le Marché commun et la lutte contre l'alcoolisme," 2.

31. BAC, 2/1965/15. CREDOC, "Conclusions de l'étude de la demande de vin dans les pays de la communauté," 13 July 1961, 4.

32. Historical Archives of the European Council (hereafter CM2)/1970/638. "Note: Propositions de règlements dans le secteur viti-vinicole," 14 November 1968, 3. See also Chen's discussion in "Wine in Their Veins," esp. 66–70.

33. BAC, 129/1983/555. General Secretariat, European Commission, "Réponse à la question écrite N141/68 posée par M. Riedel," September 1968.

34. Smith, *Vin et politique,* 82. See note 51.

35. Centre des Archives économiques et financières (hereafter CAEF), 1A/373/1. CNJA, "Que faire pour la viticulture? Positions et propositions des jeunes agriculteurs," May 1975, 2.

36. "L'Avenir de la viticulture française," sessions of 11 and 12 October 1977, *Journal officiel de la République française: Avis et rapports du Conseil économique,* 15 February 1978, 253.

37. See, for example, CM2/1970/638. "Aide-mémoire: Position de la délégation française à l'égard de l'établissement d'une politique commune viti-vinicole," 11 November 1968.

38. Quoted in Geneviève Gavignaud-Fontaine, *Le Languedoc viticole, la Méditerranée et l'Europe au siècle dernier (XXe)* (Montpellier, France: Publications de l'Université Paul-Valéry, 2000), 185.

39. On the growing number of cooperative wineries, see Leo A. Loubère, *The Wine Revolution in France: The Twentieth Century* (Princeton: Princeton University Press, 1990), 147. On the cooperative movement in the Languedoc, see Winnie Lem, *Cultivating Dissent: Work, Identity, and Praxis in Rural Languedoc* (Albany: State University of New York Press, 1999).

40. CAC, 19940020, art. 9. Letter from Léon Fleck to Charles Kroepfle, deputy-mayor of Saint-Louis (Haut-Rhin), 16 July 1963.

41. Philippe Lamour recounts this story in *Le Cadran solaire* (Paris: Robert Laffont, 1980), 341.

42. CAC, 1940020, art. 4. "Séance du HCEIA du 11 janvier 1973," 6.

43. CAC, 1940020, art. 9. Léon Fleck, "Note à l'attention de Monsieur le Premier Ministre," 23 June 1965.

44. Loubère, *The Wine Revolution in France,* 132.

45. BAC, 154/1980/1684. Pierre Viansson-Ponte, "Produire pour détruire," *Le Monde,* 14–15 mars 1976.

46. Quoted in André Talvas, "L'alcool, est un ami qui vous veut du mal," *Témoignage chrétien,* 15 May 1969.

47. Archives d'histoire contemporaine (hereafter AHC), 2DE52. "Exposé de Monsieur le Professeur Debré," session of the HCEIA, 10 January 1962, 7–8.

48. It is worth noting that, unlike the home distillers and the settlers of Algeria, the peasants of the Languedoc found some sympathy among Parisian elites. See, for example, the writings of Wladimir d'Ormesson in *Le Figaro* around 1959–1960. During the surplus crises of the early 1970s, Paris newspapers of various political leanings saw the peasants as the victims of the large merchants.

49. Kiran Klaus Patel, "The Paradox of Planning: German Agricultural Policy in a European Perspective, 1920s to 1970s," *Past and Present* 212 (August 2011): 262.

50. CAC, 19940020, art. 2. "Séance du HCEIA du 11 décembre 1963," 10.

51. CAC, 19940020, art. 2. "Séance du HCEIA du 14 février 1962," 3.

52. "The Treaty of Rome," 25 March 1957.

53. CAC, 19940020, art. 18. "Aide-Mémoire relative aux propositions du Haut Comité d'étude et d'information sur l'alcoolisme," likely February 1963, 4.

54. Gavignaud-Fontaine discusses Philippe Lamour in *Le Languedoc viticole*, especially pp. 175–177.

55. I gathered this from archival material in Archives of the Association nationale de prévention en alcoologie et addictologie (hereafter ANPAA), Box Hérault.

56. The economists had their own journal, *Le Progrès agricole et viticole*, led by Jean Branas, who also corresponded with Robert Debré.

57. On Lamour's European politics, see Gilbert Noël, *Du pool vert à la politique agricole commune: Les tentatives de Communauté agricole européenne entre 1945 et 1955* (Paris: Economica, 1988), 425–426.

58. To understand the commission's goals, see PAV, "La vigne, cette plaie," *Le progrès agricole et viticole*, 31 March 1962, 143.

59. CAC, 19940020, art. 18. "Proposition de règlement du conseil établissant des règles générales pour la désignation des vins et des moûts," no date but likely 1971 or 1972.

60. CAC, 19940020, art. 18. Letter from Edgard Pisani to the minister of economic affairs and finance, 23 April 1963.

61. "M. Pisani: La France doit remplacer sa production viticole de masse par une production de luxe," *Le Monde*, 2 April 1963.

62. François Bouchard, "L'exportation des grands vins de France," *Revue du vin de France*, February 1967, 9–10.

63. "Décret #64-453 du 26 mai 1964 relatif à l'organisation du vignoble et à l'amélioration de la qualité de la production viticole," *Journal officiel de la République française: Lois et décrets*, 27 May 1964, 4507–4508; and "Décret #64-902 du 31 août 1964 relatif à la production viticole et à l'organisation du marché du vin," *Journal officiel de la République française: Lois et décrets*, 1 September 1964, 7951–7953. For a summary of these decrees, see René Barthe, *L'Europe du vin: 25 ans d'organisation communautaire du secteur viti-vinicole (1962–1987)* (Paris: Cujas, 1989), 108–110.

64. CAC, 19940020, art. 18. M. Roche, "Note à l'attention de M. le Professeur Debré," May 1963.

65. CAC, 19940020, art. 18. Letter from Robert Debré to the prime minister, 16 April 1964.

66. CAC, 19940020, art. 18. Council of State, "Note," session of 26 November 1963.

67. "Rapport moral présenté par le Conseil d'administration de la Confédération nationale des producteurs de vins et eaux-de-vie de vin à appellations d'origine contrôlées," *Bulletin de l'Institut national des appellations d'origine des vins et eaux-de-vie*, July 1966, 70.

68. CAC, 19940020, art. 18. Letter from Maurice Seguin, president of the Center of Research on National Drinks (CRDBN), to Jacques Chaban-Delmas, 14 September 1970.

69. CAC, 19940020, art. 28. Alain Barjot, vice president of the HCEIA, "Les problèmes de la production, de la commercialisation et de la consommation des boissons alcoolisées dans la communauté économique européenne," 2.

70. More work needs to be done on the IWO. For a start, see Olivier Jacquet, "De la Bourgogne à l'international: construction et promotion des norms d'appellation d'origine ou l'influence des syndicats professionnels locaux,"*Anthropology of Food* (December 2004).

71. See, for example, R. Protin, "La politique viticole et vinicole de la Communauté économique européenne: les accords dits 'de Bruxelles,'" *Bulletin de l'Office international du vin*, March 1962.

72. Deroudille, *Le vin face à la mondialisation*, 86.

73. Delagrange, "Le vin de qualité Europe?," 17.

74. On the importance of the 1970s to the current era of globalization, see Niall Ferguson, Charles S. Maier, Erez Manela, and Daniel J. Sargent, eds., *The Shock of the Global: The 1970s in Perspective* (Cambridge, Massachusetts: The Belknap Press of Harvard University Press, 2010).

75. For a discussion of the fate of Algerian wine after French rule, see Keith Sutton, "Algeria's Vineyards: A Problem of Decolonization," *Méditerranée* 65, no. 3 (1988): 55–66.

76. "Le vin d'Evian," *Le Monde*, 24 June 1963.

77. BAC, 129/1983/215. "Communication de la Commission au Conseil concernant le régime applicable à l'importation dans la Communauté de vins et autres produits viti-vinicoles en provenance du Maroc et de la Tunisie," 24 July 1970. See annex no. 1.

78. Raoul Browne, "Soutien nouveau au marché du vin," *Combat*, 23 June 1965.

79. Archives du Ministère des Affaires étrangères (hereafter AMAE), 29QO/69. Quoted in letter from the secretary of state at the prime ministry who was responsible for Algerian affairs to the prime minister, 26 September 1964.

80. For Italy's call to create a common external tariff, see, for example, BAC, 15/1993/71. General direction of foreign relations and general direction of the internal market, "Note concernant le problème des importations en République fédérale d'Allemagne des vins de distillation d'origine hellénique et algérienne," 3 January 1967, 4–5.

81. P.E., "Les raisons de la colère," *L'Express*, 28 February 1971.

82. Phillip C. Naylor, *France and Algeria: A History of Decolonization and Transformation* (Gainesville: University Press of Florida, 2000), 80.

83. Jean Offredo, *Algérie avec ou sans la France? Quatre dossiers clés* (Paris: Les Éditions du Cerf, 1973), 53.

84. Naylor, *France and Algeria*, 106.

85. Ibid., 54.

86. Loubère, *The Wine Revolution in France*, 234.

87. AMAE, DE-CE/714. Arriving telegram from François Seydoux in Bonn, Germany, 23 April 1970. See also Chen, "Wine in Their Veins."

88. For an understanding of Jacques Chaban-Delmas's politics, see Bernard Lachaise, Gilles Le Béguec, and Jean-François Sirinelli, eds., *Jacques Chaban-Delmas en politique* (Paris: Presses Universitaires de France, 2007).

89. CAC, 19940020, art. 18. CRDBN, *Fascicule d'information*, no date (but probably the early 1970s), 5.

90. Ibid.

91. "L'avenir de la viticulture française," sessions of 11–12 October 1977, *Journal officiel de la République française: Avis et rapports du Conseil économique et social*, 15 February 1978, 251.

92. CAEF, 1A/373/1. CNJA, "Que faire pour la viticulture?," 11.

93. Christine Clerc, "Vin: Une tragédie du sous-developpement," *Le Point*, 8 March 1976.

94. BAC, 130/1983/359. Letter from Jacques Allion, president of the National Committee for Community Commerce in Wines and Spirits, to Pierre Lardinois, general commissioner

of the European Commission who was responsible for agricultural problems, 16 February 1976, 4.

95. CAEF, 1A/373/1. Letter from H. M. Ghigonis, general delegate of the National Federation of Road Transportation, to Fourcade, minister of the economy and finance, 4 April 1975.

96. CAEF, 1A/373/1. Alain Lamassoure, "Note pour le Ministre," 18 June 1975, 5.

97. CAEF, 1A/373/1. National Assembly, "Compte rendu analytique officiel: Séance du mercredi 23 avril 1975," 32–33.

98. For these figures, see Rod Phillips, A Short History of Wine (New York: Ecco, 2002), 308.

99. Leo A. Loubère, Jean Sagnes, Laura Frader, and Rémy Pech, The Vine Remembers: French Vignerons Recall Their Past (Albany: State University of New York Press, 1985), 161.

100. On the important place of the Socialist Party in the Hérault between 1945 and the early 1960s, see Olivier Dedieu, "Le 'rouge' et le vin: Le socialisme à la conquête du vignoble héraultais," in Vignobles du Sud, XVIe–XXe siècle, ed. Henri Michel and Geneviève Gavignaud-Fontaine (Montpellier, France: Publications de l'Université Paul-Valéry, 2003), 623–645. On the leftist tradition in the Languedoc and its continuation after World War II, see Jean-Philippe Martin, "Les gauches vigneronnes contestataires en Languedoc, singularités, différenciations et évolutions (1945–2000)," in Vignobles du Sud, XVI–XXe siècle, 661–679; and Jean Sagnes, Le midi rouge, mythe ou réalité: Études d'histoire occitane (Paris: Anthropos, 1982).

101. This common identity was especially pronounced in the 1970s. Several books testify to this fact. See, for example, Claude Albranq, La guerre du vin (Nîmes, France: Théâtre de la Carriera, 1973); Jaume Bardissa, Cent ans de guerre du vin (Paris: Tema-Éditions, 1976); Pierre Bosc, Le vin de la colère (Paris: Galilée, 1976); Daniel Combes, Crises d'un siècle (Narbonne, France: CGVM, 1976); Henri Fabre-Colbert, Le défi occitan (Narbonne, France: Univers, 1976); Jean-Roger Fontvieille, Pauvre Midi: La révolte des vignerons, 1970–1977 (Paris: La Courtille, 1977); Michel Le Bris, Occitanie: Volem viure al païs (Paris: Gallimard, 1974); Emmanuel Maffre-Baugé, Vendanges amères (Paris: J.-P. Ramsay, 1976); Emmanuel Maffre-Baugé, Face à l'Europe des impasses (Toulouse, France: Privat, 1979); and Claude Marti, Homme d'Oc (Paris: Stock, 1975). A recent monograph that explores this theme is Andrew W. M. Smith, Terror and Terroir: The Winegrowers of the Languedoc and Modern France (Manchester, UK: Manchester University Press, 2016).

102. P.M.D., "La tension croit dans le vignoble méridional à quelques heures des manifestations," Le Monde, 10 April 1971.

103. André Cazes, André Castéra, Jacques Mestre, Michel Romain, M. Tallavignes, Jean Vialade, Claude Marti, and J.-P. Laval, La révolte du Midi (Mayenne, France: Les Presses d'Aujourd'hui, 1976), 207.

104. J.-P. Chabrol and Claude Marti, Caminarèm (Paris. Robert Laffont, 1978), 51. Quoted in Loubère, The Wine Revolution in France, 162.

105. Quoted in Jean-Robert Pitte, Philippe Lamour, 1903–1992: Père de l'aménagement du territoire en France (Paris: Fayard, 2002), 179.

106. Jean-Philippe Martin, "Les syndicates de viticulteurs en Languedoc (Aude et Hérault) de 1945 à la fin des années 1980," (PhD Diss., Université de Paul-Valéry-Montpellier III, 1994), 15–16.

107. Gavignaud-Fontaine, Le Languedoc viticole, 336–339. This was also the title of a book by Michel Le Bris, Occitanie: Volem viure al païs.

108. P.B. and S.J., "Comme prévu," Libération, 5 March 1976.

109. Loubère, The Wine Revolution in France, 135.

110. BAC, 48/1984/1132. European Commission, "Le marché européen du vin," February 1978; and Chen, "Wine in Their Veins," 124–129.

111. On the role of this group in giving France especially adept diplomatic skills in Brussels, see N. Piers Ludlow, "The Making of the CAP: Towards a Historical Analysis of the EU's First Major Policy," *Contemporary European History* 14 (August 2005): 347–371.

112. CAC, 19940020, art. 4. "Séance du HCEIA du 8 avril 1976," 4.

113. Deroudille, *Le vin face à la mondialisation,* 88.

114. BAC, 130/1983/3. M. Libero Della Briotta, "Rapport fait au nom de la commission de l'agriculture sur les propositions de la Commission des Communautés européennes au Conseil," *Parlement européen: Documents de séance,* document no. 187/75, 9 July 1975, 13–16.

115. Quoted in Jacques Godard and René Quatrefages, "Les milieux viticoles et leur langage," in "Les actes du congrès de Strasbourg," *Alcool ou santé* 1/2 (1977): 62.

116. CAC, 19940020, art. 9. Letter from Jean Trillat, general secretary of the HCEIA, to the general secretary of the government, 1 June 1976.

117. Martin, "Les syndicates de viticulteurs en Languedoc," 139–140.

118. See, for example, Olivier Dedieu, "Raoul Bayou, député du vin: Les logiques de constitution d'un patrimoine politique," *Pôle sud* 9, no. 1 (1998): 104. For a broader discussion of the viticultural transformation of the 1970s in the Languedoc, see William Genieys and Andy Smith, "'La grande transformation viticole: Une analyse du rôle des politiques européennes," in *Vignobles du Sud, XVI–XXe siècle,* 713–735.

119. Cazes, et al., *La révolte du Midi,* 108.

120. Council of Ministers, "Le sort de l'agriculture est maintenant le plus grand problème de la France," 30 May 1962, in Alain Peyrefitte, *C'était de Gaulle: "La France redevient la France"* vol. 1 (Paris: Fayard, 1994), 302.

121. Benjamin Stora suggests that the end of the Algerian war reawakened interest among French people in their regional identities. See *La gangrène et l'oubli: La mémoire de la guerre d'Algérie* (Paris: La Découverte, 1992), 212–213.

122. James Simpson characterizes this production as "industrial" in *Creating Wine: The Emergence of a World Industry, 1840–1914* (Princeton: Princeton University Press, 2011).

123. George M. Taber, *Judgment of Paris: California vs. France and the Historic 1976 Paris Tasting That Revolutionized Wine* (New York: Scribner, 2006).

124. See, among others, Marie-France Garcia-Parpet, *Le marché de l'excellence: Les grands crus à l'épreuve de la mondialisation* (Paris: Seuil, 2009); and Olivier Torrès, *The Wine Wars: The Mondavi Affair, Globalization, and "Terroir"* (New York: Palgrave Macmillan, 2006).

125. Raymond Dumay, *La mort du vin* (Paris: Stock, 1976), 7, 8, 231. The passage is not presented in order.

Conclusion

1. For more on the Bové story, see José Bové and François Dufour, *The World Is Not for Sale: Farmers Against Junk Food,* trans. Anna de Casparis (New York: Verso, 2002).

2. Scholarly accounts include Vicki Birchfield, "José Bové and the Globalisation Countermovement in France and Beyond: A Polanyian Interpretation," *Review of International Studies* 31 (2005): 581–598; Wayne Northcutt, "José Bové vs. McDonald's: The Making of a National Hero in the French Anti-Globalization Movement," *Proceedings of the Western*

Society for French History 31 (January 2003), http://quod.lib.umich.edu/w/wsfh/0642292.00 31.020?rgn=main;view=fulltext, accessed on 29 August 2015; Sarah Waters, "Globalization, the Confédération Paysanne, and Symbolic Power," *French Politics, Culture, and Society* 28 (Summer 2010): 96–117.

3. Quoted in Northcutt, "José Bové vs. McDonald's," 1.

4. Quoted in Sarah Bowen, "Embedding Local Places in Global Spaces: Geographical Indications as a Territorial Development Strategy," *Rural Sociology* 75, no. 2 (2010): 209–210.

5. See, for example, Carlo Petrini, *Slow Food: The Case for Taste*, trans. William Mc-Cuaig (New York: Columbia University Press, 2001); and Amy B. Trubek, *The Taste of Place: A Cultural Journey into Terroir* (Berkeley: University of California Press, 2008).

6. The idea of McWorld comes from Benjamin Barber, "Jihad vs. McWorld," *The Atlantic,* March 1992.

7. For French responses to globalization since the 1970s, see Rawi Abdelal, *Capital Rules: The Construction of Global Finance* (Cambridge, Massachusetts: Harvard University Press, 2007); Emile Chabal, ed. *France since the 1970s: History, Politics, and Memory in an Age of Uncertainty* (New York: Bloomsbury, 2014); Philip H. Gordon and Sophie Meunier, *The French Challenge: Adapting to Globalization* (Washington, D.C.: Brookings Institution Press, 2001); Herman Lebovics, *Bringing the Empire Back Home: France in the Global Age* (Durham: Duke University Press, 2004); Sophie Meunier, "Globalization and Europeanization: A Challenge to French Politics," *French Politics* 2, no. 2 (2004): 125–150; and Timothy B. Smith, *France in Crisis: Welfare, Inequality, and Globalization since 1980* (Cambridge: Cambridge University Press, 2004).

8. Quoted in Elizabeth Barham, "Translating 'Terroir': Social Movement Appropriation of a French Concept," paper presented at the Workshop on "International Perspectives on Alternative Agro-Food Networks, Quality, Embeddedness, and Bio-Politics," University of California, Santa Cruz, 12–13 October 2001, 2.

9. For an explanation of how the CP has recently mobilized the international community against industrialized agriculture, see Chaia Heller, *Food, Farms, and Solidarity: French Farmers Challenge Industrial Agriculture and Genetically Modified Crops* (Durham: Duke University Press, 2013).

10. For this statistic, see "Importance du vin dans l'économie française," *Bulletin de l'Institut national des appellations d'origine des vins et eaux-de-vie*, July 1959, 27.

11. For a general overview of how Algeria inspired wine reforms within metropolitan France, see Giulia Meloni and Johan Swinnen, "The Rise and Fall of the World's Largest Wine Exporter—and Its Institutional Legacy," *Journal of Wine Economics* 9, no. 1 (2014): 3–33.

12. Historical Archives of the European Commission (hereafter BAC), 28/1980/750. General director for exterior relations to Joseph A. Greenwald, extraordinary and plenipotentiary ambassador, chief of mission for the United States to the European Communities, 30 October 1974.

13. Throughout the twentieth century, many French intellectuals on both the right and the left viewed the United States as the land of crass commercialism. See, for example, David Strauss, *The American Menace: The Rise of French Anti-Americanism in Modern Times* (Westport, Connecticut: Greenwood Press, 1978). For post–World War II French anti-Americanism, see Richard F. Kuisel, *Seducing the French: The Dilemma of Americanization* (Berkeley: University of California Press, 1993); and Kuisel, *The French Way: How France Embraced and Rejected American Values and Power* (Princeton: Princeton University Press, 2013).

14. See, for example, Kermit Lynch, *Adventures on the Wine Route: A Wine Buyer's Tour of France* (New York: Farrar, Straus, Giroux, 1988).

15. For a history of the American fascination with Provence, see Helen Lefkowitz Horowitz, *A Taste for Provence* (Chicago: University of Chicago Press, 2016).

16. For discourses on the peasantry since the 1970s, see Sarah Farmer, "Memoirs of French Peasant Life: Progress and Nostalgia in Postwar France," *French History* 25, no. 3 (2011): 362–379; and Susan Carol Rogers, "Good to Think: The 'Peasant' in Contemporary France," *Anthropological Quarterly* 60 (April 1987): 56–63.

17. For *terroir*'s growing popularity starting in the late 1960s, see Serge Wolikow, "La construction des territoires du vin et l'émergence des terroirs: Problématique et démarches," in *Territoires et terroirs du vin du XVIIIe au XXIe siècles: Approche internationale d'une construction historique*, ed. Serge Wolikow and Olivier Jacquet (Dijon, France: Éditions Universitaires de Dijon, 2011), 19–21.

18. Pierre-Marie Doutrelant, "Alcool: Le mal français," *Le Nouvel observateur*, 21 June 1980, 45.

19. Jacques Duquesne, "La France entre deux vignes," *Le Point*, 6 March 1973.

20. Eugen Weber, *Peasants into Frenchmen: The Modernization of Rural France, 1870–1914* (Stanford: Stanford University Press, 1976); and Weber, *La fin des terroirs: La modernisation de la France rurale, 1870–1914*, trans. Antoine Berman and Bernard Géniès (Paris: Fayard, 1983).

21. On this topic, see Lebovics, *Bringing the Empire Back Home*, esp. 107–114.

22. François Portet, "*Produits de terroir*: Between Local Identity and Heritage," in *Recollections of France: Memories, Identities, and Heritage in Contemporary France*, ed. Sarah Blowen, Marion Demossier, and Jeanine Picard (New York: Berghahn Books, 2000), 168–184.

23. Jacques Revel, "Histoire vs. mémoire en France aujourd'hui," *French Politics, Culture, and Society* 18 (Spring 2000): 1–12.

24. Georges Durand, "La vigne et le vin," *Les Lieux de mémoire, III. Les France, 2. Traditions*, ed. Pierre Nora (Paris: Gallimard, 1994), 785–823.

25. Marion Demossier, "Consuming Wine in France: The 'Wandering' Drinker and the *Vin-anomie*," in *Drinking Cultures: Alcohol and Identity*, ed. Thomas M. Wilson (New York: Berg, 2005), 149.

26. Olivier Jacquet, "De la Bourgogne à l'international: Construction et promotion des normes d'appellation d'origine ou l'influence des syndicats professionnels locaux," *Anthropology of Food* (December 2004): 1–15.

27. Kal Raustiala and Stephen R. Munzer, "The Global Struggle over Geographical Indications," *European Journal of International Law* 18, no. 2 (2007): 350.

28. See, for example, Raustiala and Munzer, "The Global Struggle over Geographical Indications," 340–347.

29. Daniela Benavente, *The Economics of Geographical Indications* (Geneva: Graduate Institute Publications, 2013).

30. Quoted in Raustiala and Munzer, "The Global Struggle over Geographical Indications," 350.

31. Elizabeth Barham, "Translating Terroir: The Global Challenge of French AOC Labeling," *Journal of Rural Studies* 19:1: 127–138. On the international debate about *terroir*, see Tim Josling, "The War on *Terroir*: Geographical Indications as a Transatlantic Trade Conflict," *Journal of Agricultural Economics* 57, no. 3 (2006): 337–363.

32. Quoted in Sarah Bowen, *Divided Spirits: Tequila, Mezcal, and the Politics of Production* (Oakland: University of California Press, 2015), 16.

33. Quoted in Waters, "Globalization, the Confédération Paysanne, and Symbolic Power," 108.

34. Bowen, *Divided Spirits*, 16.

35. On the relationship between the European Union's appellation advocacy and the developing world, see Hélène Ilbert, "Products with Denominations of Origin and Intellectual Property Rights—the International Bargaining Process," in *Geographical Indications and International Agricultural Trade: The Challenge for Asia*, ed. Louis Augustin-Jean, Hélène Ilbert, and Neantro Saavedra-Rivano (New York: Palgrave Macmillan, 2012), 91–116.

36. For more information on this group, see Massimo Vittori, "The International Debate on Geographical Indications (GIs): The Point of View of the Global Coalition of GI Producers—oriGIn," *Journal of World Intellectual Property* 13, no. 2 (2010): 304–314.

37. See OriGIn's website, www.origin-gi.com.

38. Quoted in Vittori, "The International Debate on Geographical Indications (GIs)," footnote 312.

39. For criticisms of the globalization of appellations, see William A. Kerr, "Enjoying a Good Port with a Clear Conscience: Geographic Indicators, Rent Seeking, and Development," *Estey Centre Journal of International Law and Trade Policy* 7, no. 1 (2006): 1–14; and Louis Augustin-Jean, "Introduction: The Globalization of Geographical Indications: The Challenge for Asia," in *Geographical Indications and International Agricultural Trade*, 6–9.

40. For examples of other place-based products, see Sarah Besky, *The Darjeeling Distinction: Labor and Justice on Fair-Trade Tea Plantations in India* (Berkeley: University of California Press, 2014); Bowen, *Divided Spirits*; Claire Delfosse, *La France fromagère (1850–1990)* (Paris: La Boutique de l'Histoire, 2007); and Susan J. Terrio, *Crafting the Culture and History of French Chocolate* (Berkeley: University of California Press, 2000).

41. See how the Old and New Worlds interact in Jonathan Nossiter, dir., *Mondovino*, 2004, DVD.

42. See Mike Veseth, *Wine Wars: The Curse of the Black Nun, the Miracle of Two Buck Chuck, and the Revenge of the Terroirists* (New York: Rowman & Littlefield, 2011).

43. Harold McGee and Daniel Patterson, "Talk Dirt to Me," *New York Times*, 6 May 2007.

44. On Parker's influence on the French wine industry, see Elin McCoy, *The Emperor of Wine: The Rise of Robert M. Parker, Jr. and the Reign of American Taste* (New York: Harper, 2005).

45. See, for example, Paul Lukacs, *American Vintage: The Rise of American Wine* (Boston: Houghton Mifflin Company, 2000), 343–350.

46. Quoted in McGee and Patterson, "Talk Dirt to Me."

47. See Eric Asimov's numerous articles in his column, "The Pour," in *The New York Times*; and Jon Bonné, *The New California Wine: A Guide to the Producers and Wines behind a Revolution in Taste* (Berkeley: Ten Speed Press, 2013).

48. On this topic, see Trubek, *The Taste of Place*.

49. Marie-France Garcia-Parpet, *Le marché de l'excellence: Les grands crus à l'épreuve de la mondialisation* (Paris: Seuil, 2009), 189–199.

50. For a study of the consequences of recent globalization on peasant production, see, for example, Walden F. Bello, *The Food Wars* (New York: Verso, 2009); and Raj Patel, *Stuffed and Starved: The Hidden Battle for the World Food System* (Brooklyn: Melville House, 2007).

51. See Bowen, *Divided Spirits*.

52. It is worth pointing out that this trend is not new. See Corinne Marache and Philippe Meyzie, eds., *Les produits de terroir: L'empreinte de la ville* (Rennes, France: Presses Universitaires de Rennes, 2015).

53. Marie-Josée Cougard, "Lactalis: le fromager aux vingt-sept AOC," www.lesechos. fr/15/10/2010/LesEchos/20785-040-ECH_lactalis--le-fromager-aux-vingt-sept-aoc. htm, accessed on 2 August 2017. Véronique Richez-Lerouge discusses how multinational

corporations have taken over appellation cheeses in *Main basse sur les fromages AOP* (Paris: Érick Bonnier, 2017).

54. Michael Steinberger, *Au Revoir to All That: Food, Wine, and the End of France* (New York: Bloomsbury, 2009), 149.

55. See, for example, Alain Chatriot, "Qu-est-ce qu'un 'grand vin'? Entre terroirs, producteurs et consommateurs, quel rôle de l'État pour réguler le marché?," unpublished paper, 2016.

56. On the role of banks and corporations in globalization, see, for example, Ngaire Woods, *The Globalizers: The IMF, the World Bank, and Their Borrowers* (Ithaca: Cornell University Press, 2006); Alfred D. Chandler Jr. and Bruce Mazlish, eds., *Leviathans: Multinational Corporations and the New Global History* (New York: Cambridge University Press, 2005); and Geoffrey Jones, *Multinationals and Global Capitalism from the Nineteenth to the Twenty-First Century* (New York: Oxford University Press, 2005).

57. Charles S. Maier discusses this concept in "Consigning the Twentieth Century to History: Alternative Narratives for the Modern Era," *American Historical Review* 105, no. 3 (2000): 807–831. Also see his *Once within Borders: Territories of Power, Wealth, and Belonging since 1500* (Cambridge, Massachusetts: The Belknap Press of Harvard University Press, 2016).

58. On the rise of industrialized agriculture in the United States, see, for example, Paul Conkin, *A Revolution Down on the Farm: The Transformation of American Agriculture since 1929* (Lexington: University of Kentucky Press, 2009); and Deborah Fitzgerald, *Every Farm a Factory: The Industrial Ideal in American Agriculture* (New Haven: Yale University Press, 2010).

59. Quoted in Petrini, *Slow Food*, 26.

BIBLIOGRAPHY

Archives

Archives nationales (AN), Paris
    Agriculture Ministry
    Commerce and Industry Ministry
    Economic Council
    Interior Ministry
    National Assembly
    Planning Commissions
    Presidential Archives
    Prime Ministry
Archives du Ministère des Affaires étrangères (AMAE), Courneuve
Archives du Sénat (AS), Paris
Archives départementales de la Gironde (ADG), Bordeaux
    Private Papers of Jean-Max Eylaud
Archives départementales de la Seine-Saint-Denis (ADSSD), Bobigny
    Archives of the French Communist Party
Archives d'Histoire contemporaine (ADC), Fondation nationale des sciences politiques
    Papers of Michel Debré

Archives of the World Health Organization, Geneva, Switzerland
Centre des Archives contemporaines (CAC), Fontainebleau
  Interior Ministry
  Justice Ministry
  Prime Ministry
  Transportation Ministry
Centre des Archives économiques et financières (CAEF), Savigny-le-Temple
Historical Archives of the European Commission (BAC), Brussels, Belgium
Historical Archives of the European Council (CM2), Brussels, Belgium
Private Archives of the Association nationale de prévention en alcoologie et addictologie
  (ANPAA), Paris
  Private Archives of the Comités départementaux de défense contre l'alcoolisme
Private Archives of the Institut Pierre Mendès France (IPMF)

Mainstream Press

Press Clippings at Sciences Po
  "Alcoolisme" (1945–1976)
  "Vin" (1945–1976)
Réalités (1950–1958)

Specialized Press

Action automobile et touristique (1954, 1958, 1959, 1964, 1965, 1970)
Alcool et dérivés (1951–1959)
Alcool ou santé (1952–présent)
Algérie agricole et viticole (1931, 1935, 1951–1962)
L'Argus des assurances (1954, 1958–1959, 1964–1965, 1970)
Le Betteravier français (1946–1960)
Le Bouilleur de France (1947–1957)
Bulletin de l'Académie de Médecine (1939–1976)
Bulletin du Conseil économique (1954, 1959)
Bulletin d'information de l'Union fédérale de la consommation (1952–1976)
Bulletin d'informations du Haut Comité d'étude et d'information sur l'alcoolisme (1956–
  1976)
Bulletin de l'Intitut national des appellations d'origine des vins et eaux-de-vie (1937–1971)
Bulletin de Liaison des Comités départmentaux et locaux (1956–1976)
Bulletin de l'Office international du vin (1945–1976)
Bulletin de presse de la Santé de la France (1958–1963)
Bulletin des transports (1950, 1953)
Cuisine de France (1947–1948)
Études anti-alcooliques (1947–1952)
Guide Michelin (1947, 1950, 1954, 1962, 1964, 1965, 1970)
La Défense des distillateurs ambulants et des bouilleurs de cru (1947–1960)
L'Hôtellerie (1950–1955, 1970)

L'Industrie hôtelière de France et d'Outre-Mer (1954–1955, 1959–1960, 1970)
La Journée vinicole (1954–1955, 1959–1960, 1970, 1978, 1991)
Midi vinicole (1953–1955)
Le Moniteur vinicole (1953, 1954–1955, 1959–1960, 1965, 1970)
Prévention routière (1952–1970)
Le Progrès agricole et viticole (1931, 1935, 1946–1976)
Revue française de l'énergie (1949, 1950, 1953)
Revue de viticulture (1931, 1935)
Revue du vin de France (1945–1976)
Sondages (1954–1955)
Touring Club de France (1945–1955, 1958–1959, 1964–1965, 1970)
La Tribune agricole (1956–1963)
La Voix des colons (1931, 1935)

Publications of *Journal officiel*

Journal officiel de la République française: Lois et décrets (1873, 1917, 1953, 1954–1955, 1958, 1959–1960, 1964, 1965, 1970)
Journal officiel de la République française: Débats parlementaires, Assemblée nationale (1950, 1951, 1952, 1953, 1954, 1955, 1959, 1960, 1965, 1970)
Journal officiel de la République française: Débats parlementaires, Sénat (1951, 1953, 1955, 1959, 1960, 1965, 1970)
Journal officiel de la République française: Documents parlementaires, Assemblée nationale (1948, 1954)
Journal officiel de la République français: Avis et rapports du Conseil économique (1948, 1950, 1952, 1953, 1954, 1959, 1961, 1968, 1977)

Reports (in chronological order)

Bonnet, Charles. "Boissons alcooliques." *Journal officiel de la République française: Avis et rapports du Conseil économique.* 30 April 1948.
Leroy, Louis. "Problème de l'orientation à donner à la production agricole et des mesures propres à organiser un nouveau statut de l'alcool." *Journal officiel de la République française: Avis et rapports du Conseil économique.* 13 July 1950.
Guyon, Jean-Raymond. *Le problème de l'alcool: Les travaux de la Commission extra-parlementaire.* Bordeaux, France: Delmas, 1952.
Tidjani, Serpos. "Fabrication, importation, vente et consommation des boissons alcooliques en AOF, AEF, Cameroun et Togo." *Journal officiel de la République française: Avis et rapports du Conseil économique.* 21 May 1952.
Taïx, Gabriel. "Étude des problèmes posés par les excédents d'alcool." *Journal officiel de la République française: Avis et rapports du Conseil économique.* 21 July 1953.
May, Étienne. "Le problème de l'alcoolisme en France." *Journal officiel de la République française: Avis et rapports du Conseil économique.* 30 January 1954.

Brunaud, Jacques-Sylvain. *Rapport sur le coût annuel et la prévention de l'alcoolisme.* Paris: Comité Central d'Enquête sur le Coût et le Rendement des Services Publics, 1955.

Groupe d'étude des relations financières entre le Métropole et l'Algérie. Algiers: Imprimerie Officielle, 1955.

High Commission for Studies and Information on Alcoholism. *Rapport au Président du Conseil des Ministres sur l'activité du Haut Comité d'étude et d'information sur l'alcoolisme.* Paris: La Documentation Française, 1958.

Ministry for Algeria. *Perspectives décennales de développement économique de l'Algérie.* Algiers: Imprimerie Officielle, 1958.

May, Étienne. "Problème de l'alcoolisme." *Journal officiel de la République française: Avis et rapports du Conseil économique.* 19 February 1959.

General Delegation for the Government in Algeria. *Plan de Constantine, 1959–1963: Rapport général.* Algiers: Imprimerie Officielle, 1960.

Rapport sur les obstacles à l'expansion économique. Paris: Imprimierie Nationale, 1960.

High Commission for Studies and Information on Alcoholism. *Rapport au Premier Ministre sur l'activité du Haut Comité d'étude et d'information sur l'alcoolisme.* Paris: La Documentation Française, 1962.

"Problèmes de sécurité routière: Étude présentée par la section des travaux publics, des transports et du tourisme sur le rapport de M. Claude de Peyron le 3 juillet 1968." *Journal officiel de la République française: Avis et rapports du Conseil économique et social.* 26 November 1968.

Ternier, Michel, Jean L'Hoste, and Jérôme Lion. "Les aspects économiques de la mise en place d'un taux légal d'alcoolémie." *L'alcoolisme en France.* Paris: La Documentation Française, 31 March 1970.

High Commission for Studies and Information on Alcoholism. *Rapport au Premier Ministre sur l'activité du Haut Comité d'étude et d'information sur l'alcoolisme.* Paris: La Documentation Française, 1972.

"L'Avenir de la viticulture française." *Journal officiel de la République française: Avis et rapports du Conseil économique et social.* 15 February 1978.

Memoirs

Debré, Michel. *Gouverner: Mémoires, 1958–1962.* Paris: Albin Michel, 1988.

Debré, Robert. *L'honneur de vivre: Témoignage.* Paris: Hermann et Stock, 1974.

Lamour, Philippe. *Le cadran solaire.* Paris: Robert Laffont, 1980.

Peyrefitte, Alain. *C'était de Gaulle: "La France reprend sa place dans le monde."* Paris: Fallois/Fayard, 1994.

——. *C'était de Gaulle: "Tout le monde a besoin d'une France qui marche."* Paris: Fallois/Fayard, 2000.

Sauvy, Alfred. *La vie en plus: Souvenirs.* Paris: Calmann-Lévy, 1981.

Primary Articles and Books

Albranq, Claude. *La guerre du vin.* Nîmes, France: Théâtre de la Carriera, 1973.

Archimbaud, Léon. *La Grande France.* Paris: Hachette, 1928.

Aubey, Catherine, and Daniel Boulet. "La consommation d'alcool en France régresse et se transforme." *Économie et statistique* 176 (April 1985): 47–56.

Augé-Laribé, Michel. *Le problème agraire du socialisme: La viticulture industrielle du Midi de la France.* Paris: V. Giard & E. Brière, 1907.

Barber, Benjamin. "Jihad vs. McWorld." *The Atlantic.* March 1992.

Bardissa, Jaume. *Cent ans de guerre du vin.* Paris: Tema-Éditions, 1976.

Barthe, Édouard. *Le combat d'un parlementaire sous Vichy: Journal des années de guerre, 1940–1943.* Introduction by Jean Sagnes. Gap, France: Editions Singulières, 2007.

Barthes, Roland. "Le vin et le lait." *Lettres nouvelles* 26 (April 1955): 636–638.

——. *Mythologies.* Paris: Seuil, 1957.

——. *Mythologies.* Translated by Annette Lavers. New York: Hill and Wang, 1972.

Bastide, Henri. "Une enquête sur l'opinion publique à l'égard de l'alcoolisme." *Population* 9, no. 1 (1954): 13–42.

Bechtel, Guy. *1907, La grande révolte du Midi.* Paris: Robert Laffont, 1976.

Bello, Walden F. *The Food Wars.* New York: Verso, 2009.

Berget, Adrien. *Les vins de France: Histoire, géographie et statistique du vignoble français.* Paris: Germer Baillière, 1900.

Bonné, Jon. *The New California Wine: A Guide to the Producers and Wines behind a Revolution in Taste.* Berkeley: Ten Speed Press, 2013.

Bonvin, Claude. *Un art de France: Le savoir-boire.* Marseille, France: La Tartane, 1948.

Borel, Jacques. *Le vrai problème de l'alcoolisme: Étude médico-sociale, ses conditions, ses limites, mensonges des statistiques, réfutation d'un mythe.* Villejuif, France: Chez l'Auteur, 1957.

Borkenstein, Robert. F. *A Practical Experiment on the Effects of Alcohol on Driving Skill: A Report on the Driving Tests Conducted by the Participants of the Seminar on Alcohol and Road Traffic at the Southern Police Institute, February 23, 1956.* Louisville: Southern Police Institute, University of Louisville, 1956.

Bosc, Pierre. *Le vin de colère.* Paris: Galilée, 1976.

Bové, José, and François Dufour. *The World Is Not for Sale: Farmers Against Junk Food.* Translated by Anna de Casparis. New York: Verso, 2002.

Bresard, Marcel. "L'opinion publique et l'alcoolisme." *Population* 3, no. 3 (1948): 544–548.

Bulletin de l'Institut national des appellations d'origine des vins & eaux-de-vie. Le vin de France dans l'histoire. Special edition, 1953.

Camus, Albert. "Réflexions sur la guillotine." In *Réflexions sur la peine capitale*, by Arthur Koestler and Albert Camus. Paris: Calmann-Lévy, 1957.

Capus, Joseph. "Le statut des vins à appellation d'origine: proposition d'une nouvelle loi." *Revue de viticulture* (2 May 1935): 278.

——. *L'Évolution de la législation sur les Appellations d'origine: Genèse des Appellations contrôlées.* Paris: Louis Larmat, 1947.

Cazes, André, et al. *La révolte du Midi.* Mayenne, France: Les Presses d'Aujourd'hui, 1976.

Cépède, Michel. "La question viticole et l'alcoolisme." *Les Cahiers économiques* (February 1955).

Charles, Georges. *Le vignoble algérien et sa reconstitution.* Algiers: Jules Carbonel, 1946.

Cholley, A. "La population de la France en 1931." *Annales de géographie* 41, no. 234 (1932): 638–640.

Combes, Daniel. *Crises d'un siècle.* Narbonne, France: CGVM, 1976.

Confédération générale des vignerons algériens. *Mise au point du problème viticole algérien.* Algiers: La Type-Litho et Jules Carbonel, 1955.

Courtin, René. "La viticulture devant les pouvoirs publiques." *Revue politique et parlementaire* 147 (10 June 1931): 454–478.

Coutaz, Colette. *Bistros, bouilleurs & cie.* Paris: Les Éditions du Centurion, 1956.

Debré, Robert, and Alfred Sauvy. *Des Français pour la France.* Paris: Gallimard, 1946.

Defossé, Gaston. *La place du consommateur dans l'économie dirigée.* Paris: Presses Universitaires de France, 1941.

Dérobert, Léon. *L'économie de l'alcoolisme.* Paris: Institut National d'Hygiène, 1953.

Dib, Mohammed. *L'incendie.* Paris: Seuil, 1954.

Direction of Roads and Traffic, Ministry of Public Works, Transportation, and Tourism. *Les accidents corporels de la circulation routière en 1954.*

Douarche, Léon. *La vigne française et l'Europe.* Paris: Rassemblement National Populaire, 1941.

———. *Le vin et la vigne dans l'économie nationale française.* Paris: Cahiers de la Réorganisation Économique, 1943.

Duhamel, Georges. *Civilisation française.* Paris: Hachette, 1944.

Dumay, Raymond. *La mort du vin.* Paris: Stock, 1976.

Dumont, René. *Le problème agricole français: Esquisse d'un plan d'orientation et d'équipement.* Paris: Les Éditions Nouvelles, 1946.

———. "Alcool, ou lait et viande? Étude technique et économique d'orientation agricole et alimentaire." *Population* 8, no. 1 (1953): 57–72.

———. "Remontons la vigne sur les coteaux." *Bulletin des transports* (February 1953).

Dussine, Pierre. *Le statut des vins délimités de qualité supérieure.* Montpellier, France: Causse, Graille, & Castelnau, 1961.

Eylaud, Jean-Max. *Vin et santé: Vertus hygiéniques et thérapeutiques du vin.* Soissons, France: La Diffusion Nouvelle du Livre, 1960.

Fabre-Colbert, Henri. *Le défi Occitan.* Narbonne, France: Univers, 1976.

Fauvet, Jacques, and Henri Mendras, eds. *Les paysans et la politique dans la France contemporaine.* Paris: Armand Colin, 1958.

Feraoun, Mouloud. *Journal, 1955–1962: Reflections on the French-Algerian War.* Translated by Mary Ellen Wolf and Claude Fouillade. Lincoln: University of Nebraska Press, 2000.

Flanner, Janet. *Paris Journal, 1944–1965.* New York: Atheneum, 1965.

Fontvielle, Jean-Roger. *Pauvre Midi. La révolte des vignerons, 1970–1977.* Paris: La Courtille, 1977.

Gaston-Pastre, J. L. "Le problème du vin." *Revue des deux mondes* (15 November 1935): 358–375.

Gendarme, René. *L'économie de l'Algérie: Sous-développement et politique de croissance.* Paris: Armand Colin, 1959.

Géralin, Henri. "Le problème de l'alcoolisme dans les territoires d'outre-mer." *Population* 8, no. 2 (1953): 291–310.

Gravier, Jean François. *Paris et le désert français: Décentralisation, équipement, population.* Paris: Le Portulan, 1947.

Gringberg, Ph. "Le régime des alcools et les branches organisées de l'économie agricole française." *Revue d'économique politique* 52 (March–April 1938): 404–429.

Gross, Eugène. *Est-il vrai de dire que l'Algérie c'est la France?* Oran, Algeria: Heintz Frères, 1933.

Guyon, Jean-Raymond. *Le régime économique de l'alcool.* Bordeaux, France: Delmas, 1950.

——. *Au service du vin de Bordeaux: Un demi-siècle de défense et d'organisation de la vini-viticulture girondine.* Bordeaux, France: Delmas, 1956.

Isnard, Hildebert. "Vigne et colonisation en Algérie (1880–1947)." *Annales: Économie, sociétés, civilisations* 2, no. 3 (1947): 288–300.

——. "Vigne et colonisation en Algérie." *Annales de géographie* 58, no. 311 (1949): 212–219.

——. *La vigne en Algérie: étude géographique.* 2 vols. Gap, France: Ophrys, 1951, 1954.

——. "La viticulture algérienne: erreur économique?" *La revue africaine* 50 (1956).

——. "Vineyards and Social Structure in Algeria." Translated by James H. Labadie. *Diogenes* 7 (1959): 63–81.

Kruger, Édouard. *Les bienfaits de l'Union douanière métropole-Algérie et la question vinicole.* Oran, Algeria: Syndicat du commerce des vins en gros du départment d'Oran, 1933.

La Gravière, Emmanuel. "L'Alcoolisation des populations d'outre-mer." In *Problèmes sociaux: La prostitution, l'alcoolisme, le logement.* Paris: Fayard, 1954.

Le Bris, Michel. *Occitanie: Volem viure al país.* Paris: Gallimard, 1974.

Ledermann, Sully. *Alcool, alcoolisme, alcoolisation: Données scientifiques de caractère physiologique, économique et social.* 2 vols. Paris: Presses Universitaires de France, 1956, 1964.

Létinier, Georges. "Éléments d'un bilan national de l'alcoolisme." *Population* 1, no. 2 (1946): 317–328.

de Lur-Saluces, Mis. "Les grands vins de France." *Revue des deux mondes* (15 March 1953).

Lynch, Kermit. *Adventures on the Wine Route: A Wine Buyer's Tour of France.* New York: Farrar, Straus, and Giroux, 1988.

Maffre-Baugé, Emmanuel. *Vendanges amères.* Paris: J.-P. Ramsay, 1976.

——. *Face à l'Europe des impasses.* Toulouse, France: Privat, 1979.

Malignac, Georges. "La consommation d'alcool en France et à l'étranger." *Population* 8, no. 4 (1953): 766–770.

Malignac, Georges, and Robert Colin. *L'alcoolisme.* Paris: Presses Universitaires de France, 1954.

Marfaing, Norbert. *Contrôle de la production de l'alcool en France.* Paris: Domat-Montchrestien, 1940.

Marres, Paul. *La vigne et le vin en France.* Paris: Armand Colin, 1950.

Marti, Claude. *Homme d'Oc*. Paris: Stock, 1975.

McGee, Harold, and Daniel Patterson. "Talk Dirt to Me." *New York Times*, 6 May 2007.

Mendès France, Pierre. *Oeuvres complètes: S'engager*. vol. 1. Paris: Gallimard, 1984.

——. *Oeuvres complètes: Gouverner c'est choisir*. vol. 3. Paris: Gallimard, 1986.

Michot, Albert. "Le problème du lait en France." *Population* 2, no. 1 (1947): 67–80.

Mignot, André. *L'alcoolisme: Suicide collectif de la nation*. Paris: Cahiers des Amis de la Liberté, 1955.

——. *Le Privilège des bouilleurs de cru . . . ou le scandale qui nous coûte plus de 50 milliards par an*. Paris: Allain SICAR Elbeuf, 1958.

Milhau, Jules. *Le problème français du vin*. Montpellier, France: Causse, Graille, & Castelnau, 1945.

——. "L'avenir de la viticulture française." *Revue économique* 4, no. 5 (1953): 700–738.

Miot, Pierre. *Le régime économique de l'alcool*. Paris: Éditions Berger-Levrault, 1962.

Nicolas, Maurice. *Avec Pierre Poujade sur les routes de France*. Les Sables-d'Olonne, France: Les Éditions de l'Équinoxe, 1955.

Offredo, Jean. *Algérie avec ou sans la France? Quatre dossiers clés*. Paris: Les Éditions du Cerf, 1973.

Patel, Raj. *Stuffed and Starved: The Hidden Battle for the World Food System*. New York: Melville, 2008.

Patouillet, Joseph. "Le problème viticole et la pénible situation des vins de crus." *L'État moderne* (3 March 1936): 173–189.

Petrini, Carlo. *Slow Food: The Case for Taste*. Translated by William McCuaig. New York: Columbia University Press, 2001.

Peynaud, Emile. *Le goût du vin*. Paris: Dunod, 1980.

Peyronnet, Francis Raymond. *Le vignoble nord-africain*. Paris: J. Peyronnet et Cie, 1950.

Pinon, René. "Les nouvelles conceptions de l'État." *Revue économique internationale* 4, no. 1 (October 1929): 7–30.

Portmann, Georges. *Son activité parlementaire, scientifique, économique et sociale*. Bordeaux, France: Delmas, 1959.

——. *Son activité parlementaire, scientifique, économique et sociale*. Bordeaux, France: Delmas, 1962.

Poujade, Pierre. *J'ai choisi le combat*. Saint-Céré, France: Société Générale des Éditions et des Publications, 1955.

Querlin, Marise. *Les chaudières de l'enfer: Le problème de l'alcoolisme en France*. Paris: Gallimard, 1955.

Richez-Lerouge, Véronique. *Main basse sur les fromages AOP*. Paris: Érick Bonnier, 2017.

Sadoun, Roland, Giorgio Lolli, and Milton Silverman. *Drinking in French Culture*. New Brunswick, New Jersey: Rutgers Center of Alcohol Studies, 1965.

Sauvy, Alfred. "Faits et problèmes du jour." *Population* 5 (1950): 5–12.

——. *Ce que serait la France sans l'alcoolisme*. December 1956.

——. *Histoire économique de la France entre les deux guerres (1931–1939)*. Vol. 2 Paris: Economica, 1984.

——. *De Paul Reynaud à Charles de Gaulle: Un économiste face aux hommes politiques, 1934–1967*. Paris: Casterman, 1972.

Servan-Schreiber, Jean Jacques. *Le défi américain*. Paris: Denoël, 1967.

Steinberger, Michael. *Au Revoir to All That: Food, Wine, and the End of France*. New York: Bloomsbury, 2009.

Taïx, Gabriel. *La faillite de la viticulture est-elle pour demain?* Bordeaux, France: Delmas, 1934.

——. *Les problèmes posés par les excédents d'alcool*. Paris: Presses Universitaires de France, 1953.

Toché, François. *L'art de bien conduire*. Paris: Flammarion, 1954.

Trémolières, Jean. *Manger pour vivre*. Paris: Éditions Jeheber, 1955.

——. *Les boissons: Physiologie, comportement, hygiène*. Paris: Institut National d'Hygiène, 1957.

Vallin, Jacques, and Jean-Claude Chesnais. "Les accidents de la route en France: Mortalité et morbidité depuis 1953." *Population* 3 (1975): 443–478.

Volck, Antoinette. *Le problème viticole franco-algérien*. Paris: Domat-Montchrestien, 1934.

Widmark, Erik M. P. *Les lois cardinals de la distribution et du métabolisme de l'alcool éthylique dans l'organisme humain*. Lund, Sweden: C.W.K. Gleerup, 1930.

——. *Principles and Applications of Medicolegal Alcohol Determination*. Davis, California: Biomedical Publications, 1981. First published in 1932.

Secondary Sources

Abdelal, Rawi. *Capital Rules: The Construction of Global Finance*. Cambridge, Massachusetts: Harvard University Press, 2007.

Abrams, L., and D. J. Miller. "Who Were the French Colonialists? A Reassessment of the Parti Colonial, 1890–1914." *Historical Journal* 19, no. 3 (September 1976): 685–725.

Ageron, Charles-Robert. *Histoire de l'Algérie contemporaine*. Vol. 2, 1871–1954. Paris: Presses Universitaires de France, 1979.

——. "Les colonies devant l'opinion publique française (1919–1939)." *Revue française d'histoire d'outre-mer* 77, no. 286 (1990): 31–73.

Anderson, Barbara Gallatin. "How French Children Learn to Drink." In *Beliefs, Behaviors, and Alcoholic Beverages: A Cross-Cultural Survey*, edited by Mac Marshall. Ann Arbor: University of Michigan Press, 1979.

Andrew, C. M., and A. S. Kayna-Forstner. "The French 'Colonial Party': Its Composition, Aims, and Influence, 1885–1914." *Historical Journal* 14, no. 1 (March 1971): 99–128.

Andrieu, Claire, Lucette Le Van, and Antoine Prost, eds. *Les nationalisations de la Libération: De l'utopie au compromis*. Paris: Presses de la Fondation Nationale des Sciences Politiques, 1987.

Augé-Laribé, Michel. *La politique agricole de la France de 1880 à 1940*. Paris: Presses Universitaires de France, 1950.

Augustin-Jean, Hélène Ilbert, and Neantro Saavedra-Rivano, eds. *Geographical Indications and International Agricultural Trade: The Challenge for Asia.* New York: Palgrave Macmillan, 2012.

Auslander, Leora. *Taste and Power: Furnishing Modern France.* Berkeley: University of California Press, 1996.

Bagnol, Jean-Marc. *Le Midi viticole au Parlement: Édouard Barthe et les députés du vin de l'Hérault (années 1920–1930).* Montpellier, France: Presses Universitaires de la Méditerranée, 2010.

Barclay, Fiona, Charlotte Ann Chopin, and Martin Evans. "Introduction: Settler Colonialism and French Algeria." *Settler Colonial Studies* (2017): 1–16.

Barham, Elizabeth. "Translating "Terroir": Social Movement Appropriation of a French Concept." Paper presented at the Workshop on "International Perspectives on Alternative Agro-Food Networks, Quality, Embeddedness, and Bio-Politics," University of California, Santa Cruz, 12–13 October 2001.

——. "Translating Terroir: The Global Challenge of French AOC Labeling." *Journal of Rural Studies* 19 (2003): 127–138.

Barrows, Susanna. "Alcohol, France, and Algeria: A Case Study in the International Liquor Trade." *Contemporary Drug Problems* (Winter 1982): 525–543.

——. "'Parliaments of the People': The Political Culture of Cafés in the Early Third Republic." In *Drinking: Behavior and Belief in Modern History*, edited by Susanna Barrows and Robin Room, 87–97. Berkeley: University of California Press, 1991.

Barthe, René. *L'Europe du vin: 25 ans d'organisation communautaire du secteur vitivinicole (1962–1987).* Paris: Cujas, 1989.

Bédarida, François, and Jean-Pierre Rioux, eds. *Pierre Mendès France et le mendésisme: L'expérience gouvernementale (1954–1955) et sa posterité.* Paris: Fayard, 1985.

Benamouzig, Daniel. *La santé au miroir de l'économie.* Paris: Presses Universitaires de France, 2005.

Benavente, Daniela. *The Economics of Geographical Indications.* Geneva: Graduate Institute Publications, 2013.

Bennoune, Mahfoud. *The Making of Contemporary Algeria, 1830–1987.* New York: Cambridge University Press, 1988.

Berlivet, Luc. "Les démographes et l'alcoolisme: Du 'fléau social' au 'risque de santé.'" *Vingtième Siècle* 95 (July–September 2007): 93–113.

Berstein, Serge, Pierre Milza, and Jean-François Sirinelli, eds. *Michel Debré: Premier ministre, 1959–1962.* Paris: Presses Universitaires de France, 2005.

Besky, Sarah. *The Darjeeling Distinction: Labor and Justice on Fair-Trade Tea Plantations in India.* Berkeley: University of California Press, 2014.

Bess, Michael. *The Light-Green Society: Ecology and Technical Modernity in France, 1960–2000.* Chicago: University of Chicago Press, 2003.

Bessaoud, Omar. "La viticulture oranaise, au coeur de l'économie colonial." In *Histoire de l'Algérie à la période coloniale*, edited by Abderrahmane Bouchène et al., 425–428. Paris: La Découverte, 2012.

Birchfield, Vicki. "José Bové and the Globalisation Countermovement in France and Beyond: A Polanyian Interpretation." *Review of International Studies* 31, no. 3 (2005): 581–598.

Birebent, Paul. *Hommes, vignes et vins de l'Algérie française, 1830–1962*. Nice, France: Jacques Gandini, 2007.

Bivar, Venus. "The Ground beneath Their Feet: Agricultural Industrialization and the Remapping of Rural France, 1945–1976." PhD Diss., University of Chicago, 2010.

Bloch-Lainé, François, and Jean Bouvier. *La France, 1944–1954: Dialogue sur les choix d'une modernisation*. Paris: Fayard, 1986.

Blondiaux, Loïc. *La fabrique de l'opinion: Une histoire sociale des sondages*. Paris: Seuil, 1998.

Bohling, Joseph. "'Drink Better, but Less': The Rise of France's Appellation System in the European Community, 1946–1976." *French Historical Studies* 37, no. 3 (Summer 2014): 501–530.

——. "The Mendès France Milk Regime: Alcoholism as a Problem of Agricultural Subsidies, 1954–1955." *French Politics, Culture, and Society* 32, no. 3 (Winter 2014): 97–120.

Bologne, Jean Claude. *Histoire morale et culturelle de nos boissons*. Paris: Robert Laffont, 1991.

Boltanski, Luc. *The Making of a Class: Cadres in French Society*. Translated by Arthur Goldhammer. New York: Cambridge University Press, 1987. First published 1982 by Minuit.

Boninchi, Marc. *Vichy et l'ordre moral*. Paris: Presses Universitaires de France, 2005.

Bourdieu, Pierre. *Distinction: A Social Critique of the Judgment of Taste*. Translated by Richard Nice. Cambridge, Massachusetts: Harvard University Press, 1984.

——. "Taste of Luxury, Taste of Necessity." In *The Taste Culture Reader: Experiencing Food and Drink*, edited by Carolyn Korsmeyer, 72–78. New York: Berg, 2005.

Boussard, Isabel. *Vichy & la corporation paysanne*. Paris: Presses de la Fondation Nationale des Sciences Politiques, 1980.

——. "Roland Maspétiol, une figure marquante de l'économie rurale." *Économie rurale* 223 (1994): 3–5.

Bowen, Sarah. "Embedding Local Places in Global Spaces: Geographical Indications as a Territorial Development Strategy." *Rural Sociology* 75, no. 2 (2010): 209–243.

——. *Divided Spirits: Tequila, Mezcal, and the Politics of Production*. Oakland: University of California Press, 2015.

Brower, Benjamin C. *A Desert Named Peace: The Violence of France's Empire in the Algerian Sahara, 1844–1902*. New York: Columbia University Press, 2009.

Brown, Bernard E. "Alcohol and Politics in France." *American Political Science Review* 51, no. 4 (December 1957): 976–994.

Brown, Megan. "Drawing Algeria into Europe: Shifting French Policy and the Treaty of Rome (1951–1964)." *Modern and Contemporary France* 25 (2017): 191–218.

Canevet, Corentin. *Le modèle agricole breton: histoire et géographie d'une révolution agro-alimentaire*. Rennes, France: Presses Universitaires de Rennes, 1992.

Cépède, Michel. *Agriculture et alimentation en France durant la deuxième guerre mondiale*. Paris: Éditions Génin, 1961.

Chabal, Emile, ed. *France since the 1970s: History, Politics, and Memory in an Age of Uncertainty*. New York: Bloomsbury, 2014.

Chandler, Jr., Alfred D., and Bruce Mazlish, eds. *Leviathans: Multinational Corporations and the New Global History.* New York: Cambridge University Press, 2005.

Chapman, Herrick. *State Capitalism and Working-Class Radicalism in the French Aircraft Industry.* Berkeley: University of California Press, 1991.

——. "Modernity and National Identity in Postwar France." *French Historical Studies* 22, no 2 (Spring 1999): 291–314.

——. *France's Long Reconstruction: In Search of the Modern Republic.* Cambridge, Massachusetts: Harvard University Press, 2018.

Chatriot, Alain. *La Démocratie sociale à la française: L'expérience du Conseil national économique, 1924–1940.* Paris: La Découverte, 2002.

——. "Renouveaux et permanence d'une institution représentative. Le Conseil économique sous la IVe République." In *Les nouvelles dimensions du politique. Relations professionnelles et régulations sociales*, edited by Laurent Duclos, Guy Groux, and Olivier Mériaux. Paris: Librairie Générale de Droit et de Jurisprudence, 2009.

——. *Pierre Mendès France: Pour une République moderne.* Paris: Armand Colin, 2015.

——. "Qu'est-ce qu'un 'grand vin'? Entre terroirs, producteurs et consommateurs, quel rôle de l'État pour réguler le marché?" Unpublished paper, 2016.

Chatriot, Alain, Marie-Emmanuelle Chessel, and Matthew Hilton, eds. *Au nom du consommateur: Consommation et politique en Europe et aux États-Unis au XXe siècle.* Paris: La Découverte, 2004.

Chatriot, Alain, Edgar Leblanc, and Édouard Lynch, eds. *Organiser les marchés agricoles: Le temps des fondateurs des années 1930 aux années 1950.* Paris: Armand Colin, 2012.

Chen, Maria X. "Wine in Their Veins: France and the European Community's Common Wine Policy, 1967–1980." PhD Diss., London School of Economics and Political Science, 2013.

Choi, Sung Eun. *Decolonization and the French of Algeria: Bringing the Settler Colony Home.* New York: Palgrave Macmillan, 2016.

Clarke, Jackie. *France in the Age of Organization: Factory, Home, and Nation from the 1920s to Vichy.* New York: Berghahn, 2011.

Cleary, M. C. *Peasants, Politicians, and Producers: The Organization of Agriculture in France since 1918.* New York: Cambridge University Press, 1989.

Collovald, Annie. "Le verre de lait de Pierre Mendès France ou l'oubli des origines politiques." In *La santé dans tous ses états*, edited by Alain Garrigou. Biarritz, France: Atlantica, 2000.

Conkin, Paul. *A Revolution Down on the Farm: The Transformation of American Agriculture since 1929.* Lexington: University of Kentucky Press, 2009.

Cooper, Frederick. "Provincializing France." In *Imperial Formations*, edited by Ann Laura Stoler, Carole McGranahan, and Peter C. Perdue, 341–377. Santa Fe: School for Advanced Research Press, 2007.

Csergo, Julia. "The Emergence of Regional Cuisines." In *Food: A Cultural History*, edited by Jean-Louis Flandrin and Massimo Montanari, 497–511. Translated by A. Sonnenfeld. New York: Columbia University Press, 1999.

Cupers, Kenny. *The Social Project: Housing Postwar France.* Minneapolis: University of Minnesota Press, 2014.

Dard, Olivier. "La technocratie." In *La France d'un siècle à l'autre, 1914–2000: Dictionnaire critique*, edited by J.-P. Rioux and J.-F. Sirinelli, 883–890. Paris: Hachette, 1999.

Dargelos, Bertrand. *La lutte antialcoolique en France depuis le XIXe siècle*. Paris: Dalloz, 2008.

da Silva Lopes, Teresa. *Global Brands: The Evolution of Multinationals in Alcoholic Beverages*. New York: Cambridge University Press, 2007.

Davis, Muriam Haleh. "Restaging Mise en Valeur: 'Postwar Imperialism' and the Plan de Constantine." *Review of Middle East Studies* 44, no. 2 (Winter 2010): 176–186.

Decreton, Séverine. "Les trois temps de la communication de sécurité routière." *Quaderni* 33, no. 1 (1997): 85–98.

Dedieu, Olivier. "Raoul Bayou, député du vin: les logiques de constitution d'un patrimoine politique." *Pôle Sud* 9, no. 1 (1998): 88–110.

——. "Le 'rouge' et le vin. Le socialisme à la conquête du vignoble héraultais." In *Vignobles du sud, XVIe–XXe siècle*, edited by Henri Michel and Geneviève Gavignaud-Fontaine, 623–645. Montpellier, France: Publications de l'Université Paul-Valéry, 2003.

Delfosse, Claire. *La France fromagère (1850–1990)*. Paris: La Boutique de l'Histoire, 2007.

Demossier, Marion. "Consuming Wine in France: The 'Wandering' Drinker and the *Vin-anomie*." In *Drinking Cultures: Alcohol and Identity*, edited by Thomas M. Wilson. Oxford: Berg, 2005.

——. *Wine Drinking Culture in France: A National Myth or a Modern Passion?* Cardiff: University of Wales Press, 2010.

Deroudille, Jean-Pierre. *Le vin face à la mondialisation: L'exception viticole contre la mondialisation des marchés?* Paris: Hachette, 2003.

Dion, Roger. *Histoire de la vigne et du vin en France: Des origines au XIXe siècle*. Paris: Clavreuil, 1959.

Dufumier, Marc. *Un agronome dans son siècle: Actualité de René Dumont*. Paris: Karthala, 2002.

Dulong, Delphine. *Moderniser la politique: Aux origines de la Ve République*. Paris: L'Harmattan, 1997.

Durand, Georges. "La vigne et le vin." In *Les Lieux de mémoire, III. Les France, 2. Traditions*, edited by Pierre Nora, 785–821. Paris: Gallimard, 1992.

Durand, Sébastien. "Négociants du Bordelais et de Bourgogne." In *Dictionnaire historique des patrons français*, edited by Jean-Claude Daumas et al. Paris: Flammarion, 2010.

Enjalbert, Henri. *Histoire de la vigne et du vin: L'avènement de la qualité*. Paris: Bordas, 1975.

Farmer, Sarah. "Memoirs of French Peasant Life: Progress and Nostalgia in Postwar France." *French History* 25, no. 3 (2011): 362–379.

Ferguson, Niall, et al., eds. *The Shock of the Global: The 1970s in Perspective*. Cambridge, Massachusetts: The Belknap Press of Harvard University Press, 2010.

Ferré, Georges. *1907, la guerre du vin: Chronique d'une désobéissance civique dans le Midi*. Portet-sur-Garonne, France: Loubatières, 1997.

Fillaut, Thierry. *Les Bretons et l'alcool (XIXe–XXe siècle)*. Rennes, France: École Nationale de la Santé Publique, 1991.

Fitzgerald, Deborah. *Every Farm a Factory: The Industrial Ideal in American Agriculture*. New Haven: Yale University Press, 2010.

Flonneau, Mathieu. *L'automobile au temps des trente glorieuses: Un rêve d'automobilisme*. Carbonne, France: Loubatières, 2016.

Ford, Caroline. *Creating the Nation in Provincial France: Religion and Political Identity in Brittany*. Princeton: Princeton University Press, 1993.

Fourastié, Jean. *Les trente glorieuses ou la révolution invisible de 1946 à 1975*. Paris: Fayard, 1979.

Fourcade, Marion. "The Vile and the Noble: On the Relation between Natural and Social Classifications in the French Wine World." *Sociological Quarterly* 53, no. 4 (2012): 524–545.

Fourquet, François, ed. *Les comptes de la puissance. Histoire de la comptabilité nationale et du plan*. Paris: Encres, 1980.

Frader, Laura Levine. *Peasants and Protest: Agricultural Workers, Politics, and Unions in the Aude, 1850–1914*. Berkeley: University of California Press, 1991.

Franche, Dominique, and Yves Léonard. *Pierre Mendès France et la démocratie locale: Actes du colloque du conseil général de l'Eure*. Rennes, France: Presses Universitaires de Rennes, 2004.

Frankel, Charles. *Terres de vignes*. Paris: Seuil, 2011.

Furlough, Ellen. "Making Mass Vacations: Tourism and Consumer Culture in France, 1930s–1970s." *Comparative Studies in Society and History* 40, no. 2 (1998): 247–286.

Gale, George D. *Dying on the Vine: How the Phylloxera Transformed Wine*. Berkeley: University of California Press, 2011.

Galtier, Gaston. *Le vignoble du Languedoc méditerranéen et du Roussillon. Études comparatives d'un vignoble de masse*. 3 vols. Montpellier, France: Causse, Graille & Castelnau, 1960.

Garcia-Parpet, Marie-France. *Le marché de l'excellence: Les grands crus à l'épreuve de la mondialisation*. Paris: Seuil, 2009.

Garrier, Gilbert. *Le phylloxéra: Une guerre de trente ans (1870–1900)*. Paris: Albin Michel, 1989.

——. *Histoire sociale et culturelle du vin*. Paris: Bordas, 1995.

Gavignaud-Fontaine, Geneviève. "L'extinction de la 'viticulture pour tous' en Languedoc, 1945–1984?" *Pôle Sud* 9, no. 1 (1998): 57–70.

——. *Le Languedoc viticole, la Méditerranée et l'Europe au siècle dernier (XXe)*. Montpellier, France: Publications de l'Université Paul-Valéry, 2000.

Genieys, William, and Andy Smith. "La grande transformation viticole. Une analyse du rôle des politiques européennes." In *Vignobles du sud, XVI–XXe siècle*, edited by Henri Michel and Geneviève Gavignaud-Fontaine. Montpellier, France: Publications de l'Université Paul-Valéry, 2003.

Gicquel, Jean, and Lucien Sfez. *Problèmes de la réforme de l'État en France depuis 1934*. Paris: Presses Universitaires de France, 1965.

Gordon, Philip H., and Sophie Meunier. *The French Challenge: Adapting to Globalization*. Washington, D.C.: Brookings Institution Press, 2001.

Gosnell, Jonathan K. *The Politics of Frenchness in Colonial Algeria, 1930–1954*. Rochester: University of Rochester Press, 2002.

Grenard, Fabrice. *La France du marché noir (1940–1949)*. Paris: Payot, 2008.

Guy, Kolleen M. *When Champagne Became French: Wine and the Making of a National Identity*. Baltimore: Johns Hopkins University Press, 2003.

———. "Culinary Connections and Colonial Memories in France and Algeria." *Food and History* 8, no. 1 (2010): 219–236.

———. "Silence and *Savoir-Faire* in the Marketing of Products of the *Terroir*." *Modern and Contemporary France* 19, no. 4 (November 2011): 459–475.

Haine, W. Scott. *The World of the Paris Café: Sociability among the French Working Class, 1789–1914*. Baltimore: Johns Hopkins University Press, 1996.

———. "Drink, Sociability, and Social Class in France, 1789–1945: The Emergence of a Proletarian Public Sphere." In *Alcohol: A Social and Cultural History*, edited by Mack P. Holt, 121–144. New York: Berg, 2006.

Hall, Peter A. *Governing the Economy: The Politics of State Intervention in Britain and France*. New York: Oxford University Press, 1986.

Hansen, Peo, and Stefan Jonsson. *Eurafrica: The Untold History of European Integration and Colonialism*. New York: Bloomsbury, 2014.

Harp, Stephen L. *Marketing Michelin: Advertising and Cultural Identity in Twentieth-Century France*. Baltimore: Johns Hopkins University Press, 2001.

———. *Au Naturel: Naturism, Nudism, and Tourism in Twentieth-Century France*. Baton Rouge: Louisiana State University Press, 2014.

Heath, Elizabeth. *Wine, Sugar, and the Making of Modern France: Global Economic Crisis and the Racialization of French Citizenship, 1870–1910*. New York: Cambridge University Press, 2014.

———. "The Color of French Wine: Southern Wine Producers Respond to Competition from the Algerian Wine Industry in the Early Third Republic." *French Politics, Culture, and Society* 35, no. 2 (Summer 2017): 89–110.

Hecht, Gabrielle. *The Radiance of France: Nuclear Power and National Identity after World War II*. Cambridge, Massachusetts: The MIT Press, 2000.

Heller, Chaia. *Food, Farms, and Solidarity: French Farmers Challenge Industrial Agriculture and Genetically Modified Crops*. Durham: Duke University Press, 2013.

Henrich-Franke, Christian. "Mobility and European Integration: Politicians, Professionals and the Foundation of the ECMT." *Journal of Transport History* 29, no. 1 (March 2008): 64–82.

Hinnewinkel, Jean-Claude. *Les terroirs viticoles: Origines et devenirs*. Bordeaux, France: Féret, 2004.

Hodeir, Catherine. *Stratégies d'empire: La grand patronat colonial face à la décolonisation*. Paris: Belin, 2003.

Hoffmann, Stanley. *Le mouvement Poujade*. Paris: Armand Colin, 1956.

———. "Paradoxes of the French Political Community." In *In Search of France: The Economy, Society, and Political System in the Twentieth Century*, edited by Stanley Hoffman et al. New York: Harper & Row, 1963.

Horne, Alistair. *A Savage War of Peace: Algeria, 1954–1962*. New York: New York Review of Books, 2006. First published 1977 by Macmillan.

Horowitz, Helen Lefkowitz. *A Taste for Provence*. Chicago: University of Chicago Press, 2016.

Howard, Sarah. "Selling Wine to the French: Official Attempts to Increase French Wine Consumption, 1931–1936." *Food and Foodways* 12, no. 4 (2004): 197–224.

——. *Les images de l'alcool en France, 1915–1942.* Paris: Centre National de la Recherche Scientifique, 2006.

——. "The Advertising Industry and Alcohol in Interwar France." *Historical Journal* 51, no. 2 (2008): 421–455.

Humbert, Florian. "L'INAO, de ses origines à la fin des années 1960: Genèse et évolutions du système des vins d'AOC." PhD Diss., Université de Bourgogne, 2011.

——. "La Champagne viticole au prisme du national, de la mise en place des AOC à la creation du CIVC." In *La construction des territoires du Champagne (1811–1911–2011),* edited by Serge Wolikow, 197–205. Dijon, France: Éditions Universitaires de Dijon, 2013.

Jackson, Julian. *France: The Dark Years, 1940–1944.* New York: Oxford University Press, 2001.

Jacquet, Olivier. "De la Bourgogne à l'international: Construction et promotion des normes d'appellation d'origine ou l'influence des syndicats professionnels locaux." *Anthropology of Food* (December 2004).

——. *Un siècle de construction du vignoble bourguignon: Les organisations vitivinicoles de 1884 aux AOC.* Dijon, France: Éditions Universitaires de Dijon, 2009.

Jacquet, Olivier, and Gilles Laferté. "Le contrôle républicain du marché: Vignerons et négociants sous la Troisième République." *Annales: Histoire, sciences sociales* 61, no. 5 (September–October 2006): 1147–1170.

——. "La route des vins et l'émergence d'un tourisme viticole en Bourgogne dans l'entre-deux-guerres." *Cahiers de géographie du Québec* 57, no. 162 (2013): 425–444.

Jayet, Marie-Claire. *Prévention du risque "alcool au volant" dans un pays producteur de vin, 1960–1990.* Arcueil, France: Institut National de Recherche sur les Transports et leur Sécurité, 1994.

Jobs, Richard Ivan. *Riding the New Wave: Youth and the Rejuvenation of France after the Second World War.* Stanford: Stanford University Press, 2007.

Jones, Geoffrey. *Multinationals and Global Capitalism from the Nineteenth to the Twenty-First Century.* New York: Oxford University Press, 2005.

Jones, Joseph. *The Politics of Transport in Twentieth-Century France.* Montreal: McGill-Queen's University Press, 1984.

Josling, Tim. "The War on *Terroir*: Geographical Indications as a Transatlantic Trade Conflict." *Journal of Agricultural Economics* 57, no. 3 (2006): 337–363.

Kalman, Samuel. *French Colonial Fascism: The Extreme Right in Algeria, 1919–1939.* New York: Palgrave Macmillan, 2013.

Kaplan, Steven Laurence. *Good Bread Is Back: A Contemporary History of French Bread, the Way It Is Made, and the People Who Make It.* Translated by Catherine Porter. Durham: Duke University Press, 2006.

Keeler, John T. S. "The Corporatist Dynamic of Agricultural Modernization in the Fifth Republic." In *The Fifth Republic at Twenty,* edited by William G. Andrews and Stanley Hoffman. Albany: State University of New York Press, 1981.

——. *The Politics of Neocorporatism in France: Farmers, the State, and Agricultural Policy-making in the Fifth Republic.* New York: Oxford University Press, 1987.

Kemp, Tom. *The French Economy, 1913–39: The History of a Decline.* New York: St. Martin's Press, 1972.

Kerr, William A. "Enjoying a Good Port with a Clear Conscience: Geographic Indicators, Rent Seeking, and Development." *Estey Centre Journal of International Law and Trade Policy* 7, no. 1 (2006): 1–14.

Kladstrup, Don, and Petie Kladstrup. *Wine and War: The French, the Nazis, and the Battle for France's Greatest Treasure*. New York: Broadway Books, 2001.

Kletzlen, Anne. *L'automobile et la loi: Comment est né le Code de la route?* Paris: L'Harmattan, 2000.

———. *De l'alcool à l'alcool au volant: La transformation d'un problème public*. Paris: L'Harmattan, 2007.

Knudsen, Ann-Christina L. *Farmers on Welfare: The Making of Europe's Common Agricultural Policy*. Ithaca: Cornell University Press, 2009.

Kuisel, Richard F. *Capitalism and the State in Modern France: Renovation and Economic Management in the Twentieth Century*. New York: Cambridge University Press, 1981.

———. "Coca-Cola and the Cold War: The French Face Americanization, 1948–1953." *French Historical Studies* 17, no. 1 (1991): 96–116

———. *Seducing the French: The Dilemma of Americanization*. Berkeley: University of California Press, 1993.

———. *The French Way: How France Embraced and Rejected American Values and Power*. Princeton: Princeton University Press, 2012.

Kurzer, Paulette. *Markets and Moral Regulation: Cultural Change in the European Union*. New York: Cambridge University Press, 2001.

Lachaise, Bernard, Gilles Le Béguec, and Jean-François Sirinelli, eds. *Jacques Chaban-Delmas en politique*. Paris: Presses Universitaires de France, 2007.

Lachiver, Marcel. *Vins, vignes et vignerons: Histoire du vignoble français*. Paris: Fayard, 1988.

Lackerstein, Debbie. *National Regeneration in Vichy France: Ideas and Policies, 1930–1944*. Burlington, Vermont: Ashgate, 2012.

Laferté, Gilles. *La Bourgogne et ses vins: Image d'origine contrôlée*. Paris: Belin, 2006.

———. "The Folklorization of French Farming: Marketing Luxury Wine in the Interwar Years." *French Historical Studies* 34, no. 4 (2011): 679–712.

Launay, Michel. *Paysans algériens: La terre, la vigne et les hommes*. Paris: Seuil, 1963.

Lavenir, Catherine Bertho. *La roue et le stylo: Comment nous sommes devenus touristes*. Paris: Odile Jacob, 1999.

Lebovics, Herman. *The Alliance of Iron and Wheat in the Third French Republic, 1860–1914: Origins of the New Conservatism*. Baton Rouge: Louisiana State University Press, 1988.

———. *True France: The Wars over Cultural Identity, 1900–1945*. Ithaca: Cornell University Press, 1992.

———. *Bringing the Empire Back Home: France in the Global Age*. Durham: Duke University Press, 2004.

Le Bras, Stéphane. "La domination du marché viticole par le négoce des vins languedociens en temps de crise (1925–1939)." *Siècles* 35–36 (2012): 1–12.

———. "Négoce et négociants en vins dans l'Hérault: Pratiques, influences, trajectoires (1900–1970)." PhD Diss., Université de Montpellier III—Paul Valéry, 2013.

Lefeuvre, Daniel. *Chère Algérie: La France et sa colonie, 1930–1962*. Paris: Flammarion, 2005.

Lem, Winnie. *Cultivating Dissent: Work, Identity, and Praxis in Rural Languedoc*. Albany: State University of New York, 1999.

Lerner, Barron H. *One for the Road: Drunk Driving since 1900*. Baltimore: Johns Hopkins University Press, 2011.

Lévy, Michel Louis. *Alfred Sauvy: Compagnon du siècle*. Paris: La Manufacture, 1990.

Loubère, Leo A. *The Red and the White: A History of Wine in France and Italy in the Nineteenth Century*. Albany: State University of New York Press, 1978.

———. *The Wine Revolution in France: The Twentieth Century*. Princeton: Princeton University Press, 1990.

Loubère, Leo A., et al., eds. *The Vine Remembers: French Vignerons Recall Their Past*. Albany: State University of New York Press, 1985.

Loubet, Jean-Louis. *Histoire de l'automobile française*. Paris: Seuil, 2001.

Luckin, Bill. "A Kind of Consensus on the Roads? Drink Driving Policy in Britain, 1945–1970." *Twentieth Century British History* 21, no. 3 (2010): 350–374.

Ludlow, N. Piers. "Challenging French Leadership: Germany, Italy, the Netherlands, and the Outbreak of the Empty Chair Crisis of 1965–1966." *Contemporary European History* 8, no. 2 (July 1999): 231–248.

———. "The Making of the CAP: Towards a Historical Analysis of the EU's First Major Policy." *Contemporary European History* 14, no. 3 (August 2005): 347–371.

Lukacs, Paul. *American Vintage: The Rise of American Wine*. Boston: Houghton Mifflin Company, 2000.

———. *Inventing Wine*. New York: Norton, 2012.

Lynch, Édouard. "Le 'moment Debré' et la genèse d'une nouvelle politique agricole." In *Michel Debré, Premier minister (1959–1962)*, edited by Serge Berstein, Pierre Milza, and Jean-François Sirinelli, 335–363. Paris: Presses Universitaires de France, 2005.

Lyons, Amelia H. *The Civilizing Mission in the Metropole: Algerian Families and the French Welfare State during Decolonization*. Stanford: Stanford University Press, 2013.

Maier, Charles S. "Consigning the Twentieth Century to History: Alternative Narratives for the Modern Era." *American Historical Review* 105, no. 3 (2000): 807–831.

———. *Once within Borders: Territories of Power, Wealth, and Belonging since 1500*. Cambridge, Massachusetts: The Belknap Press of Harvard University Press, 2016.

Marache, Corinne, and Philippe Meyzie, eds. *Les produits de terroir: L'empreinte de la ville*. Rennes, France: Presses Universitaires de Rennes, 2015.

Margairaz, Michel, ed. *Pierre Mendès France et l'économie: Pensée et action*. Paris: Odile Jacob, 1989.

Margairaz, Michel. *L'État, les finances et l'économie. Histoire d'une conversion, 1932–1952*. 2 vols. Paris: Comité pour l'Histoire Économique et Financière de la France, 1991.

Markham, Dewey. *1855: A History of the Bordeaux Classification*. New York: John Wiley & Sons, 1998.

Marseille, Jacques. *Empire colonial et capitalisme français: Histoire d'un divorce*. Paris: Albin Michel, 2005. First published 1984 by Albin Michel.

Martin, Jean-Philippe. "Les syndicats de viticulteurs en Languedoc (Aude et Hérault) de 1945 à la fin des années 1980." PhD Diss., Université de Paul-Valéry-Montpellier III, 1994.

———. "Les gauches vigneronnes contestataires en Languedoc, singularités, différenciations et évolutions (1945–2000)." In *Vignobles du sud, XVI–XXe siècle*, edited by Henri Michel and Geneviève Gavignaud-Fontaine, 661–679. Montpellier, France: Publications de l'Université Paul-Valéry, 2003.

Martin, Philippe. "Viticulture du Languedoc: Une tradition syndicale en mouvement." *Pôle sud* 9, no. 1 (1998): 71–87.

Matthews, Mark A. *Terroir and Other Myths of Winegrowing.* Oakland: University of California Press, 2015.

McCoy, Elin. *The Emperor of Wine: The Rise of Robert M. Parker, Jr. and the Reign of American Taste.* New York: Harper, 2005.

Meloni, Giulia, and Johan Swinnen. "The Political Economy of Wine Regulations." *Journal of Wine Economics* 8, no. 3 (2013): 244–284.

——. "The Rise and Fall of the World's Largest Wine Exporter—and Its Institutional Legacy." *Journal of Wine Economics* 9, no. 1 (2014): 3–33.

——. "Bugs, Tariffs, and Colonies: The Political Economy of the Wine Trade, 1860–1970." AAWE Working Paper 206 (October 2016).

Mendras, Henri, and Jacques Fauvet, eds. *Les paysans et la politique dans la France contemporaine.* Paris: Armand Colin, 1958.

Meunier, Jacob. *On the Fast Track: French Railway Modernization and the Origins of the TGV, 1944–1983.* Westport, CT: Praeger, 2002.

Meunier, Sophie. "Globalization and Europeanization: A Challenge to French Politics." *French Politics* 2, no. 2 (2004): 125–150.

Meynaud, Jean. *Les groupes de pression en France.* Paris: Armand Colin, 1958.

Milward, Alan S. *The Reconstruction of Western Europe.* Berkeley: University of California Press, 1984.

——. *The European Rescue of the Nation-State.* Berkeley: University of California Press, 1992.

Mioche, Philippe. *Le Plan Monnet: Genèse et élaboration 1941–1947.* Paris: Publications de la Sorbonne, 1987.

Moravcsik, Andrew. *The Choice for Europe: Social Purpose and State Power from Messina to Maastricht.* Ithaca: Cornell University Press, 1998.

Moulin, Annie. *Peasantry and Society in France since 1789.* Translated by M. C. Cleary and M. F. Cleary. New York: Cambridge University Press, 1991.

Mouré, Kenneth. "Food Rationing and the Black Market in France, 1940–1944." *French History* 24, no. 2 (2010): 262–282.

Muller, Pierre. *Le technocrate et le paysan. Essai sur la politique française de modernisation de l'agriculture, de 1945 à nos jours.* Paris: Les Éditions Ouvrières, 1984.

Munholland, Kim. "'Mon docteur le vin': Wine and Health in France, 1900–1950." In *Alcohol: A Social and Cultural History,* edited by Mack P. Holt, 77–90. New York: Berg, 2006.

Napo, Félix. *La révolte des vignerons.* Toulouse, France: Privat, 1971.

Naylor, Phillip C. *France and Algeria: A History of Decolonization and Transformation.* Gainesville: University Press of Florida, 2000.

——. "A Reconsideration of the Fourth Republic's Legacy and Algerian Decolonization." *French Colonial History* 2 (2002): 159–180.

Neiertz, Nicolas. *La coordination des transports en France: De 1918 à nos jours.* Paris: Comité pour l'Histoire Économique et Financière de la France, 1999.

Niederbacher, Antonio. *Wine in the European Community*. Luxembourg: Office for Official Publications of the European Communities, 1988.

Noël, Gilbert. *Du pool vert à la politique agricole commune: Les tentatives de la Communauté agricole européenne entre 1945 et 1955*. Paris: Economica, 1988.

Nord, Philip. *France's New Deal: From the Thirties to the Postwar Era*. Princeton: Princeton University Press, 2010.

Northcutt, Wayne. "José Bové vs. McDonald's: The Making of a National Hero in the French Anti-Globalization Movement." *Proceedings of the Western Society for French History* 31 (January 2003).

Nourrisson, Didier. *Le buveur du XIXe siècle*. Paris: Albin Michel, 1990.

———. *À votre santé: Éducation et santé sous la IVe République*. Saint-Étienne, France: Publications de l'Université de Saint-Étienne, 2002.

Orselli, Jean. "Usages et usagers de la route, mobilité et accidents, 1860–2008." PhD Diss., Université de Paris I, 2009.

Parker, Thomas. *Tasting French Terroir: The History of an Idea*. Oakland: University of California Press, 2015.

Patel, Kiran Klaus. "The Paradox of Planning: German Agricultural Policy in a European Perspective, 1920s to 1970s." *Past and Present* 212, no. 1 (August 2011): 239–269.

Paul, Harry W. *Science, Vine, and Wine in Modern France*. New York: Cambridge University Press, 1996.

———. *Bacchic Medicine: Wine and Alcohol Therapies from Napoleon to the French Paradox*. Amsterdam: Rodopi B. V., 2001.

Paxton, Robert O. *Vichy France: Old Guard and New Order, 1940–1944*. New York: Columbia University Press, 1972.

———. *French Peasant Fascism: Henry Dorgères's Greenshirts and the Crises of French Agriculture, 1929–1939*. New York: Oxford University Press, 1997.

Pech, Rémy. *Entreprise viticole et capitalisme en Languedoc-Roussillon: Du phylloxera aux crises de mévente*. Toulouse, France: Publications de l'Université de Toulouse-Le Mirail, 1975.

Pedigo, Nathan. "The Struggle for *Terroir* in French Algeria: Land, Wine, and Contested Identity in the French Empire." PhD Diss., Southern Illinois University, 2015.

Peer, Shanny. *France on Display: Peasants, Provincials, and Folklore in the 1937 Paris World's Fair*. Albany: State University of New York Press, 1998.

Persell, Stuart Michael. *The French Colonial Lobby, 1889–1938*. Stanford: Hoover Institution Press, 1983.

Pesche, Denis. *Le syndicalisme agricole spécialisé en France: Entre la spécificité des intérêts et le besoin d'alliances*. Paris: L'Harmattan, 2000.

Pessis, Céline, ed. *Une autre histoire des "trente glorieuses": Modernisation, contestations et pollutions dans la France d'après-guerre*. Paris: La Découverte, 2013.

Phillips, Rod. *A Short History of Wine*. New York: Ecco, 2002.

———. *French Wine: A History*. Oakland: University of California Press, 2016.

Piketty, Thomas. *Capital in the Twenty-First Century*. Translated by Arthur Goldhammer. Cambridge, Massachusetts: Harvard University Press, 2014.

Pinkard, Susan. *A Revolution in Taste: The Rise of French Cuisine.* Cambridge, UK: Cambridge University Press, 2008.

Pitte, Jean-Robert. *Philippe Lamour, 1903–1992: Père de l'aménagement du territoire en France.* Paris: Fayard, 2002.

Plack, Noelle. *Common Land, Wine, and the French Revolution: Rural Society and Economy in Southern France, c. 1789–1820.* Surrey, UK: Ashgate, 2009.

Portet, François. *"Produits de terroir*: Between Local Identity and Heritage." In *Recollections of France: Memories, Identities, and Heritage in Contemporary France,* edited by Sarah Blowen, Marion Demossier, and Jeanine Picard, 168–184. New York: Berghahn, 2000.

Prestwich, Patricia E. *Drink and the Politics of Social Reform: Antialcoholism in France since 1870.* Palo Alto, CA: Society for the Promotion of Science and Scholarship, 1988.

Pritchard, Sara. *Confluence: The Nature of Technology and the Remaking of the Rhône.* Cambridge, Massachusetts: Harvard University Press, 2011.

Prochaska, David. "The Political Culture of Settler Colonialism in Algeria: Politics in Bone (1870–1920)." *Revue de l'Occident musulman et de la Méditerranée* 48–49 (1988): 293–311.

——. *Making Algeria French: Colonialism in Bône, 1870–1920.* New York: Cambridge University Press, 1990.

Pulju, Rebecca J. *Women and Mass Consumer Society in Postwar France.* New York: Cambridge University Press, 2011.

Quennouelle-Corre, Laure. *La direction du Trésor, 1947–1967, l'État banquier et la croissance.* Paris: Comité pour l'Histoire Économique et Financière de la France, 2000.

Rabinbach, Anson. *The Human Motor: Energy, Fatigue, and the Origins of Modernity.* Berkeley: University of California Press, 1990.

Raustiala, Kal, and Stephen R. Munzer. "The Global Struggle over Geographic Indications." *European Journal of International Law* 18, no. 2 (2007): 337–365.

Reed, Eric. *Selling the Yellow Jersey: The Tour de France in the Global Era.* Chicago: University of Chicago Press, 2015.

Reggiani, Andres Horacio. "Procreating France: The Politics of Demography, 1919–1945." *French Historical Studies* 19, no. 3 (Spring 1996): 725–754.

Revel, Jacques. "Histoire vs. mémoire en France aujourd'hui." *French Politics, Culture, and Society* 18, no. 1 (Spring 2000): 1–12.

Robinson, Jancis, ed. *The Oxford Companion of Wine.* 3rd ed. New York: Oxford University Press, 2006.

de Rochebrune, Renaud and Jean-Claude Hazera. "Du riz dans le pastis: Vichy condamne Ricard à partir de zero." In *Les patrons sous l'Occupation.* Paris: Odile Jacob, 1995: 433–471.

Rogers, Susan Carol. "Good to Think: The 'Peasant' in Contemporary France." *Anthropological Quarterly* 60, no. 2 (April 1987): 56–63.

Rosanvallon, Pierre. *L'État en France de 1789 à nos jours.* Paris: Seuil, 1990.

Rosental, Paul-André. *L'intelligence démographique: Sciences et politiques des populations en France (1930–1960).* Paris: Odile Jacob, 2003.

Ross, Kristin. *Fast Cars, Clean Bodies: Decolonization and the Reordering of French Culture.* Cambridge, Massachusetts: The MIT Press, 1995.

Roudié, Philippe. *Vignobles et vignerons du Bordelais, 1850–1980.* Paris: Centre National de la Recherche Scientifique, 1988.

Rousselier, Nicolas. "Gouvernement et parlement dans l'entre-deux-guerres." In *Serviteurs de l'État: Une histoire politique de l'administration française (1875–1945),* edited by Marc-Olivier Baruch and Vincent Duclert, 112–126. Paris: La Découverte, 2000.

Rousso, Henry, ed. *De Monnet à Massé: Enjeux politique et objectifs économiques dans le cadre des quatre premiers Plans (1946–1965).* Paris: Centre National de la Recherche Scientifique, 1986.

——. *La Planification en crises (1965–1985).* Paris: Centre National de la Recherche Scientifique, 1987.

Rudolph, Nicole C. *At Home in Postwar France: Modern Mass Housing and the Right to Comfort.* New York: Berghahn, 2015.

Sagnes, Jean. *Le midi rouge, mythe ou réalité: Études d'histoire occitane.* Paris: Anthropos, 1982.

——. "Viticulture et politique dans la 1re moitié du XX siècle: Aux origines du statut de la viticulture." In *La viticulture française aux XIXe et XXe siècles,* edited by Jean Sagnes, 49–81. Béziers, France: Presses du Languedoc, 1993.

Sagnes, Jean, Monique Pech, and Rémy Pech. *1907 en Languedoc-Roussillon.* Montpellier, France: Espace Sud, 1997.

Sanders, Paul. *Histoire du marché noir.* Paris: Perrin, 2001.

Saul, Samir. *Intérêts économiques français et décolonisation de l'Afrique du Nord (1945–1962).* Geneva: Droz, 2016.

Schivelbusch, Wolfgang. *The Railway Journey: The Industrialization of Time and Space in the Nineteenth Century.* Oakland: University of California Press, 2014. First published 1979 by Urizen Books.

Sessions, Jennifer. *By Sword and Plow: France and the Conquest of Algeria.* Ithaca: Cornell University Press, 2011.

Shennan, Andrew. *Rethinking France: Plans for Renewal, 1940–1946.* Oxford: Clarendon Press, 1989.

Shepard, Todd. *The Invention of Decolonization: The Algerian War and the Remaking of France.* Ithaca: Cornell University Press, 2006.

Simmons, Dana. *Vital Minimum: Need, Science, and Politics in Modern France.* Chicago: University of Chicago Press, 2015.

Simpson, James. *Creating Wine: The Emergence of a World Industry, 1840–1914.* Princeton: Princeton University Press, 2011.

Smith, Andrew W. M. *Terror and Terroir: The Winegrowers of the Languedoc and Modern France.* Manchester, UK: Manchester University Press, 2016.

Smith, Andy, Jacques de Maillard, and Olivier Costa. *Vin et politique: Bordeaux, la France, la mondialisation.* Paris: Presses de la Fondation Nationale des Sciences Politiques, 2007.

Smith, J. Harvey. "Work Routine and Social Structure in a French Village: Cruzy in the Nineteenth Century." *Journal of Interdisciplinary History* 5, no. 3 (1975): 357–382.

Smith, Timothy B. *France in Crisis: Welfare, Inequality, and Globalization since 1980.* New York: Cambridge University Press, 2004.

Smith, Tony. "Muslim Impoverishment in Colonial Algeria." *Revue de l'Occident musulman et de la Méditerranée* 17, no. 1 (1974): 139–162.

Souillac, Romain. *Le mouvement Poujade: De la défense professionnelle au populisme nationaliste (1953–1962).* Paris: Presses de la Fondation Nationale des Sciences Politiques, 2007.

Stanziani, Alessandro. "Wine Reputation and Quality Controls: The Origin of the AOCs in 19th Century France." *European Journal of Law and Economics* 18, no. 2 (2004): 149–167.

——. *Histoire de la qualité alimentaire (XIXe–XXe siècle).* Paris: Seuil, 2005.

Stora, Benjamin. *La gangrène et l'oubli: La mémoire de la guerre d'Algérie.* Paris: La Découverte, 1992.

——. *Algeria, 1830–2000: A Short History.* Translated by Jane Marie Todd. Ithaca: Cornell University Press, 2001.

Stovall, Tyler. *The Rise of the Paris Red Belt.* Berkeley: University of California Press, 1990.

Strachan, John. "The Colonial Identity of Wine: The Leakey Affair and the Franco-Algerian Order of Things." *Social History of Alcohol and Drugs* 21, no. 2 (Spring 2007): 118–137.

Strauss, David. *The American Menace: The Rise of French Anti-Americanism in Modern Times.* Westport, Connecticut: Greenwood Press, 1978.

Sulkunen, Pekka. *À la recherche de la modernité: Consommation et consommateurs d'alcool en France aujourd'hui: le regard d'un étranger.* Report No. 178. Helsinki: Social Research Institute of Alcohol Studies, 1988.

Sutton, Keith. "Algeria's Vineyards: A Problem of Decolonization." *Méditerranée* 65, no. 3 (1988): 55–66.

Taber, George M. *Judgment of Paris: California vs. France and the Historic 1976 Paris Tasting That Revolutionized Wine.* New York: Scribner, 2006.

Talbott, John. "French Public Opinion and the Algerian War: A Research Note." *French Historical Studies* 9, no. 2 (Autumn 1975): 354–361.

Terray, Aude. *Des francs-tireurs aux experts. L'organisation de la prévision économique au ministère des Finances, 1948–1968.* Paris: Comité pour l'Histoire Économique et Financière de la France, 2002.

Terrio, Susan J. *Crafting the Culture and History of French Chocolate.* Berkeley: University of California Press, 2000.

Thoenig, Jean-Claude. *L'ère des technocrates: Le cas des Ponts et Chaussées.* Paris: Les Éditions d'Organisation, 1973.

Tiersten, Lisa. *Marianne in the Market: Envisioning Consumer Society in Fin-de-Siècle France.* Berkeley: University of California Press, 2001.

Torrès, Olivier. *The Wine Wars: The Mondavi Affair, Globalization, and "Terroir."* New York: Palgrave Macmillan, 2006.

Touchelay, Béatrice. "L'INSEE des origines à 1961: Évoluion et relation avec la réalité économique et sociale." PhD Diss., Université de Paris XII, 1993.

Trentmann, Frank. "Political Culture and Political Economy: Interest, Ideology, and Free Trade." *Review of International Political Economy* 5, no. 2 (Summer 1998): 217–251.

Tristram, Frédéric. *Une fiscalité pour la croissance: La Direction générale des impôts et la politique fiscale en France de 1948 à la fin des années 1960.* Paris: Comité pour l'Histoire Économique et Financière de la France, 2005.

Trubek, Amy. *The Taste of Place: A Cultural Journey into Terroir.* Berkeley: University of California Press, 2008.

Urry, John. *Mobilities.* Malden, MA: Polity, 2007.

Vaudour, Emmanuelle. *Les terroirs viticoles: Définitions, caractérisation et protection.* Paris: Dunod, 2003.

Verdier, Olivier. "Action politique et défense des intérêts catégoriels. André Liautey et le monde des groupes de pression (1919/1960)." PhD Diss., Université Paris X, 2009.

Vernon, James. *Hunger: A Modern History.* Cambridge, Massachusetts: The Belknap Press of Harvard University Press, 2007.

Veseth, Michael. *Wine Wars: The Curse of the Blue Nun, the Miracle of Two Buck Chuck, and the Revenge of the Terroirists.* Lanham, Maryland: Rowman & Littlefield, 2011.

Vigreux, Jean. *Waldeck Rochet: Une biographie politique.* Paris: La Dispute, 2000.

——. *La vigne du maréchal Pétain ou un faire-valoir bourguignon de la Révolution nationale.* Dijon, France: Éditions Universitaires de Dijon, 2005.

Vittori, Massimo. "The International Debate on Geographical Indications (GIs): The Point of View of the Global Coalition of GI Producers—oriGIn." *Journal of World Intellectual Property* 13, no. 2 (2010): 304–314.

Walton, Whitney. *France at the Crystal Palace: Bourgeois Taste and Artisan Manufacture in the Nineteenth Century.* Berkeley: University of California Press, 1992.

Warner, Charles K. *The Winegrowers of France and the Government since 1875.* New York: Columbia University Press, 1960.

Waters, Sarah. "Globalization, the Confédération Paysanne, and Symbolic Power." *French Politics, Culture, and Society* 28, no. 2 (Summer 2010): 96–117.

Weber, Eugen. *Peasants into Frenchmen: The Modernization of Rural France, 1870–1914.* Stanford: Stanford University Press, 1976.

——. "L'Hexagone." In *Les Lieux de mémoire*, vol. 2, *La Nation*, edited by Pierre Nora, 97–116. Paris: Gallimard, 1986.

Weiner, Susan. *Enfants Terribles: Youth and Femininity in the Mass Media in France, 1945–1968.* Baltimore: Johns Hopkins University Press, 2001.

Whalen, Philip. "'Insofar as the Ruby Wine Seduces Them': Cultural Strategies for Selling Wine in Inter-war Burgundy." *Contemporary European History* 18, no. 1 (2009): 193–224.

——. "Gastronomic Burgundy as a Regional Modernization Project." In *Place and Locality in Modern France*, edited by Philip Whalen and Patrick Young. New York: Bloomsbury Academic, 2014.

White, Owen. "The Bottle of Algiers: A Vineyard in French Algeria, 1869–1963." Paper presented at Stanford University, 26 April 2012.

——. "Roll Out the Barrel: French and Algerian Ports and the Birth of the Wine Tanker." *French Politics, Culture, and Society* 35, no. 2 (Summer 2017): 111–132.

Wilder, Gary. *The French Imperial Nation-State: Negritude and Colonial Humanism between the Two World Wars.* Chicago: University of Chicago Press, 2005.

Williams, Philip M. *Crisis and Compromise: Politics in the Fourth Republic*. London: Longmans, 1964.

Wilson, James E. *Terroir: The Role of Geology, Climate, and Culture in the Making of French Wines*. Berkeley: University of California Press, 1998.

Winnacker, Rudolph A. "Elections in Algeria and the French Colonies under the Third Republic." *American Political Science Review* 32 (April 1938): 261–277.

Wolikow, Serge, and Olivier Jacquet, eds. *Territoires et terroirs du vin du XVIIIe au XXIe siècles: Approche internationale d'une construction historique*. Dijon, France: Éditions Universitaires de Dijon, 2011.

Woods, Ngaire. *The Globalizers: The IMF, the World Bank, and Their Borrowers*. Ithaca: Cornell University Press, 2006.

Wright, Gordon. "Peasant Politics in the Third French Republic." *Political Science Quarterly* 70, no. 1 (March 1955): 75–86.

———. *Rural Revolution in France: The Peasantry in the Twentieth Century*. Stanford: Stanford University Press, 1964.

Wylie, Laurence. *Village in the Vaucluse*. Cambridge, Massachusetts: Harvard University Press, 1957, 1974.

Young, Patrick. *Enacting Brittany: Tourism and Culture in Provincial France, 1871–1939*. Farnham, UK: Ashgate, 2012.

Zdatny, Steven M. *The Politics of Survival: Artisans in Twentieth-Century France*. New York: Oxford University Press, 1990.

Znaien, Nessim. "Le vin et la viticulture en Tunisie colonial (1881–1956): Entre synapse et apartheid." *French Cultural Studies* 26, no. 2 (2015): 140–151.

Index

Milton Keynes UK
Ingram Content Group UK Ltd.
UKHW010812150624
444077UK00004B/50/J